To
Kathryn J. Skhal, whose industriousness, ingenuity, and
attention to detail greatly facilitated the completion
of this manuscript

Introduction *to* Reference Sources in the Health Sciences

Fourth Edition

Compiled and Edited By

JO ANNE BOORKMAN

JEFFREY T. HUBER

FRED W. ROPER

NEAL-SCHUMAN PUBLISHERS, INC.
NEW YORK   LONDON

Published by Neal-Schuman Publishers, Inc.
100 William Street, Suite 2004
New York, NY 10038

The paper used in this publication meets the minimum requirements of American National Standard for Informational Sciences—Permanence of Paper for Printed Library Materials, ANSI Z39.48—1992

Published in cooperation with the Medical Library Association

Printed and bound in the United States of America.

Library of Congress Cataloging-in-Publication Data

Introduction to reference sources in the health sciences /
    compiled and edited by Jo Anne Boorkman, Jeffrey T.
    Huber, Fred W. Roper.—4th ed.
        p. cm.
Includes bibliographical references and index.
ISBN 1–55570–481–6 (alk. paper)
        1. Medicine—Reference books—Bibliography. 2.
Medicine—Bibliography. 3. Medicine—Information services.
I. Boorkman, Jo Anne. II. Huber, Jeffrey T. III. Roper, Fred W.
(Fred Wilburn)

Z6658.I54 2004
[R118.6]
610.72—dc21   2003056209

TABLE OF CONTENTS

PART I The Reference Collection

Organization and Management of the Reference Collection
Jo Anne Boorkman

PART II Bibliographic Sources

Bibliographic Sources for Monographs
Jeffrey T. Huber

Bibliographic Sources for Periodicals
Fred W. Roper

Indexing, Abstracting, and Digital Database Resources
Jerry Perry, David K. Howse, and Joan Schlimgen

U.S. Government Documents and Technical Reports
Fred W. Roper

Conferences, Reviews, and Translations
Fred W. Roper

PART III Information Sources

Terminology
Fred W. Roper

List of Figures and Tables

PREFACE

Reference work is the cornerstone of public services in libraries and is fundamental to health sciences librarianship. Assisting a medical student in finding reference values for a diagnostic test, helping a secretary complete a bibliographic citation in order to finalize a grant application, identifying a drug's side effects for a nursing student, or showing a graduate student which databases to search for information on their research topic are just a few of the many types of questions that fall into the realm of providing health sciences reference services. *Introduction to Reference Sources in the Health Sciences,* Fourth Edition, provides basic information on the nature of reference work and the authors' selections of some of the most important resources for answering questions in the health sciences.

The chapters in this guide identify and describe both recommended general reference resources that are important sources for answering bibliographic reference questions as well as authoritative reference sources specific to health sciences librarianship which can be used to assist a library's clientele in finding information on medical topics. This text is designed to identify and describe the best resources available for answering questions from health professionals, students, researchers, and consumers interested in health information.

Every edition of *Introduction to Reference Sources in the Health Sciences* has included both print and electronic resources. In the first edition, most references cited and discussed were for print resources, with electronic resources focused on online bibliographic databases (e.g., MEDLINE and BIOSIS). At that time, these databases were primarily available to librarians who provided mediated searches for clientele. With the growth of the Internet, many print reference resources became available via the Web, such as *The Merck Manual of Diagnosis and Therapy* and *Enzyme Nomenclature*. Other new resources that bring together full-text of books, journals, and other information under one aggregated portal, such as MD Consult, also became available, providing the power of searching across multiple sources for information on a topic. The Web has also allowed availability to a wealth of electronic-only resources that may or may not have had a counterpart in print, such as the information from professional associations and organizations (e.g., Association of American Medical Colleges and the Malaria Foundation International), as well as collaborative ventures such as the Cochrane Library's databases with information on evidence-based medicine. These have all enriched the range of resources available to our libraries to answer reference questions for our clientele or assist them in researching their own questions.

Purpose and Scope

Our purpose remains the same—to discuss various types of bibliographic and information sources and their use in reference work in the heath sciences, regardless of format, but with an increased focus on highlighting electronic resources that have become such a fundamental part of reference services. Our library clientele has become familiar with searching the Web using search engines such as Google and Yahoo! for all types of information, so their expectations are that their libraries will be able to provide them with desktop access to information they need for their personal, patient care, research, and teaching needs as well. Health sciences librarians are now challenged to provide electronic versions of traditionally print reference sources as well as new reliable electronic-only resources, thereby creating electronic reference collections that complement the print collection for use by their clientele directly with librarian assistance. The wealth of free quality information that is available via the Web can augment a small library's collection and the librarians' resources for assisting clientele in answering questions. On the other hand, many online resources come with restrictive licenses and hefty access fees that make it difficult or impossible for some libraries to make them available to their clientele. This fourth edition of *Introduction to Reference Sources in the Health*

Sciences explores these issues. We address questions librarians need to consider in developing and maintaining their reference collections in both the print and online environments, for use by their clientele directly or with librarian assistance. We have chosen those tools that librarians may use on a daily basis in reference work in the health sciences—those that may be considered foundation or basic works. Some major specialized works have also been included when appropriate. Emphasis is placed on U.S. publications and libraries, although an attempt has been made to address Canadian publications and needs.

The Arrangement of the Material

The major portions of *Introduction to Reference Sources in the Health Sciences* present the different types of bibliographic and information sources. Each chapter contains a discussion of the general characteristics of the type of source being considered, followed by examples of the most important tools in the area. For this new edition, the former chapters on "Indexing and Abstracting Services" and "Electronic Bibliographic Databases" have been combined into a single chapter: "Indexing, Abstracting, and Digital Database Resources." The "Audiovisual, Microcomputer, and Multimedia Reference Sources" chapter has been dropped from this edition. A new chapter on "Consumer Health Sources" has been added. Emphasis is on the use of materials, and where available, a comparison with similar materials is included. If available, readings are again included for each topic.

The book is organized into three parts: *The Reference Collection*, *Bibliographic Sources*, and *Information Sources*. In Part I, the first chapter discusses the nature of reference and ways to organize and manage a reference collection. It includes results of a survey of current practices for selecting, organizing, and weeding the collection and discusses criteria health sciences librarians consider relevant for selecting both print and electronic resources.

Part II covers bibliographic sources. Chapter 2 discusses sources for verifying, locating, and selecting monographs while Chapter 3 discusses sources for verifying, locating, and selecting periodicals. Chapter 4 focuses on the rich array of databases now available in the health sciences, providing the authors' perspective on primary and secondary databases. Chapter 5 discusses U.S. government and technical report literature, and Chapter 6 discusses resources for identifying conference proceedings, reviews, and literature in translation. Citations list availability of electronic access to print resources in addition to listing new electronic resources.

Part III focuses on information sources. Chapter 7 covers terminology and dictionaries while Chapter 8 discusses handbooks, manuals, and nomenclature sources. Chapter 9 discusses drug information sources, including databases. Chapter 10 discusses consumer health resources, which has become a growing area of collecting and service in many health sciences libraries. Chapter 11 provides an extensive discussion on the types of medical and health statistics that are collected and resources where they can be found. Chapter 12 discusses directory and biographical information sources while Chapter 13 provides information on history sources. The final Chapter 14 provides information on grant sources. As with Part II, citations to print sources provide information regarding online availability along with new citations for electronic sources.

Because no absolute consensus exists as to what constitutes "basic works," the materials represent the authors' candidates for such a list. In many instances, other equally appropriate examples could have been selected. For certain groups of sources (e.g., technical report literature), materials that are considerably broader in scope than the health sciences field alone have been included to help the reader toward a clear understanding of the use of these sources in reference work in the health sciences. The text is designed for students and librarians to review sections selectively, to become familiar with resources in areas that may not be familiar to them, and possibly to discover unexpected information about familiar resources.

The URLs for Web resources are included with citations and were checked for accuracy at the time of manuscript submission; however, due to the ever-changing nature of health sciences publishing and the wide range of technical glitches that can occur, the authors cannot guarantee that these Web addresses will remain the same. Web addresses are included for both free and licensed resources.

A BRIEF HISTORY OF INTRODUCTION TO REFERENCE SOURCES IN THE HEALTH SCIENCES

In 1979, Fred Roper approached the Medical Library Association's publications program about writing a text to support a course in health sciences reference that he taught at the University of North Carolina-Chapel Hill's School of Library Science, with the idea that it would be useful for others teaching similar courses at other library schools. The Medical Library Association expressed interest and suggested that there would be a broader audience for such a text among practicing health sciences librarians and for supporting MLA's CE course in reference resources. At that time, Jo Anne Boorkman was head of public services and head of reference at the Health Sciences Library at UNC-Chapel Hill. Fred asked her to join him as a coeditor in this endeavor. They invited several librarians, some of whom were relatively new to the field and others with a wealth of experience, to participate in this publishing venture. This mix of contributors proved to be a successful collaboration.

In 1980, the first edition appeared and was met with enthusiasm. It became a familiar text for both library school courses and MLA CE courses. It also gained a broader audience than the authors expected among practicing librarians from general academic and public libraries as well as health sciences librarians. The second edition followed 4 years later and continued to receive acceptance and recognition. With major career moves for both of them to different parts of the country, their goal of regular updates slipped, and the 3rd edition did not appear until 1994.

The reception of the first three editions of *Introduction to Reference Sources in the Health Sciences* has been most gratifying. It was the editors' intention to begin work on a fourth edition soon after publication of the third edition, to keep the publication up to date to reflect the changes brought on by the growth of the Web and the expansion of electronic reference resources. It is hard to believe that almost 10 years have passed since the publication of the third edition. Needless to say, the Web availability of many traditionally print resources, the vast number of freely available health resources for both professionals and consumers, and the expectations of readers of this text have made this edition long overdue. With this edition being completed as Fred prepared for retirement, Jeff Huber was invited to assist as one of the editors and with the hope that he would continue with future editions of this book. A different mix of authors was invited to contribute to this edition for another successful collaboration. The editors hope readers and browsers will concur.

Many people have played important roles in the production of this fourth edition. The chapter authors have all shared their expertise, experience, and enthusiasm for their respective topics. New authors have revised several chapters from the third edition. These authors are indebted to Diane L. Fishman, Frieda Weise, Judith M. Johnson, Judith A. Overmier, and Pamela Broadley for the excellent groundwork that they laid for this edition in preparing the chapters in the fourth edition. Their contributions are gratefully acknowledged.

Bernadette S. Daly and Kathryn Skhal deserve thanks for assisting with the survey of academic and hospital reference services which was conducted as background for the first chapter. Thanks to Beryl Glitz for preparation of the index for this edition. Special thanks go to Kathryn Skhal at the Carlson Health Sciences Library, University of California, Davis, for assistance with final manuscript preparation.

Jo Anne Boorkman
Jeffrey T. Huber
Fred W. Roper
Editors

Part I

Chapter 1

Organization and Management of the Reference Collection

Jo Anne Boorkman

Introduction to Reference Sources in the Health Sciences introduces a number of works considered to be desirable tools in the reference collection of a health sciences library. All are appropriate, if not essential, for a large library. Smaller libraries will need to be selective in acquiring the most appropriate tools for their collections. This book introduces both print and electronic resources that are appropriately considered reference tools. Some tools are only available in print whereas others are available in both print and electronic formats; yet others are only electronically available. Many tools are freely available via the Internet. Some are only available through paid license agreements. Fortunately for the smaller libraries, there are many excellent resources that are available at no cost which can greatly expand the budgeted resources of a library and which enable librarians to assist in answering the reference questions of patrons. First, however, it seems appropriate to explore the nature of the reference collection: how it differs from other collections of a library, what characterizes the materials in it, and how these are selected, organized, and maintained.

Reference collections evolve and develop from the nature of reference work. In addition to carrying out literature searches, reference librarians are most frequently called on for assistance in answering factual and bibliographic questions. Questions such as

1

- Is Dr. James Jones board certified in surgery?
- Where did Dr. Jones get his medical training?
- Can you verify an article by Dr. J. P. Jones in the *American Journal of Surgery*? I think it was published in 2001.
- What was the incidence of antibiotic-resistant tuberculosis in Los Angeles in 2000?

should readily be answered by resources within the reference collection.

The tools most frequently used to answer these types of questions make up the reference collection. Materials in this collection are consulted for specific and immediate information instead of being read from beginning to end. To assure that these materials are available for immediate and short-term use, the reference collection is separated from the circulating collections of the library, placed in an easily accessible library service area, and made noncirculating. Some smaller libraries find it advantageous to interfile reference books with the circulating collection, marking the reference books so filed for easy identification and access [1]. It should be noted that some medical reference tools require the assistance of a trained librarian for effective use. As reference tools are progressively acquired in electronic format, this assistance takes on additional importance because the librarian becomes involved with instruction in effective use of the equipment as well as the reference material. A new dimension is added as libraries provide reference resources in print and via their Web pages.

Little has been written on the nature of the reference collection and of the policies for developing and maintaining it [2]. Clemmons and Schwartz summarized the essential elements 1) collection policy decisions, 2) types of materials, 3) selection criteria, 4) electronic reference sources, 5) selection aids, 6) weeding the collection, and 7) arrangement of the collection [3]. A written collection development policy is a very useful tool and, similar to other library policies, has a variety of uses. In a time of limited resources, the collection development policy helps to define the scope of the collection for greater selection consistency and wiser use of resources. It can be used to train new staff and to help orient them to the nature of reference work in a particular library. It can be used for evaluation of current and future needs based on user queries, new curriculum and research

2

demands, and new technological developments. The reference collection policy can also be useful in defining areas of cooperative collection building with neighboring libraries or, in large academic institutions, with other campus libraries. Web resources are increasingly becoming important components of reference service. Defining their place in the reference collection development policy can facilitate their integration into the overall reference collection.

Selection policies [4–6], while generally discussing the collection as a whole, usually define four levels of coverage for subject areas: exhaustive/comprehensive, research, reference, and skeletal. These can be described as follows.

1. *Exhaustive.* For a subject collected on the exhaustive level, the library will obtain copies of all editions of all books, journals, pamphlets, reports, and so on, dealing with the subject and published at any time in any language. All manuscript materials relating to this subject will also be acquired.

2. *Research.* For a subject collected on the research level, the library will obtain current or best editions of the books, journals, pamphlets, reports, and documents in the commonly used languages and which are necessary to permit independent research on a doctoral level.

3. *Reference.* For a subject collected on the reference level, the library will obtain a current dictionary, a current encyclopedia, the latest or best editions of several texts, a comprehensive bibliography, one or more journals, an indexing or abstracting journal, and one or more histories.

4. *Skeletal.* For a subject collected on the skeletal level, the library will obtain a current dictionary, the latest or best edition of one or two texts, and a history [7].

Regardless of the level at which the material is collected, the subject should be represented in both the reference and the general collections of the library. Therefore, simply defining a level of coverage does not adequately answer the question, "Which materials should comprise a reference collection?"

A reference collection policy should be developed as a document parallel to the overall collection development policy of the library. It

3

should be defined not only in relation to the research and educational goals of the particular institution, but also in relation to the types of materials most often used in the reference situation [8].

Consideration should also be given to the format of materials, both print and nonprint, in the reference collection. Specifically, will tools only available in microform or electronic format (e.g., online databases and portable databases on CD-ROM and diskette) be acceptable? Which types of tools will be considered for purchase in print form? in electronic formats? in which other formats? For ready-reference purposes, will access to databases or bibliographic utilities be considered in lieu of purchase of a particular print title? The author's 2003 survey of health sciences libraries reference collection selection and organization practices revealed that when print and electronic versions are both available for many types of reference resources, librarians overwhelmingly prefer to provide both formats. Electronic indexing and abstracting resources are the only reference resources that are preferred to be accessible only in electronic format. Such preferences for format should be codified in the reference collection policy statement.

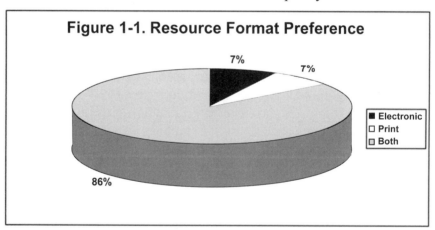

Figure 1-1. Resource Format Preference

Online and portable electronic formats—sources of both bibliographic information and factual data—can be considered a part of the reference collection and should be included as a possible format for reference access in the collection policy statement. It could be argued that online and portable electronic sources form a separate reference service; however, they are considered here as additional formats for some of the most heavily used reference tools: indexes, abstracts, and drug/chemical resources.

Full-text online searching of a number of journals provides another approach to answering reference queries. Familiar reference resources are becoming available in online versions (e.g., *American Board of Medical Specialists Directory and The Merck Manual*), and new electronic resources are appearing (e.g., Who Named It dictionary of medical eponyms). Having a well-defined written reference collection development policy will make it easier to fit these new tools and other sources into a collection.

Another area to consider is duplication of materials. Some tools, such as heavily used textbooks, should be considered for the circulating, reference, and/or online collections. Also, duplicate copies of heavily used reference books (e.g., medical dictionaries or the *Physicians' Desk Reference [PDR]*), may be needed at the reference desk and in the reference office in addition to placement in the reference collection. The need for multiple formats of bibliographic tools also needs to be considered.

In the example of a reference collection policy outline [9–11] shown in Table 1-1, consideration of formats and multiple copies are separately listed for illustrative purposes. They could be incorporated into Section V under each specific category. The richness of resources available via the Web provides an opportunity for a library to define which resources will exclusively be provided online, which will only be available in print, and which will have both print and online access.

Table 1-1. Outline for a Reference Collection Policy
I.   Introduction
     A. History of the policy
         i.   Date of the original formulation
         ii. Authority establishing the policy
     B. Present revision of the policy with the date of approval
II. Objectives of the reference collection
     A. Purpose of the collection
     B. Clientele served
III. Scope of the reference collection related to:
     A. User information needs

B. Subject coverage in relation to the overall collection policy of the library
C. Depth of collection of materials by subject
D. Subjects outside the scope of the collection
IV. Physical size of the collection
V. Categories of reference materials
  A. Information on persons, organizations, or institutions
    i. Directories of persons—biographical directories
    ii. Directories of organizations
    iii. Telephone directories
  B. Factual data
    i. Dictionaries
      1. General English-language
      2. Subject
      3. Foreign-language/polyglot
    ii. Encyclopedias
    iii. Handbooks
    iv. Drug/chemical resources
    v. Statistical sources
    vi. Legislation, regulations
      1. Federal
      2. State
      3. Local
    vii. Catalogs
      1. Educational institutions
      2. Commercial products, including laboratory equipment and supplies
    viii. Manuals and guides
      1. Writing and style manuals
      2. Online search manuals
    ix. Indexes, abstracts, and bibliographies
    x. Lists of meetings
  C. Union lists and catalogs
    i. Book catalogs
    ii. Serial sources
      1. Union lists

2. Abbreviations lists, lists of journals indexed or abstracted (included by indexing and abstracting services)
   iii. Media and software sources
      1. Catalogs from producers
      2. Union lists
   iv. Translation sources
  D. Textbooks and histories
  E. Ephemeral and pamphlet materials
VI. Format
  A. Print
  B. Nonprint
    i. Microcomputer software
    ii. CD-ROMs, diskettes, DVDs
    iii. Microforms
    iv. Online databases, Web sites, texts, and so forth
  C. Multiple copies (consider need for duplication with print format when online format is available or whether print is preferred in lieu of online due to cost, archival need, and so forth)
    i. Serials (e.g., *Index Medicus)*
      1. Determination of need
      2. Locations
    ii. Books (e.g., medical dictionary, *PDR*)
      1. Determination of need
      2. Locations: reference stacks, reference desk, reading room(s), and so forth
    iii. Online search tools
      1. Determination of need
      2. Locations: reference office, reference desk, public PCs, and so forth
    iv. Electronic resources
      1. Determination of need

Writing the reference collection policy should not be considered an academic exercise. It is a concrete means by which a collection can be measured and developed. It can also be used to orient and train new librarians and reference staff about the collection and the types of materials needed to serve the clientele of the library. The outline in Table 1-1 provides a framework for developing a policy [12] (see also Appendix 1). However, a policy, similar to a collection, must regularly be reviewed to determine if it fulfills the goals of maintaining a vital reference collection. The policy should be considered a creative tool.

Along with the collection development policy for reference, there should be a sensible weeding and retention policy. Many reference tools appear in new editions at regular intervals—annually or biennially, for example. It would be impossible to maintain a usable reference collection if all these editions were kept in the reference collection. Unlike weeding for the general collection in which materials are discarded or offered on exchange to other libraries, a reference weeding policy has the option of retiring earlier editions of reference tools to the general circulating collection. Of course, duplicate copies could be withdrawn: Two copies of the 2002 *American Hospital Association Guide to the Health Care Field* in the circulating collection would not be sensible when there are two copies of the current edition in the reference collection. In this example, one copy is sufficient for comparative or historical purposes.

In some instances, however, it is useful to keep more than one edition of a tool in the reference collection. For example, when the latest edition of a reference book drops a section and the only source of the information is the earlier edition of the book, it is advisable to keep both editions on reference.

A reference collection weeding policy could be outlined as shown in Table 1-2.

Table 1-2. Outline for a Reference Weeding Policy
I. Introduction
A. History of the policy
i. Date of original formulation
ii. Authority establishing the policy
B. Present revision of the policy with the date of approval
II. Purpose of the policy
III. Retention policy

(To be coordinated with the overall collection development policy for areas in which exhaustive collections or archival material would always be kept)

- A. Only the latest edition is kept in library on reference (primary materials that supersede themselves)
  - i. Online manuals
  - ii. Holdings lists of individual libraries
  - iii. Pamphlets
  - iv. Catalogs
- B. Latest edition kept on reference, earlier editions in circulating collection
  - i. Any Category A materials (above) found to be unique and worth retaining in the collection for historical or research purposes
  - ii. Dictionaries
  - iii. Directories
  - iv. Handbooks
  - v. Drug resources
  - vi. Textbooks
  - vii. Encyclopedias
  - viii. Writing and style manuals
  - ix. Book catalogs
- C. Earlier editions kept on reference as usefulness of reference and available space permit
  - i. Any Category B materials (above) containing unique information found useful to reference
  - ii. Indexing and abstracting services
  - iii. Bibliographies
  - iv. Statistical sources
  - v. Union lists and serials sources
  - vi. Translation sources
  - vii. Lists of meetings

Note: As traditional print resources become available on the Web with regular updates, libraries will need to consider which resources should continue to be available in both the print reference collection and online.

Although a separate outline for a weeding policy is presented here, retention information could easily be incorporated into a reference collection policy for each category of reference tool. (See Appendix 1 for an example of a combined selection-retention policy statement.)

In practice, most libraries rely on the serial nature of many reference tools to keep the collection current and "weeded," withdrawing an earlier edition or sending it to the general collection when a new edition appears. In fact, they have a continuous weeding process. However, there are many reference materials that are not necessarily updated on a regular basis to trigger the weeding process. To maintain a current relevant collection, it is advisable to have an annual or biennial review of the reference collection, following the guidelines in the reference collection policy. Other factors that prompt weeding include space limitations, material in disrepair, and subjects no longer useful for reference purposes. Adalian and Rockman [13] recommend a title-by-title review of reference materials and identify nine objectives for such a review.

1. To serve as an inventory of the reference collection, identifying missing titles and volumes.
2. To serve as a means of purging the reference collection of seldom-used or obsolete books, which would be transferred to either a storage facility or the circulating collection or entirely eliminated from the library.
3. To monitor standing orders, which require claim action by the serials department.
4. To determine the appropriateness of all standing orders to see if only the latest edition or all volumes of a continuation should be kept in the reference department.
5. To ascertain whether a standing order should be placed for a serial title that was held in the collection but for which no standing order existed.
6. To determine if a later edition of a title not published on a regular basis is needed in the reference collection.
7. To identify gaps in the reference collection.
8. To identify and order a current title comparable in subject to an earlier title of which no updated edition is available.

9. To serve as a continuing education vehicle for the reference librarians by which they could become better acquainted with the strengths and weaknesses of the collection and therefore more proficient in selecting titles for, and retrieving information from, the collection.

In practice, weeding the collection is one of those activities that is often neglected. The author's survey revealed that health sciences librarians rely on the appearance of new editions and the serial nature of many reference materials, resulting in continuous collection "weeding." A periodic review of the entire collection is done at varying intervals ranging from biennially to every five years. Table 1-3 indicates the criteria health sciences librarians use for this more thorough weeding process.

Table 1-3. Reasons for Weeding		
Response	**Count**	**Percentage**
Space	97	58.40%
New edition received	151	91.00%
Out-of-date material	154	92.80%
Material in disrepair	44	26.50%
Subject no longer useful for reference use	86	51.80%
Other	9	5.40%

Access to the tools in the reference collection is generally through the public catalog. Online public access catalogs (OPACs) provide copy location information for those libraries that have automated their holdings records and provide a means of identifying those materials in the reference collection. The OPAC has the advantage of identifying and describing electronic-only resources and print resources that are available in full-text online then including hot-links with the catalog record or holdings statement for these references.

For libraries still using a card catalog, a stamped note or plastic overlay on the card will indicate that an item is in the reference collection; similarly, adding "also in reference" on the catalog card identifies [rather than stipulates] items in the general collection that are duplicated in reference. Larger libraries may have a separate reference catalog or reference shelf list for access to the reference collection alone.

However, in libraries where the reference collection is small, items in the general collection may be used more frequently than in large libraries to answer clients' queries; in this case access to all items, including reference materials, through a single public catalog would be preferable.

Organization of the Reference Collection

How should a reference collection be organized? There are varying schools of thought on this subject. A reference collection consists of both monographic and serial publications. The monographic collection will probably be classified by means of the National Library of Medicine's (NLM) classification system or some other method. The serial collection may or may not be classified; many libraries prefer to arrange their serials alphabetically. Some additional questions may arise concerning serials in the reference collection: Are reference serials to be classified or arranged alphabetically? Which items are considered serials for reference—just the indexes and abstracts or all serials publications?

If an entirely classified arrangement is chosen, the collection is usually shelved by classified (subject) arrangement, regardless of the type of format of the material. An exception is often made for indexes and abstracts, which are arranged on index tables for ease of use. The NLM classification scheme allows for format division within subject categories. For example, directories are indicated by "22":

W 22	general medicine
WU 22	dental
WX 22	hospital

and dictionaries by "13":

W 13	general medical
WM 13	psychiatry
WY 13	nursing

A modification of the classified arrangement can also be used in which the monographic collection is classified and arranged by call number, but the serial publications are arranged alphabetically and not classified. These are primarily indexes and abstracts, but can also include other serial publications (e.g., *Unlisted Drugs, Vital and Health Statistics*) usually found in a reference collection. In practice, some libraries classify reference serials, others leave them alphabetically arranged, and others group them chronologically, as is frequently done with *Index Medicus* and its predecessors. One real problem with the alphabetically arranged serials collection arises when the title of a work changes, thus separating consecutive volumes of a work.

The monographic reference collection, while classified, may not always be arranged strictly by call number. Some reference departments prefer an arrangement by form categories [14,15] in which all dictionaries, directories, handbooks, and so on are shelved together (see list in Reference Categories, below). These categories, however, are not arranged just by form. Some provide subject groupings such as "drug lists," which include handbooks, dictionaries, manuals, and so forth, on the subject. Other libraries have a combination of a classified arrangement with a form arrangement for heavily used items such as dictionaries, directories, textbooks, and college catalogs. When such arrangements are used, proper labeling of the public catalog or the holdings statements in an online catalog and of the reference collection is essential to guide the user to the location of the material in the reference area. Pizer and Walker caution that "such a reorganization of the collection, however, required additional . . . files to indicate shelf position and that makes the user dependent upon library staff to point out locations" [16].

Reference Categories

1. Dictionaries (medical and other subjects; English and foreign; also includes nomenclature, terminology, and quotation lists).
2. Manuals and guides (style manuals, writing guides, programmed textbooks on medical terminology, and legal and ethical manuals).
3. Almanacs and statistical compilations (includes all reference material on statistics).

4. Subject handbooks and data books such as *Handbook of Chemistry and Physics, Biology Data Handbook, and Handbook of Clinical Laboratory Data*).
5. Drug lists (all reference materials on drugs, including manuals, dictionaries, and handbooks).
6. Biographical directories (includes all reference materials listing people).
7. Directories (includes listings of institutions, organizations, scholarships, educational programs, and agencies).
8. Geographical atlases (includes geographical materials such as *Webster's Atlas and Zip Code Directory and Hotel and Motel Red Book*).
9. Encyclopedias and encyclopedic works (such as *Encyclopedia Britannica, Handbook of Experimental Pharmacology, and Practice of Medicine*).
10. Library information (includes directories, handbooks, and manuals in the field of library science).
11. Bibliographies and histories (includes selected bibliographies in the health sciences and histories of medicine and nonprint media).
12. Serial information (includes union catalogs, abbreviations lists, and directories of periodicals such as *Ulrich's International Periodicals Directory*).
13. Book catalogs (includes listings of books such as *Books in Print, National Library of Medicine Current Catalog,* and *Cumulative Book Index*).
14. Lists of meetings and translations (such as *Technical Translations Index, World Meetings: United States and Canada,* and *Annual International Congress Calendar*).

Whatever arrangement is chosen, ease of use by the library user as well as the reference librarian should be of primary consideration. Jeuell, in presenting an arrangement by categories, argues that arrangement by form increases the retrievability of information from the collection because clients frequently want a *type* of information (e.g., biographical) but may not know the subject area in which to look. A classified arrangement would require looking for biographies in several subject areas. She concludes:

> Form arrangement results in efficient use of the monographic collection by making it more retrievable, in terms of the patron's information needs, than a straight call number arrangement. Arrangement by form takes into account that some vital information might be missing from a reference question, and that many patrons use a monographic reference collection by browsing through a group of similar books such as biographical directories, rather than looking for a subject or for a specific title in the card catalog [17].

On the other hand, arrangement by form can lead to arbitrary placement of books in a category. Some items have multiple uses with features of handbooks, statistical compendia, and/or directories. In which category should they be placed? How efficiently is the patron then served? Subject arrangement (classified) does scatter similar forms of publications; however, it increases "browsability" within a field of interest—ophthalmology, hospitals, nursing, and so forth.

Of course, there are times when form arrangement would have its advantages and times when subject arrangement would be more advantageous. The arrangement chosen will depend on how the reference staff uses the collection and how it perceives the majority of clients use the collection—by form or by subject.

Discussion over the medical libraries discussion list, MEDLIB-L, on the Internet revealed that this is an issue still being debated among health sciences librarians. The experience at McMaster University Health Sciences Library provides a lesson for any library contemplating a change.

> Some years ago, our small-to-medium Reference Collection was arranged so as to group all the dictionaries together, all the encyclopedias, all the handbooks, all the style manuals, on the theory that it would be easier for the patrons to find the item they wanted if all they could remember was that it was a dictionary...or

whatever.... It did not work very well in our quite small collection. You could no longer rely on your years of experience in locating material by subject throughout the NLM classification because the order in which books were found on the shelf had been totally altered. A new classification had to be learned; it was devised to be simple, but it was new, and didn't seem to be as "natural" either to users or staff as had been hoped it would be.... We had a re-arranged shelf list, and a key to show us if we knew the call number where to find it on the re-arranged shelves, but it took longer because there were two look-ups rather than one!

The patrons didn't seem to reap great benefit from the rearrangement, either...some intuited quite easily where to locate what they wanted, but others were simply not on that wavelength at all! The catalogue was of no use to them because the translation tool was at the Reference Desk, intended mainly for staff use, since it was assumed that the patrons would find the new shelf arrangements easy-to-use....

We went back to shelving according to the NLM classification about five years ago simply because our effort to make using the Reference Collection simpler didn't work.... We went back to NLM shelving in the Reference Collection for the sake of consistency and because it actually promoted the likelihood that patrons would find what they wanted in Reference. They were no more familiar with it than our new scheme! [18]

The physical arrangement of the collection will also depend to a great extent on the space available. Whether the "ideal" arrangement is considered to be by form categories, classified, or a combination of classified and alphabetic, the actual arrangement may be determined by where the collection can be housed. The author's survey revealed that the majority of health sciences libraries responding (88 percent) have their reference collections in a classified arrangement.

As core reference resources become increasingly available on the Web, the physical space for the print reference collection in a library may be reduced as the library provides more public access computer stations in the reference area. The design of the library's Web page for easy access to online reference resources then becomes an important additional consideration. Medical /Health Sciences Libraries on the Web (Available: www.uiowa.edu/~hardin/hslibs.html#ky) provides links to the Web pages of both U.S. and international health sciences libraries. Reference resources are presented in a number of different ways, illustrating the creativity and ingenuity with which librarians have organized Web resources for use by their clientele.

There is no perfect answer to how a reference collection should be arranged—each library has a collection unique in size and content, based on the use and reference demands of its clientele. How the collection is arranged should be determined by these uses and reference patterns to maximize efficient use of the collection within the space constraints of the building. Easy, logical access to the collection by the clientele and staff should be the goal for organization and physical arrangement of a collection.

Selection of Materials

Maintaining the collection is an ongoing process. Current addresses, telephone numbers, statistical data, and so forth, are often the information sought from a reference tool. To provide such information, it is important to have the latest available edition of a tool in the collection. There are several ways to keep current. These include 1) publishers' announcements, 2) acquisitions lists of other health sciences libraries, and 3) online cataloging files. Based on the author's recent survey, health sciences librarians from both academic and hospital libraries rely most heavily on publishers' announcements. However, many libraries rely on approval plans for receipt of new editions and identification of potential new titles for the reference collection. Having a book in hand to evaluate before purchase is highly valued.

Acquisitions lists from other libraries were mentioned as being helpful. As Eakin points out, these are useful because "sources of information about less common reference tools may be obscure or may be more easily missed. Another exception may be in areas of special interest, and it may be worthwhile to check the acquisitions list of a particular library for a single subject...." [19].

While not limited to reviewing reference books, health sciences journals provide regular book review sections (e.g., *Annals of Internal Medicine's* "The Literature of Note" and *JAMA's* "Books, Journals, Software"). The Web sites of publishers also provide useful information for reference collections development [20].

Many reference books are serials that appear annually in new editions. Academic libraries, more than hospital libraries, rely on standing orders with publishers or vendors for these titles, thus being assured of timely receipt of new editions or volumes. However, the convenience of approval plans and standing orders does not preclude the responsibility of a librarian for final selection decisions. "Human involvement in collection decision making is essential for developing user-responsive collections" [21].

Health sciences librarians use a variety of selection tools, with the Brandon-Hill lists being highly regarded. Receipt of fax ads and phone solicitations by sales representatives was intensely disliked, producing comments from survey respondents such as, "I hate phone & fax solicitation . . . they are not welcome."

When new reference tools are selected, the guidelines from the reference collection policy should be followed. Is the tool going to provide

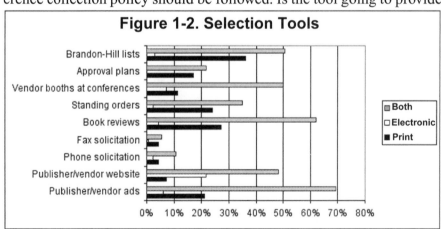

Figure 1-2. Selection Tools

new information? Does it duplicate information available in other tools? If so, is the information in a more easily retrievable format, making this new resource a desirable acquisition? Often, this information is not discernible from the announcement of a publisher. If the reference resource is not available through the approval plan, it may be advisable to wait until a review is published in a library journal such as the *Journal of the Medical Library Association* (*JMLA*) or *Medical Reference Services Quarterly* (*MRSQ*). These two sources were most frequently cited in the survey as having helpful reviews for selecting reference materials. Other sources for reviews of new reference works are the various National Network of Libraries of Medicine (NN/LM) library newsletters. These are aimed at hospital and small academic libraries and can provide guides for such collections.

Using the cataloging databases as aids in selection can also be helpful. Both the National Library of Medicine's *LOCATORplus* file and the Online Computer Library Center's (OCLC) *WorldCat* database can be used in ascertaining the latest edition of a particular work.

Selection of materials for the reference collection is generally a team effort. While in smaller libraries the library director is responsible for selection, all staff that uses the collection is encouraged to identify titles and make recommendations. In larger libraries, public services staff members are expected to contribute suggestions or make recommendations, with the ultimate decisions left to the library director, the head of public services, the head of collections/acquisitions, or a combination of all the above. In some larger libraries, one of the reference librarians is responsible for identifying appropriate materials for the reference collection and then soliciting comments from fellow librarians.

When it comes to selection of electronic reference sources, a broader group, including the library director, the head of systems, the head of audiovisuals, and the head of public services/reference, generally makes the decisions. In larger institutions and when the health sciences library has close ties to the general campus, campus-wide committees make such decisions. This is especially true for databases installed locally on servers and shared on local area network (LAN) facilities. The cost of many databases and electronic resources has led many libraries to join consortia in order to negotiate licenses and leverage subscription costs among several institutions.

Criteria for Evaluation of New Material (and New Formats)

Once identified, these new reference tools need to be measured against the existing collections in accordance with the reference collection development policy. Criteria for evaluating new material include [22,23]:

1. Significance and usefulness of the title.
2. Authority and reputation of the author, publisher, or database producer.
3. Age and currency of the work and its contents.
4. Favorable reviews in the professional literature.
5. Inclusion of the title in reference guides.
6. Difficulty level of the contents.
7. Language of the publication.
8. Price of the publication or database in relation to
   a. Availability of the information contained,
   b. Quality and physical production of the title, and
   c. Length of use.
9. Anticipated frequency of use (judge in relation to cost, available format[s], and space).
10. Appropriate format (print vs. microform vs. electronic).

The above criteria are also useful for maintaining and weeding the existing collection. Materials in some areas are particularly difficult to keep current. Directories of specialized societies are often published once, then abandoned or sporadically published. Statistical sources can also be a problem. A study may be done once and then never updated. Keeping an eye out for a useful new reference tool is aided by having a good working knowledge of the reference collection and the policy guidelines. When looking at specific reference tools, librarians use a combination of measures for evaluation, with a definite focus on their usefulness for the audience who will use these tools. The ideal combination of criteria includes authoritative material that is in scope for the subject focus of the primary clientele of a library and that presents the information in an easy-to-read format. Because budgets are frequently limited, librarians aim to select materials that are most appropriate to the collection and clientele of *their* particular library. They look for new tools that will fill the gaps in their collection. Other evaluative criteria used for selecting reference materials include good indexes, uniqueness of presentation, clear tables and illustrations, logical organization, and clarity of presentation.

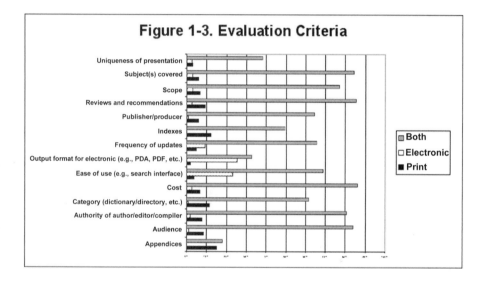

Criteria for selecting electronic reference sources require the same scope and subject coverage considerations used for print sources. Additional factors to consider include search features offered, a single vendor for consistent format when offering multiple databases, and price. Tenopir outlines evaluation criteria for both online sources and CD-ROMs [24]:

For online sources consider:

1. Connecting to the system
2. Search language
3. Effectiveness of search program
4. Contents quality
5. Search aids

For CD-ROMs consider:

1. Scope
2. Content
3. Quality
4. Accessibility

Anderson and McKnight suggest some key questions when considering electronic resources [25]:

- Does the library own the equipment necessary to use the electronic version of the product?
- Do the advantages of the electronic format offset its higher purchase price compared to the print product?
- Is the online equivalent of a print product actually less expensive to access because it is available on a pay-per-use basis?
- Can the content be searched using the Boolean operators AND, OR, and NOT?
- How many different access points are available for locating information in the electronic product?
- Can the library accommodate the licensing restrictions that apply to the product?

Library Journal's survey of use of CD-ROMs by public, academic, and special libraries noted, "the most important criterion in the selection of a CD-ROM database was . . . accuracy/authority. Ease of use and value for cost came in second and third, and most of the libraries felt that 'depth and breadth' of the product (scope or years and titles covered) were important" [26].

Because many of the electronic reference sources also have print counterparts, a decision must be made whether or not to duplicate formats. Often, electronic formats are only available for lease; consequently, libraries are reluctant to give up print versions when their collections serve an archival role. Often, producers and vendors will give a "discount" price for the electronic format when a library also has a subscription to the print version, providing additional incentive to duplicate formats. In addition, library archivists do not, as yet, consider the electronic formats archival. Survey respondents had a strong preference for providing both print and electronic versions of reference resources (see Fig. 1-1).

Electronic versions of bibliographic sources have widely been accepted by health sciences libraries, with print versions also maintained for the most heavily used indexing and abstracting services. However, the lesser-used sources for a particular library are increasingly being made available in electronic format only and often for the first time in health sciences libraries (e.g., Wilson indexes and ERIC). Academic libraries frequently provide campus-wide access to a number of sources not available in the health sciences library while hospital libraries are forming consortia or affiliating with academic libraries to make such sources available to their clientele. LANs are increasingly being abandoned for Web-based resources that are not platform specific and can offer various output formats (e.g., HTML, PDF, and hand-held devices).

As part of the evaluation process for licensed electronic resources, libraries prefer to offer trials for library clientele and librarians to evaluate fully the resource. At least a 4-week trial period is preferred (74.7 percent of survey respondents), with up to 3 months considered preferable to allow enough time for user responses. Often, the vendor will determine the length of a trial. Most libraries that use trials request evaluation responses from both librarians and users (69.3 percent).

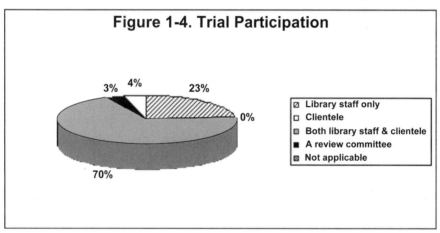

While electronic versions of reference resources are often desired, if not preferred, there are barriers that prevent libraries from acquiring access to them. The most frequently cited barrier was cost (91.6 percent), followed by already having licensed resource(s) with similar content (54.2 percent) and general licensing restrictions (53.6 percent). Thirty-seven percent of survey respondents also consider the inability to provide remote access an important barrier. Comments revealed that some organizations have firewalls that prevent offering Web-based resources to users.

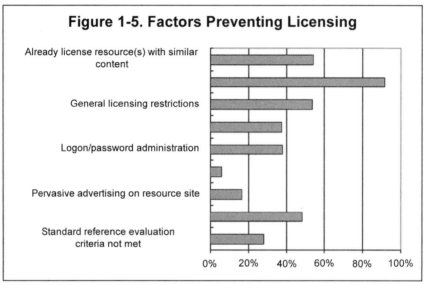

Figure 1-5. Factors Preventing Licensing

Budgetary considerations often dictate choices. The University of North Carolina, Chapel Hill recently evaluated their reference collection, asking "Electronic, Print, or Both?" [27] The following criteria were used:

- Compare cost of each format (sometimes electronic is free!).
- Arrange for trial access before purchasing an electronic product.
- Consider both user and librarian demand for a particular format.
- Test ease and speed of use of electronic versus print.
- Compare the ability to search and to browse for information.

- Compare the currency of the information in each format.
- Consider the labor involved in print loose-leaf services.
- Monitor use of print copies of electronic titles and stop purchasing those that are seldom used, except for titles of archival value.
- Evaluate the archival value of print in your collection.

When electronic-only is chosen, the library keeps the last edition and/or volume(s) in the reference collection when it has been replaced by an electronic version as an aid in transition to the electronic-only content.

Based on the author's survey, about 5–9 percent of the budget is spent on reference materials, regardless of library size. Few libraries maintain a separate budget for reference materials, with the serial publications for reference funded most often through the serials budget of a library. Many libraries also fund electronic reference tools through the serials budget as well. Sources other than the regular acquisitions budget (grants, gifts, and endowments) are frequently used to fund expensive electronic reference tools. Additional funding outside the acquisitions budget must be sought to purchase and maintain the equipment needed to use electronic sources. Funding sources vary among libraries. Some are able to fund such purchases from regular equipment budgets whereas other libraries must seek alternative funding, such as capital requests, grants, and gifts and endowments. Many libraries use a combination of funding sources.

The author's survey was conducted in early 2003 prior to the release of subscription prices for the coming year. Subsequently, library budgets, including those for all types of health sciences libraries, have been strained due to budget cutbacks and unanticipated increases in costs for library resources. Prices are high for library access to the online versions of traditional reference tools, such as electronic encyclopedias. This has especially been true for electronic resources. As libraries have made more decisions to cut print resources and rely on electronic access only, publishers have substantially increased the costs for electronic licenses and have changed the business models for these licenses. This is especially evident for journals. Society publishers have increasingly looked to library subscriptions, now electronic licenses, to sustain the activities of their organizations, not just to sustain their publications. Pricing models for access to electronic resources are shifting as publishers move to sustain a defined level of income for their organizations. As libraries have moved to electronic access only, these electronic costs to libraries that negotiate institutional and remote access for their primary clientele have significantly increased; this due in part to revenue lost by publishers from (real and/or anticipated) loss of individual subscriptions and reduced income from sale of advertisements. While many of these increased costs are for journals, both individual titles and big publisher packages rather than reference resources per se, the exponential increase in costs affect the entire collections budget. Difficult choices will need to be made as health sciences libraries and their institutions address meeting their obligations to provide the most current health information resources to their clientele. In the area of reference selection, librarians will need to make hard choices. Using the criteria listed above, comparing and evaluating resources for best value and at times being very selective, librarians will need to allocate judiciously their reference collection dollars. Fortunately, there are a number of reliable resources on the Internet which are freely available and which can also be "selected" for access via a library's OPAC and/or Web page to augment the reference collection.

The purpose of this chapter has not been to provide answers. It is intended to present the issues relating to the way a reference collection is developed and maintained. There are many factors to consider. The questions raised here are meant to lead to thoughtful consideration of how best to organize a new collection or an existing one or to assess how an existing collection came to be the way it is. The important question is: How can the collection best serve the user?

The following sections of this book will introduce the reader to representative bibliographic sources (Part II) and to information sources (Part III) for the health sciences library.

References

1. Strub JE. *Summary: shelving of reference and circulating books*. Message to: Multiple recipients of list MEDLIB-L <MEDLIB-L@LISTSERV.BUFFALO.EDU>. 2003 April 3.
2. Neeley J, ed. *Reference collection development: a bibliography*. Chicago, IL: Reference and Adult Services Division, American Library Association, 1991.
3. Clemmons NW, Schwartz DG. Management of reference services. In: Wood MS, ed. *Reference and information services in health sciences libraries*. Metuchen, NJ: Medical Library Association and The Scarecrow Press, Inc., 1994:210–21.
4. Beatty WK. Technical processes: part 1. Selection, acquisition, and weeding. In: Annan GL and Felter JW, eds. *Handbook of medical library practice*, 3rd ed. Chicago, IL: Medical Library Association, 1970:71–92.
5. National Library of Medicine (U.S). *Collection development manual of the National Library of Medicine*, 3rd ed. Bethesda, MD: U.S. Department of Health and Human Services, Public Health Service, National Institutes of Health, National Library of Medicine, 1993.
6. Eakin D. Health science library materials: collection development. In: Darling L, ed. *Handbook of medical library practice*, 4th ed. Chicago, IL: Medical Library Association, 1983:36–8.
7. Beatty WK. Technical processes: part 1. Selection, acquisition, and weeding. In: Annan GL and Felter JW, eds. *Handbook of medical library practice*, 3rd ed. Chicago, IL: Medical Library Association, 1970:73.
8. England JW. Library collection development policy. Philadelphia, PA. In: Taborsky T, Lenkowski P, and others. Collection development policies for college libraries. Chicago, IL: American Library Association, 1989:68–83. (Clip Note No. 11).
9. Beatty WK. Technical processes: part 1. Selection, acquisition, and weeding. In: Annan GL and Felter JW, eds. *Handbook of medical library practice*, 3rd ed. Chicago, IL: Medical Library Association, 1970:73–4.

10. Lehocky B. *Academic reference collection development policy statement*. Arlington, VA: ERIC Document Reproduction Service, 1979. (ERIC document ED 190160).
11. Kwan JK. *Reference collection policy*. Los Angeles: UCLA Biomedical Library, 1983 (unpublished manuscript).
12. See: Other Criteria: Thomas Jefferson Univ; Johns Hopkins Univ. In: Morse DH and Richards DT, comps. *Collection development policies for health sciences libraries*. Chicago, IL: Medical Library Association, 1992:128037 (MLA DocKit #3).
13. Adalian PT, Jr., Rockman IF. Title-by-title review in reference collection development. *Ref Serv Rev* 1984 Winter; 12:86.
14. Jeuell CA. The reorganization of a monograph reference collection. *Bull Med Lib Assoc* 1976 July; 64:293–8.
15. Truelson SD, Jr., The totally organized reference collection. *Bull Med Lib Assoc* 1976 July; 50:184–7.
16. Pizer IR, Walker WD. Physical access to resources: the reference collection. In: Darling L, ed. *Handbook of medical library practice*, 4th ed. Chicago, IL: Medical Library Association, 1982:25.
17. Jeuell CA. The reorganization of a monograph reference collection. *Bull Med Lib Assoc* 1976 July; 64: 298.
18. Flemming T. *Arrangement of reference collection*. Message to: Multiple recipients of list MEDLIB-L. <MEDLIB-L@LISTSERV.BUFFALO.EDU>. 1992 June 18.
19. Eakin D. Health science library materials: collection development. In: Darling L, ed. *Handbook of medical library practice*, 4th ed. Chicago, IL: Medical Library Association, 1983: 46–7.
20. Holmberg M. Using publishers' Web sites for reference collection development. *Issues in Sci and Tech Librarianship*. 2000 Winter. Available: www.istl.org/00-winter/article3.html.
21. Hattendorf LC. The art of reference collection development. *RQ* 1989; 29(2):220.
22. Kwan JK. *Reference collection policy*. Los Angeles: UCLA Biomedical Library, 1983: 23-4 (unpublished manuscript).
23. Lehocky B. *Academic reference collection development policy statement*. Arlington, VA: ERIC Document Reproduction Service, 1979: 61.. (ERIC document ED 190160).

24. Tenopir C. Evaluation criteria for online, CD-ROM. *Lib J* 1992 Mar. 1; 117:68.
25. Anderson SF, McKnight M. Information resources. In: Holst R and Philips SA, eds.*Medical Library Association guide to managing health care libraries*. New York: Neal-Schuman, 2000:214–5.
26. Berry J. CD-ROM: the medium of the moment. *Lib J* 1992 Feb. 1; 117:46.
27. McGraw K, McKenzie D, Hayes B. *The evolving reference collection: examining turbulent waters*. (April 30, 2003). Poster presented at the Medical Library Association Annual Meeting, San Diego, CA, May 2–5, 2003.

Readings

1. Cassell KA. *Developing reference collections and services in an electronic age*. New York: Neal-Schuman,.1999. (How-to-Do-It Manuals for Librarians, No. 95).
2. *Creating the digital medical library*. New York: Primary Research Group, 2003.
3. Lee SD. *Electronic collection development: a practical guide*. New York: Neal-Schuman in association with Library Association Publishing, London, 2002.
4. Nolan CW. *Managing the reference collection*. Chicago, IL: American Library Association, 1999.
5. Pierce SJ. *Weeding and maintenance of reference collections*. New York: The Haworth Press, 1995.

PART II

CHAPTER 2

BIBLIOGRAPHIC SOURCES FOR MONOGRAPHS

Jeffrey T. Huber

Monographs have historically played a significant role in the dissemination of health sciences information. "The seventeenth century saw the culmination of medical bibliography predicated on the publication of medical works in monographic form and the first appearance of bibliographies taking into account publication of advances in medicine in periodicals" [1]. While periodicals grew to become the preferred biomedical and scientific communication forum for current research and opinion, monographs continued to serve as an important means for conveying basic background information, such as a narrative description of a disease, pathophysiology, diagnostic techniques, common therapeutic regimens, and so forth. This trend remains true today, whether the monograph is in print or electronic format. Like the monograph itself, the materials used for bibliographic control of monographs continue to serve as an integral component of a reference collection.

Over time, bibliographies have been developed to bring order out of chaos by providing information that identifies works within a particular discipline or group of disciplines [2,3]. These bibliographies serve as verification, location, and selection tools. *Verification* refers to standard information contained in bibliographic citations such as author, title, edition, and place of publication. It may be necessary to consult multiple sources in order to verify all of the needed information about a particular monograph, often moving from a general source to a particular one with a more narrow subject area. *Location* indicates which library or other information agency owns a particular title or the vendor from which it may be purchased. Location also specifies where a title can be found in a particular library or information agency. Online bibliographic databases are the primary resources for identifying institutional holdings. Trade bibliographies, available in both print and electronic formats, are used to determine basic purchasing data. Because collection development is an essential function within a library or information setting, the *selection* function presupposes bibliographies that indicate the availability of titles within a particular subject domain, by a specific author, or in a given format.

Bibliographies in the health sciences often fulfill more than one of these three functions and typically contain entries for multiple types of materials (e.g., monographs, periodicals, government documents, and so forth).

Current Sources

While print resources have historically been a mainstay for bibliographic data, the generic growth in electronic information resources is reflected in current sources for monograph information. Many print bibliographic resources for monograph titles have been replaced by electronic ones.

The National Library of Medicine (NLM) is the leading authority concerning current coverage of health science monographs.

2.1 LOCATORplus. Bethesda, MD: National Library of Medicine. Available: www.locatorplus.gov.

LOCATORplus is the National Library of Medicine's (NLM) online catalog accessed on the Internet. In 1999, LOCATORplus replaced NLM's telnet-based online catalog, LOCATOR, and replaced the catalog databases CATLINE, SERLINE, and AVLINE. Prior to 1999, CATLINE was a primary bibliographic source for monograph records. LOCATORplus is continuously updated and includes over 800,000 catalog records for books, audiovisuals, journals, computer files, and other materials in NLM's collections. Records from the CATLINE, SERLINE, and AVLINE databases are available via

LOCATORplus. LOCATORplus contains a mixture of cataloged and uncataloged materials and includes records created by contributing special producer organizations as well as NLM. LOCATORplus contains only records that are available in machine-readable format. A user may need to consult retrospective sources for early works covering the biomedical sciences. LOCATORplus is available free of charge on the World Wide Web. The National Library of Medicine's cataloging records are also available from other vendors, such as Online Computer Library Center (OCLC) and Research Libraries Information Network (RLIN).

2.2 *WorldCat.* Dublin, OH: Online Computer Library Center (OCLC). Available: www.oclc.org/worldcat.

2.3 *Research Libraries Information Network (RLIN).* Mountain View, CA: Research Libraries Group. Available: www.rlg.org/rlin.html.

Online Computer Library Center and RLIN provide shared cataloging records and bibliographic descriptions through their respective international network systems. Cataloging records are included for a variety of materials, including monographs, in all subject domains. In addition to NLM, sources of cataloging information include the Library of Congress, National Agriculture Library, British Library, and member libraries. Both OCLC and RLIN are major sources of bibliographic information for monographs. They also provide location information, as cataloging records indicate the holding libraries for items included in their respective databases.

Online Computer Library Center is a nonprofit membership organization serving some 42,489 libraries in 86 countries and territories worldwide. The WorldCat database serves as the core for all OCLC services. WorldCat includes more than 48 million cataloging records contributed by libraries around the world.

RLIN is an international cooperative bibliographic information system. The acronym "RLIN" refers to an interface and system used to view and work with Research Libraries Group (RLG) bibliographic records. Research libraries, special libraries, and archival repositories have used RLIN for authority work and cataloging, processing manuscripts, and interlibrary loan.

2.4 *Doody's Health Sciences Book Review Journal.* Oak Park, IL: Doody Publishing, 1993–. Cumulated with additional reviews in *Doody's Health Sciences Book Review Annual.* See also: *Doody's Rating Service: A Buyer's Guide to the 250 Best Health Sciences Books.* Oak Park, IL: Doody Publishing, 1994–. Annual. Available: www.doody.com.

Doody's Health Sciences Book Review Journal and other general bibliographic resources, such as the *National Union Catalog* and *American Book Publishing Record*, are useful tools for verifying health science monograph information as well as identifying their location. However, these sources are not likely to be available in many health sciences libraries, particularly those outside of large academic settings.

Founded in 1993, Doody Publishing is a medical publishing company devoted to producing information products for health care professionals. Doody Publishing maintains a database of more than 65,000 health sciences titles. Doody's provides expert reviews for some 11,000 of those titles as well as Doody's Star Ratings. The expert reviews and star ratings are printed and published in *Doody's Heath Sciences Book Review Journal.* The star ratings are used to generate *Doody's Rating Service: A Buyer's Guide to the 250 Best Health Sciences Books.* Doody commissions original expert reviews for select titles. Reviews feature the byline of the reviewer and consist of a general description of the book, intended audience, purpose, features, assessment, and a star rating. Doody's star rating is derived from a questionnaire completed by the expert reviewer during the course of completing a review. Bibliographic and descriptive information is contained in each entry for in-print and forthcoming books. Bibliographic information is supplied by Login Brothers Book Company. Pricing and availability information is updated daily in the Doody database. Access to the database is available via the Web. Books may be ordered directly from the Web site.

2.5 *Brandon-Hill Selected Lists.* New York: Gustave L. and Janet W. Levy Library, Mount Sinai School of Medicine. Available: www.brandon-hill.com.

2.6 *National Union Catalog.* Washington, DC: Library of Congress, 1983–. Monthly. Microfiche. Continues: *National Union Catalog: A*

Cumulative Author List. Washington, DC: Library of Congress, 1956–1982.

2.7 *American Book Publishing Record.* New York: R. R. Bowker, 1960–. Monthly; annual cumulation with quinquennial cumulations.

2.8 *Publishers Weekly.* New York: Reed, 1987–.

Originally published in the *Journal of the Medical Library Association* (formerly titled *Bulletin of the Medical Library Association*), the Brandon-Hill Selected List of Print Books and Journals for the Small Medical Library, Brandon-Hill Selected List of Print Books and Journals in Allied Health, and Brandon-Hill Selected List of Print Books and Journals in Nursing are widely recognized collection development tools. The selected lists are the brainchild of Alfred N. Brandon who first published the Selected List of Books and Journals for the Small Medical Library in 1965. The selected list for nursing followed in 1979 and the selected list for allied health in 1984. The lists are now electronically available via the Web. Each list is categorized by subject. An author/editor index is included for book entries. Daggers and asterisks are used to designate level of significance for purchase.

Published by the Library of Congress (LC), the *National Union Catalog* (*NUC*) provides a cumulative record of materials currently cataloged by LC and participating libraries for imprints published in 1956 and later. The *NUC* is a vast bibliography that is frequently consulted because its holdings represent the broad scope of the world's output of monographs and other types of materials.

The microfiche *National Union Catalog* is published in multiple sections using a register/index format. The five sections of *NUC. Books* include the register, name index, title index, LC series index, and LC subject index. Item records include all bibliographic elements traditionally found on LC printed cards. Because entries appear in *NUC* only if a participating library has acquired and cataloged a title, *NUC* serves as a location source as well as a verification tool.

Monographs included in *NUC* with a publication date of 1968 or later are accessible in the CD-ROM/online arena. Primary access is available via OCLC or RLIN. DIALOG provides access as well through the Library of Congress MAchine-Readable Cataloging (MARC)-Books database.

The *American Book Publishing Record* cumulates the listings in *Publishers Weekly*. This ongoing resource provides bibliographic information about English-language publications in all subject areas. The primary goal of this bibliographic resource is to list books that can be purchased from publishers and to provide enough information to order any given title. This resource is important to the health sciences librarian because the health sciences arena is affected by disciplines outside of health and biomedicine. In addition, the *American Book Publishing Record* and *Publishers Weekly* provide a historical account of books published in the United States.

2.9 *Books in Print.* New York: R. R. Bowker, 1948–. Annual. *Books in Print Supplement.* New Providence, NJ: R. R. Bowker, 1972/73–. Annual. Available: www.booksinprint.com.

2.10 *Medical and Health Care Books and Serials in Print.* New York: R. R. Bowker, 1985–, 2 vols. Continues *Medical Books and Serials in Print,* 1978–1984.

2.11 *Canadian Books in Print. Author and Title Index.* Toronto: University of Toronto Press, 1975–. Continues *Canadian Books in Print.* 1967-1974.

An ongoing task for a librarian is to determine the availability of a given title for purchase. The librarian must first identify whether or not a title is still in print and subsequently if it is for sale. The following resources are designed to assist with this process.

Books in Print (*BIP*) is a broad resource that covers all subject areas. *Books in Print* is indexed by *Subject Guide to Books in Print, 1957–1987/88* and *Books in Print. Subject Guide, 1988/89–. BIP* is kept updated by the annual publication of *Books in Print Supplement, 1972/73–.* Each entry includes bibliographic elements, cost information, and source(s) from which the book can be purchased. Although the print version of *BIP* remains useful, Web access is becoming more common. Bowker's *Books in Print* Web site provides the same resources as the print version but with many enhanced features. For example, the Web site includes resource guides, publisher spotlights, and new features. Whereas the print version supports author and title access, the Web site allows for keyword, author, title, and ISBN/UPC access. The Web site also allows the user to browse by subject area or by index. Booksinprint.com includes the full *Books in Print* database of U.S. titles as well as *Books Out-of-Print* and *Forthcoming Books*.

Also produced by R. R. Bowker, *Medical and Health Care Books and Serials in Print* continues *Medical Books and Serials in Print*. This title serves as an index to literature in the health sciences and is of obvious interest to health sciences librarians. *Medical and Health Care Books and Serials in Print* lists more than 95,000 books under 8,000 health and biomedical subject areas. Ordering and publisher information is included in each entry to facilitate acquisitions.

Canadian Books in Print. Author and Title Index continues *Canadian Books in Print*. This work serves as a companion resource to *Books in Print* and *Whitaker's Books in Print* (formerly *British Books in Print*). *Canadian Books in Print. Author and Title Index* includes entries for titles produced by Canadian publishers. It is issued each year in one clothbound edition and in three complete microfiche editions.

2.12 Amazon.com. Seattle, WA: Amazon.com, Inc. Available: www.amazon.com.

2.13 Barnesandnoble.com. New York: Barnes & Noble, Inc. Available: www.barnesandnoble.com.

Commercial Internet vendors such as amazon.com and barnesandnoble.com have become recognized bibliographic information sources. Their customer rating and related purchases features are useful collection development tools.

Amazon.com is perhaps one of the most popular Internet vendors. Originally focusing on the book and music markets, Amazon.com has grown to include books, music, videos, DVDs, magazine subscriptions, office products, apparel, electronics, toys, games, housewares, hardware, home and garden supplies, gift items, and registries among its retail offerings. To locate monograph titles, users may perform a keyword search or browse by subjects. Records may be sorted by featured title, bestsellers, customer ratings, price, publication date, or alphabetically. Monograph records include bibliographic elements, ordering information, and purchase availability. Records also include customer ratings and reviews as well as published editorial reviews. Links are provided to authors of similar works that were purchased by individuals who purchased a particular title. Amazon.com supplies new and used books.

Another popular Internet vendor of books, textbooks, music, videos, and DVDs, barnesandnoble.com offers many of the same features as amazon.com. Users may search for monograph titles by keyword or browse by subject. Titles may be sorted by bestsellers. Entries include ordering information and note title availability for purchase. Customer reviews with ratings are included as are notes from the publisher. Records also indicate related titles purchased by individuals who purchased a particular book. In addition to new books and used books, barnesandnoble.com provides access to select out-of-print titles.

Retrospective Sources

Using clay tablets, papyrus, parchment, and, ultimately, paper, man has sought to record information for future reference. Development of the printing press in the fifteenth century forever changed the communication process. Society moved farther away from oral tradition to the printed word. Subsequently, the printed book reigned as the primary source of information until the mid-nineteenth century. By that time, the periodical had grown in use and popularity as the preferred means for disseminating scientific information.

Prior to the mid-nineteenth century, bibliographies containing entries for medical works were published, but they were not all-inclusive in subject coverage. In addition, these bibliographies were primarily concerned with medical works in monographic form. For a detailed account of early medical bibliography, the reader should consult *The Development of Medical Bibliography* by Estelle Brodman [1]; for a detailed account of medical bibliography since World War II, the reader should consult *Medical Bibliography in an Age of Discontinuity* by Scott Adams [4].

2.14 *Index-Catalogue of the Library of the Surgeon-General's Office.* Ser. 1–5. Washington, DC: U.S. Government Printing Office, 1880–1961, 61 vols.

2.15 *Index Medicus: A Monthly Classified Record of the Current Medical Literature of the World.* Ser. 1–3. Various publishers, 1879–1927, 45 vols.

John Shaw Billings, librarian of the Surgeon General's Library (forerunner of the National Library of Medicine) is considered the founding father of medical bibliography. Billings was responsible for the creation of the *Index-Catalogue of the Library of the Surgeon-General's Office* as well as the original *Index Medicus*. These two publications marked the beginning of a systematic attempt to provide bibliographic coverage of medical works worldwide.

First published in 1880, the *Index-Catalogue* contained a list of all monographic and periodical literature received by the Library of the Surgeon-General's Office (which became the Army Medical Library, the Armed Forces Medical Library, and, ultimately, the National Library of Medicine).

The *Index-Catalogue* was published in five series from 1880 to 1961, with a total of 61 volumes. Each series was intended to contain author and subject entries in dictionary form within a single alphabet. Monographic entries were listed under names of authors as well as under subject headings; entries for periodical articles were only listed under subject headings. Publication of the fourth series contained only alphabetical entries A through M, and series five did not include subject entries. Despite omissions, the *Index-Catalogue* was more comprehensive in coverage than any previous medical bibliography. Items were included as they were acquired by the library rather than by date of publication. Therefore, older items may be found in more recent series of the *Index-Catalogue*. Because the *Index-Catalogue* comprises only those items acquired by the library, it is not a comprehensive bibliography of medical works. However, the extent of the library's collection—a collection that eventually became the National Library of Medicine—makes the *Index-Catalogue* the most comprehensive listing of medical literature of the period. The *Index-Catalogue* continues to serve as a valuable retrospective bibliography and historical source.

Given that the *Index-Catalogue* was published as a series during many years, Billings developed the *Index Medicus* (*IM*) as a bibliographic updating tool. The *Index Medicus* was published from 1879 to 1927, with publication suspended from May 1899 to 1902. *IM* was published monthly from 1879 to 1920 and then quarterly from 1921 to 1927. Entries for books and journal articles were arranged by subject with an author index. The reader is referred to Chapter 4 for further discussion of *Index Medicus*.

Because the original *Index Medicus* ceased publication in 1927 and the *Index-Catalogue* contained entries for only those works purchased by the library, users should consult multiple resources in locating monograph titles published between 1927 and 1948 when the Army Medical Library *Catalog* began publication. These sources should not be limited to those specifically covering the health sciences, but should also include more general ones such as those compiled by the Library of Congress.

2.16 National Library of Medicine (U.S.). *Catalog.* Washington, DC: Library of Congress, 1956–1960/65. Issued annually with quinquennial cumulation (1955–1959) and a sexennial cumulation (1960–1965). Continues Armed Forces Medical Library (U.S.). *Catalog of the Army Medical Library,* 1952–1955. Continues Army Medical Library (U.S.). *Catalog,* 1948–1951.

From 1948 to 1965, these volumes were published as supplements to the printed catalogs published by the Library of Congress. They also serve as a bridge to *Index-Catalogue* series as well as the *National Library of Medicine Current Catalog*, which began publication in 1966. Each volume contains bibliographic information for monographs cataloged during this period, regardless of date of publication.

2.17 *National Union Catalog, Pre-1956 Imprints.* Chicago, IL: Mansell, 1968–1980, 685 vols. *Supplement,* 1980–1981, vols. 686–754.

National Union Catalog, Pre-1956 Imprints, compiled and edited with the cooperation of the Library of Congress and the National Union Catalog Subcommittee of the Resources and Technical Services

Division of the American Library Association, is a centerpiece for verification of books and other materials prior to 1956. This work is also used to verify serials titles that closed prior to 1956. *Pre-1956 Imprints* consists of an alphabetical listing of materials published prior to January 1, 1956, which have been cataloged by the Library of Congress or by one of the *NUC* participating libraries.

2.18 *The American Book Publishing Record Cumulative, 1876–1949.* New York: R. R. Bowker, 1980, 15 vols. *The American Book Publishing Record Cumulative, 1950–1977,* 1978, 15 vols.

2.19 *Health Science Books, 1876–1982.* New York: R. R. Bowker, 1982.

Essentially, the two *American Book Publishing Record Cumulative* works contain bibliographic data for every book published and distributed in the United States between 1876 and 1977. More than 1.5 million titles, with full bibliographic and cataloging information, are included in these resources.

Health Science Books, 1876–1982 contains bibliographic and cataloging information from the Library of Congress for more than 133,000 titles published and distributed in the United States between 1876 and 1982. All areas of the health sciences are represented in this work.

References

1. Broadman E. *The development of medical bibliography.* Baltimore, MD: Medical Library Association, 1954:53.
2. Katz WA. *Introduction to reference work*, 7th ed. New York: McGraw-Hill, 1997.
3. Gaskell P. *A new introduction to bibliography.* New York: Oxford University Press, 1972.
4. Adams S. *Medical bibliography in an age of discontinuity.* Chicago: Medical Library Association, 1981.

CHAPTER 3

BIBLIOGRAPHIC SOURCES FOR PERIODICALS

Fred W. Roper

The periodicals collection constitutes the major element of the holdings of most health sciences libraries. Thus, there is a strong need for tools that assist in the identification and verification of periodical titles. The terms *periodical, journal, serial,* and *magazine* are often used interchangeably, creating a certain amount of confusion. In this chapter, the term *periodical* will be used, but it may include any or all of the other terms.

Because no single library can ever acquire enough materials to be self-sufficient, bibliographic sources with locations for periodicals are essential. In addition, the health sciences librarian is continually concerned with collection development and the selection of titles to be added to or dropped from the holdings of the library. Unfortunately, the current economic climate most often dictates dropping periodical titles. Thus, the need for locations where access to titles may be gained becomes even more critical.

To perform these functions, the reference collection must contain a variety of bibliographic sources—both those that specialize in the health sciences and those of a more general nature—that deal primarily or in part with periodicals. Included among these sources are bibliographies of periodicals, both print and electronic, and union catalogs.

43

Historical Note

It was not until 1665 that the scientific periodical as a publishing form came into existence. The *Journal des Scavans*, first published on January 5, 1665, is considered the first learned journal. Soon after the initial appearance of the *Journal*, the Royal Society (London) began publication of the *Philosophical Transactions of the Royal Society*. The *Journal* was aimed at the amateur, while *Philosophical Transactions* was intended to serve as a "means of communication between practicing scientists, as well as a journal of interesting and curious knowledge" [1].

Since those beginnings in the seventeenth century, the number of scientific periodicals has increased at an extremely rapid rate, particularly since the mid-twentieth century. The periodical, in both print and electronic format, is now the most common vehicle for first publication of research results and for timely communication with colleagues. The book, on the other hand, has been relegated the task of "the formal and proper publication of mature reflections or a completed opus . . . ." rather than the reporting of work currently in progress [2].

Current Sources

Information about the status of currently published periodicals is provided by a variety of sources. Previously, print resources were necessary for maintaining current information on current periodicals. The growth of electronic resources has completely changed that situation, and today a wide range of electronic information sources is available for coverage. Products from the National Library of Medicine are of primary importance to health sciences librarians and are the major resources for maintaining health sciences periodicals collections.

3.1 *LOCATORplus.* Bethesda, MD: National Library of Medicine. Available: http://locatorplus.gov.

3.2 *NLM Gateway.* Bethesda, MD: National Library of Medicine. Available: http://gateway.nlm.nih.gov.

LOCATORplus is the National Library of Medicine's (NLM) online catalog accessed free of charge on the Internet. According to the fact sheet, it is continuously updated and includes:

- Over 800,000 catalog records for books, audiovisuals, journals, computer files, and other materials in the NLM's collections
- Holdings information for journals and other materials
- Links from catalog records to Internet resources, including online journals
- Circulation status information for materials, including those on-order or in-process at NLM.

In 1999, LOCATORplus replaced the CATLINE, SERLINE, and AVLINE databases.

The NLM Gateway is a Web-based system that lets users search simultaneously in multiple retrieval systems at NLM. It allows users of NLM services to initiate searches from one Web interface, providing "one-stop searching" for many of NLM's information resources or databases. The gateway will provide phased access to information found in an increasing number of NLM retrieval systems.

3.3 *Ulrich's Periodicals Directory.* New Providence, NJ: R. R. Bowker, 2001–. Continues *Ulrich's International Periodicals Directory.* Available: http://ulrichsweb.com/ulrichsweb.

3.4 *Medical and Health Care Books and Serials in Print.* New York: R. R. Bowker, 1985–. 2 vols. Continues *Medical Books and Serials in Print,* 1978–1984. Available: http://ulrichsweb.com/ulrichsweb.

Ulrich's Periodicals Directory provides information on more than 150,000 periodicals currently being published throughout the world. It includes serials published more frequently than once a year and publications issued annually or less frequently than once a year, or irregularly. The Ulrich's database can be searched on CD-ROM or online. Both the print publication and the electronic database cover all subject areas.

Medical and Health Care Books and Serials in Print is another Bowker product and provides international coverage of some 15,000

45

selected titles of health care periodicals in addition to monographs. The entries are taken from the same database used to compile Bowker's *Ulrich's Periodicals Directory* and can be searched in the Ulrich's database.

Lists from Indexing and Abstracting Services

The major indexing and abstracting services in the health sciences provide lists of the periodicals they index and abstract on a regular basis. In some instances the lists are issued in both print and electronic format. These lists serve as important supplements to the more inclusive bibliographies of current periodicals.

3.5 *List of Journals Indexed in Index Medicus.* Bethesda, MD: National Library of Medicine. 1960–. Available: www.nlm.nih.gov/tsd /serials/lji.html.

The *List of Journals Indexed in Index Medicus* is designed to provide bibliographic information for serials from which articles are indexed with the *Medical Subject Headings* (*MeSH*) vocabulary and cited in MEDLINE. The journals being indexed for *Index Medicus* are listed in four sections: 1) alphabetic listing by abbreviated title, followed by full title; 2) alphabetic listing by full title, followed by abbreviated title; 3) alphabetic listing by subject field; and 4) alphabetic listing by country of publication. It contains ceased titles, changed titles, titles no longer indexed, and titles currently indexed. More detailed bibliographic data and information about indexing coverage can be found in LOCATORplus, NLM's online catalog.

3.6 *EMBASE List of Journals Indexed.* Amsterdam: Excerpta Medica Foundation, 1993–. Continues: *List of Journals Abstracted,* 1964–1992.

This list is an annual publication listing more than 4,000 serial titles. The abbreviated title section gives the full title and publisher and also indicates if the journal is indexed cover-to-cover or selectively.

3.7   *BIOSIS Serial Sources.* Philadelphia, PA: BioSciences Information
        Service. 1995–. Continues: *Serial Sources for the BIOSIS Previews
        Database, 1989–1994; Serial Sources for the BIOSIS Database,
        1978–1988.*   Available: www.biosis.org/products_services
        /bss.html.

BIOSIS Serial Sources includes a listing of 5,000 current titles as
well as the 13,000 archival titles reviewed by the BioSciences
Information Service (BIOSIS). For each title, the full title, frequency,
history notes, ISSN, and publisher address are included. An indicator is
included for each of the approximately 2,300 serials from *BIOSIS
Previews* and *Biological Abstracts* which are being indexed cover to
cover.

3.8   *Master Journal List.* Philadelphia, PA: Institute for Scientific
        Information (ISI). Available: www.isinet.com/isi/journals.

This online guide includes all journal titles covered in Institute for
Scientific Information (ISI) products. Periodicals can be searched by
title, keyword, and ISSN. There is a list of all titles and a list of all journal changes for the past 12 months.

3.9   *Chemical Abstracts Service Source Index.* Columbus, OH: Chemical
        Abstracts Service. Available: http://info.cas.org/ONLINE/CD
        /CASSI/cassicd.html.

The *Chemical Abstracts Service Source Index* (*CASSI*) includes
information on the publications indexed by Chemical Abstracts (CA) in
the various Chemical Abstracts Service sources since 1907 and provides a variety of other types of information, including bibliographic
information and libraries holding copies of the titles. The information
available in the printed source is also available on CD.

Periodicals Holdings Information

Sources that reveal library holdings of periodicals are essential in
locating the nearest centers for borrowing or for photocopying
desired articles. Although printed union lists continue to be useful for

identifying libraries that hold a particular item, online systems are usually the first sources consulted with searching for this information. Many of the previous sources in this chapter will also provide holdings information.

Libraries may have individual lists, either in published or electronic format, with variations to the intent of each list and the amount of information offered. These lists will range from current subscription lists to catalogs of all titles held by the library, ceased and current, with complete holdings information. Union lists range from national lists to regional and local union catalogs that reveal holdings within an area. As aids to bibliographic verification and location, they are indispensable in a reference collection, and the reference librarian needs to be aware of both print and electronic union lists that can be of immediate assistance.

3.10 DOCLINE. Bethesda, MD: National Library of Medicine. Available: www.nlm.nih.gov/docline/newdocline.html.

DOCLINE (Documents Online) is NLM's automated interlibrary loan request routing and referral system, which provides improved document delivery service among libraries in the National Network of Libraries of Medicine by linking journal holdings to route efficiently the requests to potential lending libraries on behalf of the borrower. Access to DOCLINE is through the National Network of Libraries of Medicine (NN/LM).

A major component of DOCLINE is SERHOLD; NLM's database of holdings for biomedical serial titles held by U.S. members of NN/LM as well as Canadian and Mexican libraries. The SERHOLD (Serials Holdings) module of the DOCLINE system is available to participating DOCLINE libraries, which may add, update, or delete their own holdings.

3.11 *Union List of Serials in Libraries of the United States and Canada*, 3rd ed. New York: H. W. Wilson, 1965. 5 vols.

3.12 *New Serial Titles: A Union List of Serials Commencing Publication After December 31, 1949; 1950–1970 Subject Guide*. New York: R. R. Bowker, 1975. 2 vols.

3.13 *New Serial Titles.* Washington, DC: Library of Congress, 1953–1999.

Union List of Serials in Libraries of the United States and Canada and its successor, *New Serial Titles*, give extensive coverage to periodicals from all countries, in all languages, and in all subject areas as long as the periodicals are held by a library in the United States or Canada which reports its holdings. Because of their age, these publications are today most useful for history and cataloging information. Even so, with information available through 1999, they will be indicators for periodicals.

3.14 *World List of Scientific Periodicals Published in the Years 1900–1960*, 4th ed. Washington, DC: Butterworths, 1963.

3.15 *British Union-Catalogue of Periodicals.* New York: Academic Press, 1955. Supplement to 1960. Washington, DC: Butterworths, 1962.

3.16 *Serials in the British Library.* London: British Library, 1981–. Continues: *British Union-Catalogue of Periodicals: New Periodical Titles*, 1964–1980.

In Great Britain, two titles of importance are the *World List of Scientific Periodicals* and the *British Union-Catalogue of Periodicals* and its successors.

The fourth edition of the *World List* covers scientific, technical, and medical periodicals published from 1900 to 1960 which are held in British Libraries.

The *British Union-Catalogue of Periodicals* and its successors cover periodicals from the seventeenth century to 1960, from all over the world and in all subject areas, as long as they are held in reporting British libraries. *New Periodical Titles* and *Serials in the British Library* united the *British Union-Catalogue of Periodicals* with the *World List of Scientific Periodicals.*

Another important union list in the sciences is the *Chemical Abstracts Service Source Index* (see 3.9, above), which identifies the holding libraries of periodicals indexed by the Chemical Abstracts Service.

Abbreviations

The reference librarian is often asked to help in the identification of abbreviations of serial/periodical titles which are usually from a bibliography in a monograph or periodical article. The major problem associated with this type of request is the lack of standardization that is observed in the formulation of abbreviations. Although standards have been developed by the American National Standards Institute (Z39 Subcommittee on Periodical Title Abbreviations), actual practice continues to vary.

Lack of regard for standardization has led to similar abbreviations for different titles and to varied abbreviations for the same title. All of the major indexing and abstracting services include an approach by abbreviated periodical title in their lists of titles indexed. In addition to these titles, *World List of Scientific Periodicals* and the *British Union-Catalogue of Periodicals* also offer access by abbreviation.

When the same abbreviation is used for multiple titles, further detective work is required to determine which title is needed. The publishing history of the titles will have to be examined, and a source that provides complete bibliographic information will need to be consulted. LOCATORplus (see 3.1, above), *Ulrich's Periodicals Directory* (see 3.3, above), *Chemical Abstracts Service Source Index* (see 3.9, above), *New Serial Titles* (see 3.12, above), *Union List of Serials* (see 3.11, above) and its successors, and the *British Union-Catalogue of Periodicals* (see 3.15, above) will be of particular value when verifying an abbreviated title.

Changes

Another challenge of periodicals work is keeping up with the changes that take place in the bibliographic record of a periodical. The most common changes are new periodicals (births), cessations (deaths), and title changes. Obviously, any element in the bibliographic record may change, but these are the major problem areas.

Sources that have special sections to note changes in periodical information include *Ulrich's Periodicals Directory* (see 3.3, above), *New Serial Titles* (see 3.12, above), and *Chemical Abstracts Service Source Index* (see 3.9, above).

References

1. Brodman E. *The development of medical bibliography.* Baltimore, MD: Medical Library Association, 1954:49–50.
2. Grogan D. *Science and technology: an introduction to the literature*, 4th ed, rev. London: Clive Bingley, 1982:131.

Readings

1. Houghton B. *Scientific periodicals: their historical development, characteristics and control.* London: Clive Bingley, 1975.
2. Katz WA. Bibliographies: national library catalogs and trade bibliographies. In: *Introduction to reference work. Volume one: basic information sources*, 7th ed. New York: McGraw-Hill, 1992:118–26.
3. Walker RD, Hurt CD. Journals. In: *Scientific and technical literature: an introduction to forms of communication.* Chicago, IL: American Library Association, 1990:1–78.

CHAPTER 4

INDEXING, ABSTRACTING, AND DIGITAL DATABASE RESOURCES

Jerry Perry, David K. Howse, and Joan Schlimgen

Introduction

On June 2, 2001, previously healthy clinical trial volunteer Ellen Roche, a 24-year-old technician at the Johns Hopkins Asthma and Allergy Center, died from progressive hypertension and multiple organ failure. The Johns Hopkins University trial she was participating in involved the use of the known lung toxin hexamethonium. Ellen's death resulted in an extensive review and a 3-day shutdown of research using human subjects at the prestigious university. According to a report in *Lancet*, among the findings of the U.S. Office of Human Research Protection, which conducted the review, was that the university's internal review board (IRB) approved the trial without adequate evidence of hexamethonium's safety, specifically noting that, ". . . the investigators and the [Hopkins] IRB failed to obtain published literature about the known association between hexamethonium and lung toxicity. Such data was readily available via routine MEDLINE and Internet searches, as well as recent textbooks on pathology of the lung" [1].

Health sciences librarians responded rapidly to Ellen's death. In August 2001, then-president of the U.S. Medical Library Association

(MLA) and director of the University of North Carolina, Chapel Hill, Health Sciences Library, Carol G. Jenkins, released a statement to the press, noting, "MLA recommends that better guidelines or standard practices be developed to assist research review boards in evaluating whether searches are sufficient and will work" [2]. The MLA board later created an Expert Searcher Task Force to promote the development of guidelines to assist local IRBs and librarians in promoting best practices in conducting literature searches.

The biomedical and life sciences literature—that mass of scholarly communications and, in particular, peer-reviewed published journal articles—represents in aggregate our collective knowledge about human health. That knowledge is accessible through indexing, abstracting, and, more recently, digital database resources. Ellen's death reminds health sciences librarians of their ongoing crucial role in supporting the health care enterprise by providing the timely and contextual delivery of the best information available to help answer clinical questions, to support relevant administrative decisions, and to move health care research forward. That role rests on having a thorough knowledge of the essential tools used to organize and manage the world's biomedical and life sciences peer-reviewed published journal literature.

This chapter will describe those tools with the greatest utility for the practicing health sciences librarian, first looking at how these tools are currently deployed, followed by a brief historical survey of the development of abstracting and indexing tools through current digital databases. Key resources will then be described in detail, followed by a representation of secondary resources in tabular format, organized to provide quick access to the most pertinent information needed by practitioners. The chapter concludes with a discussion of access issues offering historical perspective and a general review of options for providing optimal end user and librarian access.

Contemporary Practice

The biomedical and life sciences information universe is radically changed from 1994, when the 3rd edition of *Introduction to Reference*

Sources for Health Sciences Librarians [3] was published. The ubiquity of the Internet and, in particular, the World Wide Web, has rendered even the least Net-savvy user a database searcher. We now routinely search databases without even necessarily knowing that is what is happening. The simple purchase of airline tickets on the Web involves a complex though transparent database search. That ubiquity and the sheer degree of access to free and easy-to-use databases for locating information has led to a tendency to disregard the nature of true excellence in using and manipulating databases. A cavalier attitude toward information, for example, may have been a contributor to Ellen Roche's death, as noted earlier. There is an opportunity in this environment for health sciences librarians to reassert their preeminence as experts in the use and manipulation of databases.

Database searching is in fact a key feature of emerging roles for progressive practitioners of health sciences librarianship. In 2000, Davidoff and Florance wrote an editorial in the *Annals of Internal Medicine* calling for the creation of a new health information professional that they termed an *informationist* [4]. This person would deliver appropriate in-context information services based on an expertise balanced in the clinical and/or research domain as well as the domain of the librarian-informatician. Central to that role is the ability to search, locate, filter, and synthesize biomedical information to meet contextual needs. Florance, Giuse, and Ketchell have described some of the knowledge components for information professionals working in clinical and research settings, citing skills with using bibliographic and specialized information resources [5].

The rise in the 1990s of the evidence-based health care movement, like the delivery of in-context information services, presupposed advanced skills in the searching and culling of the biosciences knowledge base. The key service provided by the Cochrane Collaboration, probably the most widely recognized proponent of evidence-based practice in medicine, is their Cochrane Library, a database of systematic reviews and meta-analyses of the literature, and a registry of randomized clinical trials reported in diverse forums but including the journal literature.

The magnitude—the sheer volume—of information available to the practitioner and researcher is overwhelming, giving rise to informationists and "meta" resources that summarize the extent and quality of evidence available to support biomedical decision making. Increasingly, that evidence is now available on mobile technology devices, such as personal digital assistants (PDAs), allowing "extreme" in-context delivery of evidence-based knowledge resources. The advent of tools such as InfoRetriever, a Web and PDA-accessible database of clinical practice recommendations, begs the question of what constitutes a database in contemporary practice [6].

What Is a Database?

Merriam-Webster defines a database as "a usually large collection of data organized especially for rapid search and retrieval (as by a computer)," and dates usage beginning in 1962. Librarians have traditionally, and functionally, classified databases as either bibliographic, full-text, or numeric. By 2003, University of Illinois online industry expert Martha E. Williams, in the *Gale Directory of Databases*, offered an updated classification view. According to Williams, "Databases can be classed in many ways. One method is by form of data representation. Data may be in the form of words, numbers, images or sounds. . . ." [7] This view clearly acknowledges conceptual shifts that encompass the ability of data systems to represent digital objects of any format.

The databases most familiar to health sciences librarians remain those with a "word" focus, being bibliographic or full-text. Numeric and visual object databases, however, are increasingly of use, particularly in the realms of organic chemistry, genomics, and proteomics, where multidimensional graphic representations are essential for advancing knowledge.

Clean distinctions among word-based databases—between those deemed bibliographic and those full-text—have significantly blurred, however, in the past 5 to 10 years, particularly with the advent of Web-based portals and data aggregators such as the popular clinical resource MD Consult, which combines with one search interface the purely bibliographic (MEDLINE) with links to digitized full-text article content and digitized full-text reference books.

Abstracts and Indexes: The Precursors to Digital Databases

Nearly all of the key databases routinely searched by health sciences librarians had their origin as a print-based abstracting and/or indexing service. MEDLINE began life as the *Index Medicus*, CINAHL began as the *Cumulative Index to Nursing and Allied Health*, HealthSTAR began as the *Hospital Literature Index*, and what we know now as Web of Science began as the Institute for Scientific Information's *Science Citation Index*.

Indexes provide the essential bibliographic information needed to identify an article or other publications and nominally include information related to the author of the work, source journal or other publication, volume, issue, and pagination. Abstracting tools include the same key elements but also a summary of the work, perhaps author-generated, perhaps provided by an editor or reviewer. Most indexing and abstracting services permit access to their content by way of subject and author indexes; each tool varies in how data is presented and the nature by which access is organized. Key indexing tools permit access by lead and perhaps additional authors and by subject term or phrase, usually based on a controlled vocabulary tool or keyword in context listing. It is important to note that controlled vocabularies evolve over time and so a contemporary term or concept may not exist as one proceeds back through time.

Lest any health sciences librarian assume that print abstracts and indexes are no longer relevant to contemporary practice, consider the death of Ellen Roche. In reviewing the Johns Hopkins tragedy, *Lancet*, in an August 25, 2001, article titled "1966 and all that—when is a literature search done?", noted that, "The pulmonary complications of hexamethonium have indeed been reported," going on to list studies dating from the mid-1950s and early 1960s. "How were these articles missed? The answer, it seems, is that all were published before 1966. As a result, none appears in a search of the PubMed [MEDLINE] database of the U.S. National Library of Medicine" [1]. A hand search of the print *Index Medicus* by a well-trained, qualified librarian should have located the relevant literature.

The history of MEDLINE is in itself a useful review of the general history of databases with their origins in print abstracting and indexing tools. MEDLINE essentially began life in the late nineteenth century when in 1879, the Library of the Surgeon-General's Office began publishing *Index Medicus*, a periodical index of medical articles, books, reports, and other relevant literature. In 1927, *Index Medicus* merged with the publication *Quarterly Cumulative Index* to create the *Quarterly Cumulative Index Medicus*. In 1941, the library, then named the Armed Forces Medical Library, started publishing *The Current List of Medical Literature* intended to be a "rapid finding aid" for current journal articles. In 1956, legislation was passed whereby the Armed Forces Medical Library was renamed the National Library of Medicine. In 1959, the library began considering how to employ computer technology to publish the *Index Medicus*. NLM hired General Electric's Defense Systems Department, which developed MEDLARS (Medical Literature Analysis and Retrieval System), which, by 1964, was producing the print index but also provided a platform for executing Boolean searches against the bibliographic data. By 1971, NLM began loading the MEDLARS database on its computer in Bethesda, Maryland, and the system was renamed MEDLINE [8].

In most biomedical library environments, MEDLINE is the premier bibliographic information resource. Its print precursors admittedly gather dust in many libraries and yet remain crucial tools for verifying citations and tracing the scholarly record prior to the advent of online access.

Boorkman, in the 1994 edition of this book, described the key print abstract and index resources of greatest utility to the practicing biomedical librarian. Table 4-1 lists those key tools and their producers and describes years of coverage and scope. Readers are encouraged to consult Boorkman's "Indexing and Abstracting Services" chapter of the 3rd edition of *Introduction to Reference Sources in the Health Sciences* for additional details [3].

Table 4-1. Key Print Abstracts and Indexes			
Title	**Years**	**Producer**	**Scope**
Index Medicus	1960–.	U.S. National Library of Medicine	The primary print index to the bio-medical periodical literature, published monthly and, through 2000, cumulated annually. International in scope, *Index Medicus* provides subject and author access to articles in 3,923 journals, as of March 2003, in all areas of biomedicine and health care including biomedical aspects of technology, the humanities, and the physical, life, and social sciences. Utilizes the *Medical Subject Headings* (*MeSH*), a controlled vocabulary featuring a highly structured and hierarchical schematic permitting the application of standardized subheadings for more precise concept delineation. *MeSH* is updated annually and appears in four iterations: as an alphabetic list of terms; an annotated alphabetic version; a permuted list; and as a tree structure depicting the hierarchical organization of concepts. See Boorkman [3] for a review of the scope of coverage for *Index Medicus'* precursors, which include *Index Medicus*, series I (1879–1899), series II (1903–1920), series III (1921–1927); *Index Catalogue*, 1st series (1880–1895), 2nd series (1896–1916), 3rd series (1918–1932), 4th series A-MEZ (1936–1948), 4th

Table 4.1 *continued*			
Title	**Years**	**Producers**	**Scope**
			series Mh-Mn (1955), 5th series (1959, 1961); *Quarterly Cumulative Index* (published by the American Medical Association) (1916–1926); *Quarterly Cumulative Index Medicus* (*AMA*) (1927–1956), and *Current List of Medical Literature* (1941–1959). *Index Medicus'* digital counterpart is MEDLINE.
Excerpta Medica	1947–.	Excerpta Medica (Reed Elsevier)	An important biomedical clinical and basic sciences abstracting tool, international in scope but particularly strong in the pharmaceutical literature. Covers 4,500 journals with some monographs and dissertations. *Excerpta Medica* includes 40 subject domain sections, with issue frequency based on section. Provides author and detailed subject access, and is the print basis for the online EMBASE database. In 1991, the *EMTREE Thesaurus* (controlled vocabulary) was introduced; previously (1974–1990), the *Master List of Medical Indexing Terms* (*MALIMET*) was used.
International Nursing Index	1966–2000	American Journal of Nursing Company and U.S. National Library of Medicine	Discontinued quarterly index, cumulated annually, which utilized the *Nursing Thesaurus* (a supplement to *MeSH*). Covered nearly 300 international journals, predominately nursing titles but also relevant citations from non-nursing journals culled from MEDLINE

Table 4.1 *continued*			
Title	**Years**	**Producers**	**Scope**
			and HealthSTAR. Relevant content can now be found in MEDLINE (PubMed) and *CINAHL*.
Cumulative Index to Nursing and Allied Health Literature (CINAHL)	1977–.	Cinahl Information Systems	A key nursing literature index covering nearly 1,600 journals, published quarterly and cumulated annually. Formerly (1956 to 1976) the *Cumulative Index to Nursing Literature*, the scope now includes allied health subjects including librarianship. Utilizes the *CINAHL Subject Heading List*, similar in structure to *MeSH* with many common terms. Includes nursing dissertations, standards of practice, educational software, audiovisuals and select nursing monographs and conference proceedings. *CINAHL* indexes American Nursing Association and National League for Nursing series titles. Complemented the now discontinued International Nursing Index, with overlap of the core nursing literature.
International Pharmaceutical Abstracts (IPA)	1964–.	American Society of Health Systems Pharmacists	International Pharmaceutical Abstracts, published semimonthly, indexes the pharmaceutical literature and covers nearly 700 pharmaceutical, medical, herbal, cosmetics, and health-related publications worldwide. Topical areas include the practice of pharmacy, pharmaceutical technology, pharmacoeconomics, and drug testing, analysis,

Table 4.1 *continued*			
Title	**Years**	**Producers**	**Scope**
			and chemistry, among others. IPA includes abstracts from the American Society of Health Systems Pharmacists' various meetings and state pharmacy journals.
Index to Dental Literature (IDL)	1962–1999	American Dental Association and the U.S. National Library of Medicine	Discontinued primary index to the dental literature. Quarterly, cumulated annually. The *Index* utilized a list of dental descriptors with reference to *MeSH*. Covered international dental journals but also relevant citations from nondental periodicals culled from MEDLINE. Included indexes of recent monographs and dissertations. See Boorkman [3] for a review of the scope of coverage for the precursor to the *IDL*, the *Index of the Periodical Dental Literature* (1839–1964). Relevant content can now be found in MEDLINE (PubMed).
Dental Abstracts: A Selection of World Dental Literature	1956–.	American Dental Association	Bimonthly abstracting index covering over 1,000 dental articles published internationally.
Hospital and Health Administration Index (HHAI)	1995–1999	American Hospital Association and the U.S. National Library of Medicine	Discontinued quarterly index to English-language journal articles published on the administration and management of health care services. Cumulated annually. Scope included quality assurance, legislative and public policy, and eco-

Table 4.1 *continued*			
Title	**Years**	**Producers**	**Scope**
			nomic aspects of the delivery of health care. Utilized *MeSH*, with supplemental domain terms. See Boorkman [3] for a review of the scope of coverage for the precursors to the HHAI: *Hospital Periodical Literature Index* (1945–1954) and Hospital Literature Index (1955–1995). Citations from the HHAI were included in the HealthSTAR database and relevant citations can now be found in MEDLINE (PubMed).
Biological Abstracts	1926–.	BIOSIS	Semimonthly abstracting service covering articles on original research in all aspects of the life sciences, culled from over 4,000 journals. Both Biological Abstracts and Biological Abstracts/RRM (Reports, Reviews and Meetings) provide access through author, subject, and organism indexes.
Biological Abstracts/RRM (Reports, Reviews and Meetings)	1982–.	BIOSIS	Monthly complementary index to Biological Abstracts covering research reports, symposia, book chapters, and select government reports. Both Biological Abstracts and Biological Abstracts/RRM provide access through author, subject, and organism indexes. See Boorkman [3] for a review of the scope of coverage for this title's precursors, including: *Bioresearch Titles* (1965–1966), *BioResearch*

Table 4.1 *continued*			
Title	**Years**	**Producers**	**Scope**
			Index (1967–1979), and *Biological Abstracts/RRM* (monthly) (1980–1981).
Chemical Abstracts	1907–.	Chemical Abstracts Service	A weekly international abstracting index to over 14,000 periodicals, proceedings, symposia, reports, dissertations, and monographs. The abstracts are organized into 80 sections, including biochemistry and macromolecular and organic chemistry. Indexes include author, patentees, alphabetic keyword (titles, abstracts and texts), numeric patent, and patent concordance. Volume indexes include subject, substance, and formula. The Chemical Abstracts Service assigns CAS Registry Numbers to unique chemical substances, and these numbers are tracked in the *CA Registry Handbook*, which provides substance and formula information that can be used to access the appropriate indexes.
Science Citation Index (SCI)	1961–.	Institute for Scientific Information (Thomson Corp.)	An interdisciplinary, bimonthly index to about 3,700 source publications, including journals but also monographic series, with nearly half of it coverage within the life sciences including clinical practice. Along with alphabetic author and permuted subject (keyword) indexes, the real utility of this resource lies in its Citation Index,

Table 4.1 *continued*			
Title	**Years**	**Producers**	**Scope**
			which allows the searcher to search cited references included in those citations listed in the Source Index. Cumulated annually and in 5-year increments. *SCI*, expanded in scope, is available via ISI's Web of Science.
Psychological Abstracts	1927–.	American Psychological Association	An excellent tool for locating information on the psychological aspects of illness, disease, and behavior, this monthly abstracting index covers over 1,800 titles including journals, monographs, and reports and is international in scope. Includes dissertations, though without abstracts. Includes author and subject indexes, utilizing the *Thesaurus of Psychological Index Terms*, also from the APA. *Psychological Abstracts* is cumulated annually and is available as PsycINFO.
Current Contents: Clinical Practice	Variable	Institute for Scientific Information (Thomson Corp.)	A weekly service providing tables of contents from current domain journals, usually within a week of publication. *Current Contents* is in fact a series, two of which will be of primary interest: *Clinical Medicine* and *Life Sciences*. Includes author and keyword subject indexes.

A Brief History of Online Searching

Electronic databases first emerged in the mid-1960s with the National Library of Medicine's MEDLARS service, which was introduced in 1964 as the machine-readable version of *Index Medicus*. Initially this was a batch system, which required the librarian to send a written description of the search request to NLM, where information specialists executed the search and sent the results back. The powerful search capabilities of the system considerably reduced the time it took to complete a comprehensive search despite the lag time for mail transmission. The searcher was now able to construct complex queries to produce a single list of retrieved bibliographic citations. In just a few years, the service grew from 62 requests processed in the first year to 24,000 in 1970 [9].

Things sped up considerably with NLM's first online system in 1971. Other online systems had also become available, including Dialog and SDC Orbit. Searchers dialed into remote databases stored on large mainframe computers via telephone lines using modems running at slow baud rates. There was significant training required to master these rigid systems, each of which required the use of a unique command language. Training on NLM's Elhill online system entailed a 1-week course in Bethesda, Maryland. Charges for online usage were based on connections to the system in real time, so that searches needed to be prepared offline in advance in order to avoid running up high costs. A complete history of online searching is described elsewhere [10].

Mediated Searching

The need for a high level of searching expertise ushered in the era of mediated searches. Librarians took on the role of the expert searcher, or intermediary, which proved to be efficient in terms of cost and labor savings. It also highlighted librarians' knowledge of information organization and structures and their ability to identify relevant sources in response to clinical and research needs. This model was executed by librarians conducting extensive reference interviews, preparing complex search strategies, searching multiple databases, and finally delivering the results, generally bibliographic citations and abstracts, to users.

In the medical library, these users were often clinicians who needed access to the medical literature for patient care. Some libraries established clinical medical library programs, which moved librarians closer to the hospital bedside and provided an early model for today's informationist. One study, conducted in a clinical setting, showed that including an information specialist on a clinical team increased efficiencies, exposed clinicians to the library and medical literature, and enhanced patient care [11]. Literature Attached to Charts (LATCH), developed at the Washington Hospital Center, took the trend a step further. Key articles were selected from literature searches, performed by librarians on some aspect of the patient's illness, and placed into the patient's hospital record [12]. Later studies revealed that physicians who had access to the medical literature frequently made changes in the care they provided to their patients, which resulted in improved patient care, reduced mortality, and fewer readmissions [13].

Librarians proved their value by using their knowledge of print and electronic resources along with their searching expertise to provide literature searches that were authoritative and comprehensive. In recent years, demand has increased for information professionals who are not only skilled in retrieving relevant clinical information, but who have experience and training across a broad expanse of disciplines and clinical work, including medicine, clinical epidemiology, biostatistics, and medical informatics, in order to function effectively as a member of a clinical care or research team [4].

End User Searching

By the mid-1980s, pressure was building to give end users access to a vastly larger array of online databases. Gateway systems, such as Grateful Med, were built to facilitate a less structured command language, but it was the appearance of databases on CD-ROM that finally made end user searching more affordable as subscriptions replaced online usage fees. Graphical user interfaces and natural language searching also made it easier for end users. Many libraries built complex CD-ROM networks, but users still needed to be at a workstation in the library to do their own searches.

The end user revolution required librarians to reposition themselves as their role as intermediary receded, particularly in the academic environment. Instead, there were now multitudes of end users to educate about controlled vocabularies, keywords, and proper searching technique. Librarians quickly adapted to their new teaching role, both in the classroom and at the reference desk. A typical end user training session covered such points as defining the topic, formulating the search strategy, choosing the appropriate database, evaluating the results, and revising the strategy. Studies showed that end users often relied on simple search strategies, did not always follow all the formal steps suggested by librarians, and used few and/or poor search terms [14]. As search interfaces have improved, so has end user searching, but interfaces still have a long way to go in adequately assisting the user in obtaining search results that are both high in recall and precision.

Internet Access

As Internet access has grown ubiquitous, nearly all online systems have been converted for Web access. This has provided clinical and research enterprises such as universities and hospitals with the ability to provide access to information throughout their institutions. Emphasis has moved away from access to individual bibliographic databases to the creation of gateways or portals to full-text content. The National Library of Medicine has continued to be on the forefront: NLM's Entrez search and retrieval system, which replaced Elhill, is one of the most sophisticated database searching portals. Entrez acts as a gateway to a vast array of biomedical information and is available free on the Internet. One of its components is PubMed, whose primary data source is MEDLINE. A major feature of PubMed is LinkOut, which provides access to full-text content by linking directly to publishers, databases of full-text content, or Web sites. Entrez also hosts a variety of nonbibliographic databases that include GenBank, the nucleotide sequence database and PubMed Central, a digital archive of full-text journal literature. In addition, NLM developed MEDLINEPlus, which organizes consumer- and patient-focused links to full-text information on hundreds of diseases and conditions.

Likewise, commercial publishers have made electronic journals and books available on the Web. Aggregators, such as MDConsult, bundle selected full-text journal and book content in databases, which are searchable using both controlled vocabularies and natural language. Other publishers, such as OVID, sell full-text journals and books, which are linked to bibliographic citations in the databases that they deliver.

Digital Databases: Primary and Secondary Resources

Digital bibliographic databases, with or without links to full-text, are critical resources for the contemporary health sciences librarian, representing the latest iteration of often already familiar abstracting and indexing tools. The following section of this chapter provides information on the primary digital databases of greatest utility. Individual database products are described, including database title, indexing information, dates of coverage, producer with brief contact information, vendor data, key hallmarks, and scope notes.

Primary Digital Databases

4.1   *MEDLINE.* Bethesda, MD: National Library of Medicine. Available: www.pubmed.gov.

MEDLINE is the most important of all bibliographic biomedical databases, containing over 12 million citations going back to the mid-1960s and covering nearly 4,600 journals published in the United States and in more than 70 other countries. MEDLINE is produced by the MEDLARS Management Section of the U.S. National Library of Medicine. Its print equivalent is *Index Medicus*, which has been published since 1879. Note that *Index Medicus* presently indexes approximately 3,900 journals whereas MEDLINE includes nearly 4,600 titles. Computer-based access to the data from *Index Medicus* began in 1964, with NLM's Medical Literature Analysis and Retrieval System *(*MEDLARS), and subsequently evolved into MEDLINE (MEDlars onLINE) in 1971.

The subject scope of MEDLINE is biomedicine and health, broadly defined to encompass those areas of the life sciences, behavioral sciences, chemical sciences, and bioengineering needed by health professionals and others engaged in basic research and clinical care, public health, health policy development, or related educational activities. The majority of the publications covered are scholarly journals; a small number of newspapers, magazines, and newsletters considered useful to particular segments of NLM's broad user community are also included.

New citations are added weekly and are assigned descriptor terms and publication type designations from NLM's controlled vocabulary, the *Medical Subject Headings*, or *MeSH*. A key hallmark of MEDLINE is its highly structured and rigorously managed subject indexing, derived from a selection of *MeSH*-related tools and which makes searching relatively easy and comprehensive. Over 50 percent of MEDLINE's bibliographic records include abstracts. Time span covered is from 1966 to the present.

NLM offers free Internet access to MEDLINE through PubMed, searchable via the National Center for Biotechnology Information's (NCBI) Entrez retrieval system, which is the search and retrieval system used at NCBI for a selection of major databases including PubMed, Nucleotide, Protein Sequences, Protein Structures, Complete Genomes, Taxonomy, OMIM (Online Mendelian Inheritance in Man), and many others.

Several vendors offer MEDLINE on a fee basis, including OVID, Dialog, EBSCO, JICST Online Information System, STN International, ProQuest, Aries Systems Corporation, and OCLC FirstSearch. Time coverage and update schedules vary from vendor to vendor (see Table 4-3 for contact information). MEDLINE is also available for free as an enhancement to various physician community-directed portal services, such as MEDSCAPE and BioMedNet.

MEDLINE is the "lingua franca" of biomedicine and, as such, some agents who provide access have enhanced its utility by offering options for linking directly from the MEDLINE record to full-text content, with the most widely recognized example being the LinkOut program available via NLM using the PubMed/Entrez platform. Commercial vendors such as OVID have their own versions. This interlinking, from database record to online full-text, and in some cases from the citations of online full-text content to additional bibliographic records and on to additional full-text, is a critical service enhancement for customers.

The PubMed iteration has additional useful content outside of the journal literature indexed in MEDLINE, and it remains to be seen whether vendors selling MEDLINE will try to include this extra material in the future. Librarians originally critical of Entrez have noted that it has recently improved insofar as multiple keywords are automatically linked using the Boolean AND operator, a useful feature for inexperienced users. The PubMed Clinical Queries feature is also an excellent utility for finding evidence-based studies, using a search filter developed by researchers at McMaster University in Canada.

4.2 *MEDLINEPlus*. Besthesda, MD: National Library of Medicine. Available: www.medlineplus.gov.

MEDLINEPlus is designed to deliver authoritative and easily accessible health information to the consumer and the health professional. Unlike bibliographic databases that index highly structured records, MEDLINEPlus is a free Web portal that pulls together information from a wide variety of sources. Produced by the U.S. National Library of Medicine, it made its debut on the Internet in October of 1998 with only 22 health topics. Updated daily, this searchable database now has extensive information from the National Institutes of Health (NIH) and other trusted sources on over 600 diseases and conditions.

Sources include links to preformulated searches on NLM databases, such as on MEDLINE and ClinicalTrials.gov, which provide the latest references to the medical literature and to NIH research studies. Other content comes from a database of full-text drug information, an illustrated medical encyclopedia, a medical dictionary, interactive health tutorials, and the latest health news. In addition, MEDLINEPlus links to other established and dependable Web sites after they have been evaluated by an advisory board for accuracy and quality as well as for the appropriateness of the presentation of the information. There are also lists of hospitals and physicians, extensive information on prescription and nonprescription drugs, health information from the media, and links to thousands of clinical trials.

The utility of MEDLINEPlus as a service for health consumers cannot be overestimated. Freely accessible and with a Spanish language version, librarians in any enterprise, be it biomedical, general academic, public, or corporate, will find utility in its contents. And, because delivering access to its resources has been a high priority for its parent, the U.S. National Library of Medicine, MEDLINEPlus continues to evolve with regular enhancements. For example, as of May 2003 there were over 150 interactive online tutorials with slides and sound features to assist site users. The extensive collection of medical images in the A.D.A.M. Health Illustrated Encyclopedia provides a powerful complement to the text, assisting the layperson in obtaining a deeper understanding of complex medical conditions and procedures.

4.3   *CINAHL.* Glendale, CA: Cinahl Information Systems, a division of EBSCO Publishing. Available: www.cinahl.com.

The CINAHL database indexes journal and other literature related to the nursing and allied health fields, additionally providing some coverage of biomedicine, alternative/complementary medicine, consumer health, and health sciences librarianship. Aside from journals, CINAHL also provides citation access to health care books, pamphlets, nursing dissertations, conference proceedings, standards of professional practice, educational software, and audiovisual materials. The time span covered is from 1982 to the present.

CINAHL specifically includes citations from over 2,200 journals, of which over 1,500 are currently indexed. Abstracts are available for more than 1,200 of these titles. More than 7,000 records in the database include full-text access, and 1,200 records are replete with images.

Over 10,000 CINAHL subject headings facilitate searching, with approximately 70 percent also appearing in NLM's *MeSH.* CINAHL supplements these MEDLINE descriptors with 2,000+ terms designed specifically for the nursing and allied health fields.

CINAHL was originally available as a printed index, which began in the early 1960s as the *Cumulative Index to Nursing Literature*, and later as the *Cumulative Index to Nursing and Allied Health*.

Although primarily a bibliographic resource, the CINAHL database, as noted, includes selected original and full-text materials. Full-text has rapidly expanded over the past several years and currently includes selected state nursing journals and some newsletters, standards of practice, practice acts, government publications, research instruments, and patient education materials.

A key hallmark of the database is the ability to zero in on highly specific publication delimiters, including the ability to limit to peer-reviewed journal articles and various other publication types, journal subsets, or special interest categories. These delimiters greatly enhance the utility of the database for both researchers, interested in highly specific content formats and subsets, and for novice users, looking for "a few good articles."

Commercial vendors of CINAHL include its producer, Cinahl Information Systems, as well as OVID, Dialog, Aries Systems Corporation, EBSCO, ProQuest, and OCLC FirstSearch.

4.4   HealthSTAR/OVID Healthstar. Sandy, UT: OVID Technologies. Available: www.ovid.com.

HealthSTAR (Health Services Technology, Administration, and Research) is a bibliographic database covering all aspects of administration and planning of health care facilities; health insurance and financial management; licensure and accreditation; personnel management; quality assurance; health maintenance organizations; evaluation of patient outcomes; effectiveness of procedures, programs, products, services and processes; health policy; health services research; health economics; and laws and regulations. Although clinical literature is included, the focus is mostly on nonclinical aspects of health care delivery.

HealthSTAR's print equivalent, *Hospital and Health Administration Index*, dates back to 1945 under a number of different titles and was discontinued in 1999. It was produced by the American Hospital Association (AHA), which joined the NLM in 1977 to create the online version, initially called Health Planning and Administration, then

HSTAR, and finally HealthSTAR. It was offered by a number of commercial vendors for years and was available for free from the U.S. National Library of Medicine from February 1994 until December 2000, at which time NLM and AHA decided to discontinue producing the online version as well.

OVID now offers OVID HealthSTAR as a continuation of this database. OVID HealthSTAR retains all existing back files of HealthSTAR citations and is updated with new journal citations culled from MEDLINE using the NLM's original HealthSTAR search strategy. While only citations from the journal literature are currently being added to HealthSTAR, earlier years include indexing to select monographs, technical reports, meeting abstracts and papers, book chapters, government documents, and newspaper articles. Citations are indexed with the National Library of Medicine's *Medical Subject Headings* (*MeSH*) in order to ensure compatibility with other NLM databases. OVID HealthSTAR's coverage is from 1975 to the present.

Searchers who routinely need to locate information about health care policy, the impacts of legislation, literature comparing national health care delivery systems, and quality service enhancements appreciate the accessibility of this database via OVID, now that it is no longer accessible as a separate file from the U.S. National Library of Medicine. It is also useful for finding scholarly works on the increasingly important subjects of computing and automation in medicine, both from the administrative and clinical perspectives.

4.5 *International Pharmaceutical Abstracts.* Bethesda, MD: American Society of Health-System Pharmacists. Available: www.ashp.org.

The International Pharmaceutical Abstracts (IPA) database provides worldwide coverage of pharmaceutical science and health-related literature. Comprehensive information is included for articles on drug therapy and toxicity as well as legislation, regulation, technology, utilization, biopharmaceutics, information processing, education, economics, and ethics as related to pharmaceutical science and practice. While MEDLINE indexes much of the same journal content, examples of unique coverage include the indexing of state pharmacy journals, references about drug legislation, abstracts of presentations from major pharmacy meetings, and citations to alternative and herbal medicine literature. International Pharmaceutical Abstracts is particularly good for finding materials relating to pharmacy practice.

The extensive indexing of International Pharmaceutical Abstracts includes drug trade names linked to generic names, with an underlying hierarchical pharmacological/therapeutic classification scheme that allows searches by drug classes. Other features include a human-studies limiting option, tagged continuing education articles, and the identification of review articles. Searchable fields include standard bibliographic information, controlled terms, abstracts, drug names, and CAS registry numbers. International Pharmaceutical Abstracts is updated monthly, with content from over 800 journals. The time span covered is from 1970 to the present. A printed index with the same title began publishing in 1964.

International Pharmaceutical Abstracts is produced by the American Society of Health-System Pharmacists. The database is additionally available from OVID, Dialog, and in CD-ROM format from Cambridge Scientific Abstracts.

4.6   *Cochrane Database of Systematic Reviews.* Vista, CA: Update Software Inc. Available: www.update-software.com.

The Cochrane Database of Systematic Reviews is the major product of the Cochrane Collaboration, an international network of individuals and institutions committed to preparing, maintaining, and disseminating systematic reviews of the effects of health care. The Cochrane Collaboration consists of groups of experts in over 40 clinical specialties who authoritatively review hundreds of studies on topics in their specialty, select those that meet strict evidence-based medicine criteria, perform meta-analyses when possible on all the included studies, and then write detailed, structured reviews of the topic and the findings. The database is marketed as part of The Cochrane Library and is also available through other database vendors such as OVID and EBSCO.

Cochrane reviews are full-text articles, usually reviewing all relevant randomized control trials. The reviews are highly structured and systematic, with evidence included or excluded on the basis of explicit quality criteria, to minimize bias. The reviews are presented in two types: complete reviews, which are regularly updated by Collaborative

Review Groups; and protocols, for reviews currently being prepared (all include an expected date of completion). Data included in reviews are often combined statistically (with meta-analyses) to increase the power of the findings of numerous studies. The search interface is simple and easy to use. Content is searchable by keyword and can also be browsed using subject-specific Cochrane Groups.

Users are often disappointed when they cannot find evidence-based Cochrane material on a specific subject. This is not a criticism of the database for lacking content, but rather an endorsement of the value and popularity of the evidence-based Cochrane Reviews.

4.7 *Web of Science.* Philadelphia, PA: Thomson ISI. Available: www.isinet.com.

Web of Science provides access to the Institute for Scientific Information's (ISI) citation databases and enables users to search current and retrospective multidisciplinary information from approximately 8,500 high-impact research journals worldwide. Users can search for specific articles by subject, author, journal, and/or author address. Its most impressive feature, however, is a unique search method that permits cited reference searching. Because the information stored about each indexed article includes the article's cited reference list, working from a known author or work, the searcher can retrieve citations to all articles cited by that author or work. This capacity means that Web of Science is a key database for individuals and institutions looking to measure the impact of an author's or corporate entity's scholarship. It additionally has great utility for biomedical professionals, librarians, and information scientists looking to locate the most influential journals in given disciplines.

Web of Science is in fact a concatenated database that encompasses three citation databases: the Science Citation Index Expanded, Social Sciences Citation Index, and Arts & Humanities Citation Index. Dates of coverage for each segment are: Science, 1945 to the present (note that the print "parent" index, the *Science Citation Index*, dates from 1961); Social Sciences, 1956 to the present; and Arts and Humanities, 1975 to the present. The database is updated weekly.

Web of Science is a complex database with a well-designed, simple-to-use interface. Because the user can search through cited references, many of which are older than the period cover by MEDLINE, this tool can especially be useful when searching older journal literature. A significant weakness for general subject searching is the lack of a controlled vocabulary.

The primary vendor for Web of Science is ISI. Alternatively, Dialog and STN International both offer SCISEARCH (Science Citation Index Expanded from 1974 to the present).

4.8 *PsycINFO.* Washington, DC: American Psychological Association. Available: www.apa.org.

PsycINFO, produced by the American Psychological Association, abstracts and indexes the scholarly literature in the behavioral sciences and mental health. It includes material of relevance to psychologists and professionals in related fields such as psychiatry, neuroscience, general medicine, social work, sociology, nursing, pharmacology, physiology, linguistics, anthropology, education, management, business, and law.

Historical sources for citations in PsycINFO include *Psychological Abstracts* (1927–1966), *Psychological Bulletin* (1921–1926), the *American Journal of Psychology* (1887–1966), all other American Psychological Association journals back to their first issues, the *Psychological Index* (1894–1935), and the *Harvard Book Lists* (1938–1971). The retrospective conversion of *Psychological Abstracts* has been completed, and searchers may now locate all records back to the inception of the print index in PsycINFO. It also contains records from the now defunct PsycLIT database. In addition to journal articles, PsycINFO indexes book chapters, books, dissertations, and technical reports. Over 60,000 references are added annually through weekly updates selected from more than 1,800 periodicals, including many international titles. All records from 1967 to the present are indexed using the *Thesaurus of Psychological Index Terms* and nearly all contain nonevaluative summaries.

Approximately 75 percent of the content is from journals, almost all of which are peer-reviewed. There is comprehensive coverage of more than 650 journal titles ("cover to cover"), while 300 additional journals have every article selected ("total select"). For the remaining titles, articles are specially selected for psychological relevance.

Current chapter and book coverage includes worldwide English-language material published from 1887 to the present.

Searchers looking for information about psychological aspects of patient care, diseases, and medical therapies as well as information on psychological tests will find PsycINFO quite useful. Care should be taken in choosing indexing terms from the *Thesaurus of Psychological Index Terms* as there are conceptual differences between these terms and the U.S. National Library of Medicine's *Medical Subject Headings* (*MeSH*).

PsycINFO can be accessed from a large number of commercial vendors, including OVID, Dialog, EBSCO, Elsevier, OCLC FirstSearch, ProQuest, ISI, and National Information Services Corporation (NISC).

4.9 *BIOSIS/Biological Abstracts.* Philadelphia, PA: BIOSIS. Available: www.biosis.org.

A not-for-profit organization, BIOSIS produces several databases covering life sciences literature, the most important of which is the highly comprehensive Biological Abstracts. Subject scope includes all aspects of animal (including human), plant, and microorganism life, including aerospace and underwater biological effects, agronomy, allergy, anatomy and histology, animal production, bacteriology, behavioral biology, biochemistry, biophysics, blood and body fluids, botany, medical and clinical microbiology, paleobiology, soil science, veterinary science, and many other areas.

Subscribers to the larger BIOSIS Previews database get additional content beyond the journal article records included in Biological Abstracts, such as references to meetings, reports, review articles, books and monographs, and other unique references. This added content comes from another key BIOSIS database, Biological Abstracts/RRM (Reports, Reviews, Meetings).

In total, Biological Abstracts contains more than 7.7 million bibliographic records for life science articles indexed from over 4,000 biological and medical research journals, and nearly 90 percent of these records include abstracts. Indexing by author, organism, and subject allows retrieval by descriptive subject term, taxonomic name, and related concepts. The database is updated quarterly. Electronic coverage is available back to 1969. Its progenitor was the *Biological Abstracts* print index.

BIOSIS/Biological Abstracts is available from Dialog, DIMDI, EBSCO, OVID, Elsevier, STN International, and NISC (National Information Services Corporation).

4.10 *MD Consult.* St. Louis, MO: MD Consult. Available: www .mdconsult.com.

MD Consult, now a division of Elsevier, was launched in 1997 as a Web portal for clinicians. It provides access to a variety of practical knowledge-based resources intended to support the clinician as well as additional services such as health news and continuing medical education resources. MD Consult integrates a suite of content, including 40 medical reference books; over 50 medical journals; a search interface for MEDLINE; comprehensive drug information for over 30,000 medications; more than 1,000 clinical practice guidelines; and over 3,500 customizable patient education handouts. MD Consult is updated daily, although this depends on nature and origin of the content.

As a practical "one-stop-shop" online service for clinicians, MD Consult has been phenomenally successful, garnering a significant and enviable market share. Health sciences librarians typically find fault with its limited search interface, particularly when used to search the service's journals access feature. It is important to note, however, that the primary users of this service, clinicians, do not necessarily have the same set of expectations in terms of precision versus recall, and many are happy with the results from their queries.

Secondary Digital Databases

There is substantial diversity among health sciences libraries. Staff members at each strive to match their resources and services with the local and immediate needs of their constituencies. Following is a table of secondary digital database resources that supplement the previously noted primary tools, but are more narrowly focused in scope, coverage, and target users.

Table 4-2. Secondary Databases					
Title	**URL**	**Producer**	**Vendors**	**Scope**	**Contact**
AIDSinfo Clinical Trials Information Service	http://aidsinfo.nih.gov/	U.S. Department of Health and Human Services	Free	A central resource for information about federally and privately funded HIV/AIDS clinical trials.	AIDSinfo, P.O. Box 6303, Rockville, MD 20849-6303
Alt-Health Watch	www.epnet.com	EBSCO Publishing	EBSCO Publishing	Citations and full text articles on complementary, alternative, holistic, and integrated approaches to health and wellness, from over 170 journals plus pamphlets and book excerpts.	EBSCO Publishing (World Headquarters), 10 Estes Street, Ipswich, MA 01938
Arctic Health	http://arctichealth.nlm.nih.gov/	U.S. National Library of Medicine	Free	An information portal on issues affecting the health and well-being of our planet's northern-most inhabitants, who have to cope with extreme climatic conditions and are subject to a unique set of health and environmental challenges.	Specialized Information Services, U.S. National Library of Medicine, 8600 Rockville Pike, Bethesda, MD 20894

Table 4.2 *continued*					
Title	**URL**	**Producer**	**Vendors**	**Scope**	**Contact**
CATbank	www.cebm.net	Centre for Evidence-Based Medicine	Free	A database of CATs (critically appraised topics) developed for the Web by the National Health Service (U.K.) Research and Development Centre for Evidence-Based Medicine. A CAT is a summary of findings including an appraisal of the validity and applicability of evidence identified in response to an answerable clinical question.	Centre for Evidence-Based Medicine, University Department of Psychiatry, Warneford Hospital, Headington, Oxford, OX3 7JX, United Kingdom
Clinical Evidence	www.clinical evidence.com	BMJ Publishing Group	BMJ Publishing Group, OVID	The well-designed online version of the print compendium with the same title. Users can browse by topic or use a search engine to peruse regularly updated summaries of evidence on the effects of	Clinical Evidence, BMJ Publishing Group, BMA House, Tavistock Square, London, WC1H 9RJ, United Kingdom

Title	URL	Producer	Vendors	Scope	Contact
Table 4.2 *continued*					
				common clinical interventions. Content is pulled from multiple evidence-based sources, including the Cochrane Library.	
Clinical Trials.gov	http://clinical trials.gov/	U.S. National Institutes of Health	Free	Database providing easy access to information on clinical trials for a wide range of diseases and conditions.	National Institutes of Health (NIH), 9000 Rockville Pike, Bethesda, MD 20892
Combined Health Information Database	http://chid.nih.gov/	Several collaborating health-related agencies of the U.S. Federal Government	Free	CHID is a bibliographic database of health information and health education resources produced by health-related agencies of the U.S. Federal Government. Updated quarterly, CHID lists materials and program descriptions not indexed elsewhere.	CHID Technical Coordinator, 7830 Old Georgetown Road, Bethesda, MD 20814

Table 4.2 *continued*

Title	URL	Producer	Vendors	Scope	Contact
CRISP (Computer Retrieval of Information on Scientific Projects)	http://crisp.cit.nih.gov/	Office of Extramural Research at the U.S. National Institutes of Healthe	Free	CRISP is a searchable database of federally funded bio-medical research proj-ects conducted at universities, hospitals, and other research institutions.	National Institutes of Health (NIH), 9000 Rockville Pike, Bethesda, MD 20892
Database of Abstracts of Reviews of Effectiveness (DARE)	http://nhscrd.york.ac.uk/darehp.htm	NHS Centre for Reviews and Dissemination (U.K.)	Free	Includes struc-tured abstracts of systematic reviews, criti-cally appraised by reviewers at the (U.K.) National Health Service Centre for Reviews and Dissemination at the University of York, England. Reviews are assessed according to quality criteria. Also contained in the Cochrane Library, this version of DARE is avail-able for free on the Internet	NHS Centre for Reviews and Dissemination, University of York, York, YO10 5DD, United Kingdom

Table 4.2 *continued*

Title	URL	Producer	Vendors	Scope	Contact
DIRLINE (Directory of Health Organizations Online)	http:// dirline.nlm. nih.gov/	US National Library of Medicine	Free	Information about a wide variety of organizations, research resources, projects, and databases.	US National Library of Medicine, 8600 Rockville Pike, Bethesda, MD 20894
EMBASE	www. embase .com	Elsevier Science	Dialog DataStar, Dialog, DIMDI, LEXIS/ NEXIS, Ovid, Science-Direct, and STN International	Over 4,000 international medical serial titles from over 65 countries are currently indexed in EMBASE. Includes coverage of unique international titles not indexed in MEDLINE. Subfiles include EMDRUGS, EMCANCER, EMFOREN-SIC, EMHEALTH, and EMTOX.	Elsevier Web Technical Support Team, 360 Park Avenue South, New York, NY 10010-1710
Encyclopedia of Life Sciences	www. els.net	Nature Publishing Group	Nature Publishing Group	Spans the entire range of life sciences research, with updates every month.	Offices worldwide. In the U.S.A.: 345 Park Avenue South, 10th Floor, New York, NY 10010-1707

Table 4.2 *continued*					
Title	**URL**	**Producer**	**Vendors**	**Scope**	**Contact**
Entrez	www.ncbi. nlm.nih. gov/Entrez	National Center for Biotechnology Information, U.S. National Library of Medicine	Free	Entrez is a retrieval system for searching several linked databases: PubMed, GenBank, Protein Sequence Database, and more.	National Center for Biotechnology Information, U.S. National Library of Medicine, 8600 Rockville Pike, Bethesda, MD 20894
Hazardous Substances Data Bank (HSDB)	http:// toxnet.nlm. nih.gov/	U.S. National Library of Medicine	Free	Toxicology data file on the National Library of Medicine's (NLM) Toxicology Data Network (TOXNET), focusing on the toxicology of potentially hazardous chemicals. HSDB's 4,500 individual chemical records contain information on human exposure, industrial hygiene, emergency handling procedures, environmental fate, regulatory requirements, and related areas.	U.S. National Library of Medicine, 8600 Rockville Pike, Bethesda, MD 20894

Table 4.2 *continued*

Title	URL	Producer	Vendors	Scope	Contact
HazDat	www.atsdr. cdc.gov/haz dat.html	Agency for Toxic Substances and Disease Registry (U.S.A.)	Free	HazDat contains scientific and administrative information on the release of hazardous substances from Superfund sites or from emergency events. Also provides data on the effects of hazardous substances on the health of human populations.	Agency for Toxic Substances and Disease Registry, U.S. Department of Health and Human Services, Ariel Rios Building, 1200 Pennsylvania Avenue NW, M/C 5204G, Washington, DC 20460
HCUPnet (Healthcare Cost and Utilization Project)	www.ahcpr. gov/data/ hcup/ hcupnet .htm	Agency for Healthcare Research and Quality (U.S.A.)	Free	A tool for identifying, tracking, analyzing, and comparing statistics on hospitals at the national, regional, and state level.	Agency for Healthcare Research and Quality, Executive Office Center, Suite 600, 2101 East Jefferson Street, Rockville, MD 20852
Health and Wellness Resource Center	www.gale-group.com	Gale Group	Gale Group	Provides an integrated collection of general interest and fitness magazines, medical and professional periodicals, reference	Gale Group, 27500 Drake Road, Farmington Hills, MI 48331

Table 4.2 *continued*					
Title	**URL**	**Producer**	**Vendors**	**Scope**	**Contact**
				books, and pamphlets. Records are available in a combination of indexing, abstracts, or full-text formats. Designed for nursing and allied health students as well as consumer health researchers.	
Health Business FullTEXT Elite	www. epnet.com	EBSCO Publishing	EBSCO Publishing	Provides full text for nearly 450 periodicals detailing all aspects of health care administration and other non-clinical concerns.	EBSCO Publishing, P O Box 682, Ipswich, MA 01938
healthfinder	www. health finder.gov	Office of Disease Prevention and Health Promotion, U.S. Department of Health and Human Services	Free	Includes lists of consumer health information Web sites, selected online publications, databases, self-help groups, government agencies, and non-profit organizations.	healthfinder, P.O. Box 1133, Washington, DC 20013-1133

Table 4.2 *continued*

Title	URL	Producer	Vendors	Scope	Contact
Medical Matrix	www. med matrix.org	Medical Matrix L.L.C.	Medical Matrix L.L.C.	Medical Matrix is a comprehensive, clinically oriented database designed to be a "home page" for physicians. Sites are authoritative, peer-reviewed, annotated, frequently updated, and ranked according to a five-star rating system. Editorial board members are drawn from the American Medical Informatics Association's Internet Working Group.	Medical Matrix, c/o SLACK Incorporated, 6900 Grove Road, Thorofare, NJ 08086-9447
Molecular Modeling Database (MMDB)	www.ncbi. nlm.nih. gov /Structure	The National Center for Biotechnology Information (NCBI) Structure Group	Free	MMDB is a database of macromolecular 3D structures as well as tools for their visualization and comparative analysis. MMDB contains experimentally determined biopolymer structures obtained from the Protein Data Bank (PDB).	National Center for Biotechnology Information, U.S. National Library of Medicine, 8600 Rockville Pike, Bethesda, MD 20894

Title	URL	Producer	Vendors	Scope	Contact
Table 4.2 *continued*					
National Guideline Clearing-house	www. guidelines .gov /index.asp	Agency for Healthcare Research and Quality (AHRQ), in partnership with the American Medical Association (AMA) and the American Association of Health Plans (AAHP)	Free	A searchable database of evidence-based clinical practice guidelines.	Agency for Healthcare Research and Quality, Executive Office Center, Suite 600, 2101 East Jefferson Street, Rockville, MD 20852
Protein Data Bank (PDB)	www. rcsb.org /pdb	Research Collaboratory for Structural Bioinformatics (RCSB) consortium, which includes Rutgers, the San Diego Supercomputer Center (SDSC), and the Center for Advanced Research in Biotech-nology (CARB)	Free	The single international repository for the processing and distribution of 3D biological macromolecular structure data.	Rutgers, The State University of New Jersey, Department of Chemistry and Chemical Biology, 610 Taylor Road, Piscataway, NJ 08854-8087
PDQ (Physician Data Query)	www. cancer.gov /Cancer Information/pdq	U.S. National Cancer Institute	Free	An NCI database that contains the latest information about cancer treatment, screening, prevention,	NCI Public Inquiries Office, Suite 3036A, 6116 Executive Boulevard, MSC8322, Bethesda, MD 20892-8322

Table 4.2 *continued*					
Title	**URL**	**Producer**	**Vendors**	**Scope**	**Contact**
				genetics, and supportive care, plus clinical trials.	
Rare Disease Database	www. rare diseases .org	National Organization for Rare Disorders (NORD)	National Organiza tion for Rare Disorders (NORD)	The National Organization for Rare Diseases (NORD) maintains an alphabetical index of rare disease names and three searchable databases: the Rare Diseases Database, an Organizational Database for locating support groups, and an Orphan Drug Designation Database to find out about new and experimental orphan products.	National Organization for Rare Disorders, 55 Kenosia Avenue, PO Box 1968, Danbury, CT 06813-1968
Retroviru ses	www. ncbi.nlm .nih.gov /retro viruses	National Center for Biotechnolo gy Information (NCBI), U.S. National Library of Medicine	Free	A collection of resources designed for retroviral research, including a genotyping tool that uses the BLAST algorithm to identify the genotype of a query sequence; an alignment tool that provides a global alignment of multiple	National Center for Biotechnology Information, U.S. National Library of Medicine, 8600 Rockville Pike, Bethesda, MD 20894

Table 4.2 *continued*					
Title	**URL**	**Producer**	**Vendors**	**Scope**	**Contact**
				sequences; HIV-1 automatic sequence annotation, which generates a report in GenBank format for one or more query sequences; and genome maps, which provide graphical representations of 50 complete retrovirus genomes.	
TOXNET	http:// toxnet. nlm.nih .gov/	U.S. National Library of Medicine	Free	TOXNET is a cluster of databases from the National Library of Medicine on toxicology, hazardous chemicals, and related areas.	U.S. National Library of Medicine, 8600 Rockville Pike, Bethesda, MD 20894

Included in Table 4-2 are details covering database title, URL, producer, vendor(s) (if applicable), scope, and contact information.

Vendors

Print abstracting and indexing tools may be purchased by subscription directly from the producer or through a serials vendor or agent. Digital databases may also be purchased, subscribed to, or licensed—depending on scale of need for access—directly from the producer, but often from a search system interface vendor. Many key resources are, however, available for free on the Internet (PubMed), requiring only Internet access and your favorite browsing software.

Table 4-3 provides a listing of key vendors who deliver access to the primary and secondary digital databases previously noted.

Pricing and Access Issues

Web distribution of information resources has forged significant changes in pricing and how users access resources. Complex site license agreements have replaced subscriptions, flat fee, and pay-as-you-go pricing, putting demands on librarians to negotiate provisions such as the potential user base, number of simultaneous users, methods of authenticating eligible users, and remote access. Librarians must work with their systems or information technology (IT) departments to deal with some of the technical issues of accessing Web-based databases. Many questions need to be answered. For example, should authentication, the method of verifying eligible users to the network, be done using Internet protocol (IP) addresses on the computers at their site or by other methods such as usernames and passwords? Users are demanding remote access from their home computers. Should proxy servers—software applications that authenticate remote users without the need for passwords—be installed? Will the institution's firewall for security protection interfere with access to the library's digital resources? While librarians may not need to be experts in network security, they should be familiar with the fundamental issues in order to partner effectively with their counterparts in systems and in IT.

Consortia

Librarians are expert at partnering and have formed consortia for decades. Many continue to do so in order to benefit from joint purchasing agreements with vendors. This allows them to pool their expertise in negotiating contracts, which often results in significant cost savings and provides them with opportunities to benefit from a

Table 4-3. Key Database Vendors

Vendor	URL	Contact	Key Health Databases
American Society of Health-System Pharmacists	www.ashp.org	American Society of Health-System Pharmacists, 7272 Wisconsin Avenue, Bethesda, MD 20814	IPA (International Pharmaceutical Abstracts)
Aries Systems Corporation	www.kfinder.com /newweb	Aries Systems Corporation, 200 Sutton Street, North Andover, MA 01845	CINAHL, EMBASE Alert, MEDLINE
Cinahl Information Systems	www.cinahl.com	Cinahl Information Systems,1509 Wilson Terrace, Glendale, CA 91206	CINAHL
Dialog	www.dialog.com	Dialog, 11000 Regency Parkway, Suite 10, Cary, NC 27511	Biological Abstracts, CINAHL, IPA, MEDLINE, SCISEARCH, PsycINFO
EBSCO	www.epnet.com	EBSCO Subscription Services, P.O. Box 1943, Birmingham, AL 35201-1943	Alt-HealthWatch, Biological Abstracts, CINAHL, Cochrane Collection, Health Business Elite, MEDLINE, PsycINFO
Elsevier	www.elsevier.com	Elsevier Customer Service Department, 360 Park Avenue South, New York, NY 10010-1710	Biological Abstracts, EMBASE, MD Consult, PsycINFO

Table 4-3. *Continued.*

Vendor	URL	Contact	Key Health Databases
Gale Group	www.galegroup .com	Gale Group, 27500 Drake Road, Farmington Hills, MI, 48331	Health and Wellness Resource Center
ISI	www.isinet.com /isi	ISI, 3501 Market Street, Philadelphia, PA 19104	Biological Abstracts, Web of Science
NISC (National Information Services Corporation)	www.nisc.com	NISC International, Inc., Wyman Towers, 3100 St. Paul Street, Baltimore, MD 21218	Biological Abstracts, PsycINFO
OCLC FirstSearch	www.oclc.org	OCLC Online Computer Library Center, Inc., 6565 Frantz Road, Dublin, OH 43017-3395	CINAHL, MED-LINE, PsycINFO
Ovid	www.ovid.com	Ovid Technologies, Inc., 9350 South 150 East, Suite 300, Sandy, UT 84070	Biological Abstracts, CINAHL, Cochrane Database of Systematic Reviews, MEDLINE, PsycINFO
ProQuest	www.umi.com	Proquest Information and Learning, 300 North Zeeb Road, P.O. Box 1346, Ann Arbor, MI 48106-1346	CINAHL, MED-LINE, PsycINFO

Table 4-3. *Continued.*

Vendor	URL	Contact	Key Health Databases
STN International	www.cas.org /stn.html	CAS, 2540 Olentangy River Road, Columbus, OH 43202	Biological Abstracts, EMBASE, MED- LINE, SCISEARCH
Update Software	www.update 0-software.com	Update Software Inc., 1070 South Santa Fe Avenue, Suite 21, Vista, CA 92084	Cochrane Database of Systematic Reviews, Cochrane Library

shared technological infrastructure. Two examples of consortia of health libraries are the Arizona Health Information Network (AZHIN) and the Library Consortium of Health Institutions in Buffalo (LCHIB) [15]. AZHIN provides its members with a Web portal, which delivers licensed commercial and locally developed information via the Internet at the point of need. An added benefit is the ability to customize the portal to reflect an institution's individual holdings. For many small health organizations in rural communities, belonging to a consortium such as AZHIN is the only way they can afford access to expensive knowledge-based information products.

The need for consortia continues to grow as library budgets tighten, the pricing of resources climbs, and the demand of users for access to knowledge-based information continues to increase. More information on library consortia can be found in the literature [16, 17].

The Future: Handhelds, Wireless . . .?

Health sciences librarians have, as with consortia, established a long and proud tradition of leveraging their assets in service to customer needs. Those customers are increasingly turning to advanced and miniaturized technologies to manage their information needs. Handheld computers, also known as personal digital assistants (PDAs), are rapidly being adopted by health care professionals to assist them in a variety of tasks, including management of the vast amount of medical information. Because handhelds fit in the palm or coat pocket, they are much more convenient than even the lightest laptop for providing access to medical information at the bedside or in the classroom. Significant health-related content, including general medical reference databases, pharmacopoeias, medical calculators, and patient-tracking software, are being developed for handhelds. Content is downloaded into the device from the Internet using a method called "hotsynching" in which the handheld is connected to a Web-enabled computer. The ease of hotsynching makes updating content fairly painless, though it can be time-consuming over slow Internet connections.

Just as users expect their medical libraries to be their source for print and digital databases and full-text content, they are now turning to their libraries as the source for content and support for their handhelds. Some libraries are providing synching stations and pointing users to free resources, such as ePocrates. Others are licensing medical resources, such as the 5-Minute Clinical Consult series, Inforetriever, or eMedicine, and making them available to their users.

Although the memory capacity of handhelds has expanded with the use of memory stick and secure digital expansion card slots, the amount of information that can be stored and accessed on a handheld is finite. Advances in the area of wireless technologies, such as Bluetooth, will bypass this limitation, allowing handhelds and other devices to link quickly and effortlessly to databases with the latest medical information, eliminating the need to store large files directly on the handheld and to hotsynch. Improvements in security will also ensure confidentiality of patient records accessed by the handheld [18, 19].

Conclusions

There has been tremendous change during the last several decades in the way medical information is stored, accessed, searched, and retrieved. Not only have indexing and abstracting services moved from print to digital formats, but these tools are now delivered through a number of different platforms, most recently via the Internet and on

PDA devices and often with the full-text of documents embedded with citations. Librarians have embraced each new advance in information technology and have made many significant contributions to the technology's evolution. By quickly adapting their services to take full advantage of increased functionalities in each new advance, librarians have made sure their users receive all the benefits possible. No doubt this trend will continue well into the future.

References

1. McLellan F. 1966 and all that—when is a literature search done? *Lancet* 2001 Aug. 25; 358 (9282):646.
2. Jenkins CG. Press statement, 2001 Aug. Available: www.mlanet.org/press/2001/aug01.html.
3. Boorkman JA. Indexing and abstracting services. In: Roper FW, Boorkman JA, eds. *Introduction to reference sources in the health sciences*, 3rd ed. Metuchen, NJ: Scarecrow Press, 1994:53–95.
4. Davidoff F, Florance V. The informationist: a new health profession? *Ann Intern Med* 2000 June 20; 132(12):996–8.
5. Florance V, Giuse NB, Ketchell DS. Information in context: integrating information specialists into practice settings. *J Med Libr Assoc* 2002 Jan.; 90(1):49–58.
6. Howse D. Software review: InfoRetriever. *J Med Libr Assoc* 2002 Jan.; 90(1):121–2.
7. Williams ME. The state of databases today: 2003. In: *Gale directory of databases*. Detroit: Gale Research, 2003:xxi.
8. American Society of Information Scientists (ASIS). *Pioneers of information science in North America: National Library of Medicine: a project of SIG/HFIS* (*History and Foundations of Information Science*). Available: www.asis.org/Features/Pioneers/nlm.htm.
9. Weaver CG, McGoogan LS. The impact of on-line search availability on literature retrieval patterns of researchers. *Bull Med Libr Assoc* 1982 Oct.; 70(4):389.

10. Saffady W. Online searching. *Libr Technol Rep* 2000; 36:67–100.
11. Roach AA, Addington WW. The effects of an information specialist on patient care and medical education. *J Med Educ* 1975; 50(2):176–180.
12. Sowell SL. LATCH at the Washington Hospital Center, 1967–1975. *Bull Med Libr Assoc* 1978 Apr.; 66(2):218–22.
13. Marshall JG. The impact of the hospital library on clinical decision making: the Rochester study. *Bull Med Libr Assoc* 1992 Apr.; 80(2):169–78.
14. Sutcliffe AG, Ennis M, Watkinson SJ. Empirical studies of end-user information searching. *J Am Soc Inf Sci* 2000; 51(13):1211–31.
15. Riordan ML, Perry GJ. Interlibrary cooperation: from ILL to IAIMS and beyond. *Bull Med Libr Assoc* 1999 July; 87(3): 251–5.
16. Schlimgen J, McCray JC, Perry GJ, Flance L. Considering a consortium? Practical advice to hospital librarians from the Arizona Health Information Network (AZHIN). *Med Ref Serv Q* 2001; 20(3):67–73.
17. McCray JC. Delivering health information statewide via the Internet in a collaborative environment: impact on individual member institutions. *Bull Med Libr Assoc* 1999 July; 87(3):264–9.
18. Stoddard MJ. Handhelds in the health sciences library. *Med Ref Serv Q* 2001; 20(3):75–81.
19. Adatia FA, Bedard PL. Palm reading: 1. Handheld hardware and operating systems. *Can Med Assoc J* 2002; 167(7):775–80; and Palm reading: 2. Handheld software for physicians. *Can Med Assoc J* 2003; 168(6):727–34.

CHAPTER 5

U.S. GOVERNMENT DOCUMENTS AND TECHNICAL REPORTS

Fred W. Roper

U.S. Government Documents

Government documents offer an often untapped potential as reference and information sources for health sciences libraries. Most topics of interest to researchers and practitioners in the health sciences are treated to some degree somewhere in a government publication. Unfortunately, these sources have the reputation of being difficult to work with. This perception derives from a lack of understanding both of our government's organizational structure and the bibliographic tools that provide access to the publications. Consequently, U.S. government documents are often underused.

Government documents, which appear in print and electronic formats, are the materials that have been issued by the authority of a government, even if the government has not borne the expense of printing or producing the publications. Although there are many printing offices connected with the various government agencies, the U.S. Government Printing Office (GPO) is the major supplier of U.S. government documents. The GPO (Available: www.gpoaccess.gov/index.html) does not print the majority of publications, but it does serve as the major distribution source for publications coming from the various agencies.

The National Technical Information Service (NTIS) (discussed in the "Technical Reports" section, below) is another major distribution center for U.S. government documents. In addition, there are hundreds of government Web sites filled with reliable information.

Government publications are divided into three groups that roughly correspond to the three branches of government. *Congressional* publications relate to work or proceedings of Congress, printed by the order, or for the use of, either the Senate or the House of Representatives. Court decisions published by the United States make up the bulk of *judicial* publications. *Executive* publications are published by the departments or the independent agencies of the executive branch of the government.

Under the Federal Depository Library Program (Available: www.access.gpo.gov/su_docs/fdlp/libpro.html), libraries that request and qualify for depository library status can select the categories of publications most appropriate for their collections, unless designated as a regional depository library. Regional depository libraries serve as complete depositories. Academic health sciences libraries are often associated with institutions whose main libraries have depository status and may receive depository materials in the health sciences on that basis. Libraries without depository status must select and acquire government publications from the GPO or other distribution outlets.

A major problem in dealing with government documents is the frequent changes that take place in government organizations. As agencies are abolished, created, or merged, their publications may also change. Organizational changes result in variations in bibliographic entry, which create difficulties for the librarian in locating the publications in appropriate catalogs and indexes. The secret of successful reference use of government documents lies largely in mastering the bibliographic sources that list them and in keeping up with organizational changes.

5.1   Morehead J. *Introduction to United States Government Information Sources*, 6th ed. Englewood, CO: Libraries Unlimited, Inc., 1999.

5.2   Hernon P, et al. *U.S. Government on the Web: Getting the Information You Need.* Englewood, CO: Libraries Unlimited, Inc., 1999. Available: www.lu.com.

5.3   Robinson JS. *Tapping the Government Grapevine: The User-Friendly Guide to U.S. Government Information Sources*, 3rd ed. Phoenix, AZ: Oryx Press, 1998.

Now in its 6th edition, *Introduction to United States Government Information Sources* is the standard text relating to U.S. government publications. "The purpose of this text is to provide an account of the general and specialized sources, in print and nonprint formats, that make up the bibliographic and textual structure of federal government information" [Introduction]. Included are discussions of the migration of federal government sources to the Internet, overviews of the three branches of government and their sources, and reviews of selected departments and agencies in various critical disciplines, including many relating to the health sciences. The emphasis is on the current situation, and the user is urged to refer to earlier editions for more detailed historical information.

U.S. Government on the Web is intended to provide a "road map" for conducting an Internet search for government information. The guide begins with an overview of government structure and types of publications and moves on to discussions of specific agencies and their sources plus a discussion of important subject areas. Between updates, Internet address changes are provided on the publisher's home page.

Tapping the Government Grapevine "is a guided tour of the government information landscape" [Preface]. It is filled with Internet resources and serves as a complement to *Introduction to United States Government Information Sources* as a text. Although U.S. government resources are emphasized, information about international, foreign, state, and local information sources is also provided.

5.4   Office of the Federal Register. *U.S. Government Manual*. Washington, DC: U.S. Government Printing Office, 1935–. Annual. Available: www.gpoaccess.gov/gmanual/index.html.

This is the official handbook of the federal government, and it furnishes on an annual basis information on all government entities as well as quasi-official entities and selected international organizations in which the United States participates. Agency responsibilities are summarized, and directory information is given. Appendices include

101

abolished and transferred agencies and provide a historical perspective. Since 1995–1996, it has been available online.

5.5   *Catalog of United States Government Publications.* Washington, DC: U.S. Government Printing Office, 1994–. Available: www .access.gpo.gov/su_docs/locators/cgp/a_catalog.html.

5.6   *Monthly Catalog of United States Government Publications.* Washington, DC: U.S. Government Printing Office, 1895–. (Print Format) Monthly; annual cumulative indexes.

The *Catalog of United States Government Publications* indexes print and electronic government information products created by federal agencies. Many of these products are distributed through the Federal Depository Library Program. The database contains authoritative bibliographic records generated since January 1994 and is updated daily.

The online environment provides an opportunity to enhance the features of the print and CD-ROM versions of the *Catalog.* Many records for government information products available from agency Web sites are included, with direct links to the electronic text of the document. GPO has established criteria for inclusion and treatment of Internet-accessible resources in the *Catalog.*

For earlier indexing, it is necessary to consult the print counterpart, *Monthly Catalog of United States Government Publications,* which has been issued by the Superintendent of Documents since 1895. The *Catalog of Public Documents* was the primary index of documents until it ceased publication in 1940. Since that time, the *Monthly Catalog* has become increasingly more comprehensive, and improved indexes have made it easier to use.

In 1974, the Library Division of the Superintendent of Documents Office joined the online cataloging network of the Online Computer Library Center (OCLC), converted to the MARC format, and began cataloging according to Anglo-American Cataloging Rules (AACR). In 1976, citations in the *Monthly Catalog* appeared in a new format that made it a considerably improved source for cataloging information.

The basic arrangement of the entries in the *Monthly Catalog* is by Superintendent of Documents Classification Scheme. This arrangement is typically by agency because of the interdependence of the scheme with the organization of the federal government. Author, title, subject, and series/report indexes provide additional access to the documents. Cumulative indexes are published annually.

In addition to the general listing of government documents contained in the *Catalog of United States Government Publications* and in the *Monthly Catalog*, individual agencies and departments may provide their own bibliographies and catalogs. These catalogs should be consulted for specific items published by a government unit.

Technical Reports

Health sciences librarians generally use technical reports less often than other types of materials. Reports are not easy to work with or locate and may be difficult to identify properly in some instances. To use technical reports effectively, librarians must become familiar with both the reference sources that maintain bibliographic control of reports and the primary acquisition and distribution centers.

Technical reports have achieved the potential for greater use in health sciences research with their increased availability through distribution centers and enhanced Internet access. Since World War II, technical reports, like other types of materials in the sciences, have been used more frequently as a vehicle of communication. In the early period of extensive use, technical reports were considered only one step in the process of publication of a journal article or chapter in a monograph. Today they are often considered the final step in the publication process, although portions of many reports appear eventually in more formal literature. Their frequent citation in bibliographies and reading lists is evidence of increasing use; librarians must be prepared to respond to growing pressure to verify and locate the cited reports.

A technical report normally is prepared for the agency for whom an investigation has been carried out. In general, a technical report either gives progress of the investigation currently being carried out or indicates the results of a completed investigation. The duration of the research project will determine the necessity for continuing progress reports or for one final report that covers all stages of the investigations.

Quality of the content of technical reports tends to vary, because there is usually little, if any, quality control present in the form of refereeing. Material submitted to a journal, for example, undergoes much closer scrutiny than that in a technical report. However, the lack of restrictions on length and amount of material that can be included means the researcher might obtain considerably greater detail from a technical report than that found in a journal article.

Tallman [1] has characterized technical reports in the following manner:

1. There are many titles being published from a great many different agencies and organizations. Although there are not many distributing agencies, there is still enough complexity and variance to cause confusion.
2. There is a great range of quality in both form and content of the reports, ranging "from poorly written, brief, minor items of ephemeral value, to near print, well-organized, and comprehensive reports of relatively permanent value."
3. Distribution is often limited and may be based on an established need to have access to the material contained in the report.
4. The reports are not available from the usual book trade sources; they normally have to be obtained from special distribution centers.
5. Bibliographic control of technical reports has been confined, for the most part, to specialized sources; more conventional sources usually ignore them.
6. No union list exists of individual library holdings.
7. Handling is difficult once the reports are acquired because they may have multiple personal authors, several different identification numbers assigned to them, and formats that require binding or reinforcement for library use.
8. In many instances, the data contained in reports may be of great value to the public and may be the only detailed source of information available on the topic.

Although Tallman's list of characteristics dates from 1961, it is still pertinent today. The main difference is that access both to citations and to full-text is much easier today for publications of the last 15 or 20 years. For earlier publications, it may still be necessary to use early printed bibliographies in order to locate a citation.

The major collection and distribution centers for technical reports in the United States are government agencies: National Technical Information Service (NTIS), National Aeronautics and Space Administration (NASA), Department of Energy (DOE), and Educational Resources Information Center (ERIC). The principal collection and distribution center in the United Kingdom is the British Library Document Supply Centre (BLDSC).

5.7   *National Technical Information Service.* Springfield, VA: U.S. Department of Commerce, Technology Administration. Available: www.ntis.gov.

Established in 1945 as the Publication Board in the U.S. Department of Commerce, NTIS has successively been known as the Office of Technical Services, the Clearinghouse for Federal Scientific and Technical Information, and the National Technical Information Service. Although its scope has changed with its name changes, the center's basic purpose of supplying copies of unclassified government technical reports has remained. Today NTIS serves as the central source for the sale of government-sponsored research and development reports and other analyses prepared by federal agencies, their contractors and grantees. The NTIS database is a collection of more than 3 million titles, each of which is available for purchase.

5.8   National Aeronautics and Space Administration. *Scientific and Technical Aerospace Reports.* Washington, DC: Scientific and Technical Information Branch, National Aeronautics and Space Administration. Available: www.sti.nasa.gov.

The Scientific and Technical Information database of NASA consists of more than 3.5 million references in the areas of aeronautics, space, and the supporting disciplines. Included are NASA reports, patents, conference proceedings, journal articles, and nonprint materials, as well as other aerospace-related NASA, United States, and international information. The materials cited may be ordered from the NASA Center for AeroSpace Information. Reports included in this database are abstracted in the NASA publication, *Scientific and Technical Aerospace Reports.*

5.9 Department of Energy. *Scientific and Technical Information.* Oak Ridge, TN: U.S. Department of Energy, Office of Scientific and Technical Information. Available: www.osti.gov.

The Department of Energy's Office of Scientific and Technical Information provides access to energy, science, and technology research and development information from the Manhattan Project to the present.

5.10 Educational Resources Information Center. Rockville, MD: ERIC. Available: www.eric.ed.gov.

The Educational Resources Information Center (ERIC) is composed of a series of sixteen subject-specific clearinghouses throughout the United States, each specializing in a different aspect of education. The clearinghouses are responsible for collecting and abstracting reports and other nonjournal literature. The ERIC database contains more than 1 million bibliographic records of journal articles, research reports, curriculum and teaching guides, conference papers, and books. Thousands of libraries around the world offer access to the ERIC database, the ERIC microfiche collection, and various ERIC publications.

5.11 British Library Document Supply Centre. Boston Spa, UK: The British Library. Available: www.bl.uk/services/document/dsc.html.

The British Library's Document Supply Centre is located at Boston Spa in Yorkshire. Among its extensive collections is a large report collection dating back to World War II. The BLDSC currently attempts to receive as many British reports as possible and has extensive holdings from other countries.

References

1. Tallman J. History and importance of technical reports. *Sci-Tech News* 1961 Summer; 15:46.

Readings

U.S. Government Documents

1. Katz WZ. Government documents. In: *Introduction to reference work. Volume one: basic information sources*, 8th ed. New York: McGraw-Hill, 2002:447–74.
2. Moorehead J, Fetzer M. *Introduction to United States government information sources*, 6th ed. Englewood, CO: Libraries Unlimited, 1999:373–86.

Technical Reports

1. McClure CR. The federal technical report literature: research needs and issues. *Gov Inf Q* 1988; 5(1):27–44.
2. Morehead, J. Scientific research and development. In: *Introduction to United States government information sources*, 6th ed. Englewood, CO: Libraries Unlimited, 1999:373–93.
3. Robinson, J. Scientific information. In: *Tapping the government grapevine: the user-friendly guide to U.S. government information sources*, 3rd ed. Phoenix, AZ: Oryx Press, 1998:50–68.

CHAPTER 6

CONFERENCES, REVIEWS, AND TRANSLATIONS

Fred W. Roper

Conferences

Since World War II, meetings, conferences, and congresses have emerged as an increasingly important means of communication in the sciences. Similarly, the meeting has taken on a more important role in the social sciences as well. This situation has equally been true in the health sciences, and in recent years the number of meetings has greatly increased.

These meetings are considered a major means for the exchange of information with colleagues and for the establishment of lines of professional communication. For the librarian, they pose several challenges. Patrons frequently want to know what, where, and when future meetings are planned. They might ask about the availability of papers that were presented or discussed at past meetings. Two major types of reference materials are needed to provide the information posed by these queries: calendars or lists of meetings to be held and bibliographies of the published proceedings of meetings.

Calendars

Information on future meetings is available from a variety of sources. At a minimum, these sources should provide the sponsoring organization, name or topic of the meeting, the inclusive dates, the location, and, if possible, the name and address of a contact for further information.

6.1 *JAMA: the Journal of the American Medical Association.* Chicago, IL: American Medical Association, 1848–. Weekly. Available: http://jama.ama-assn.org/

6.2 *World Meetings: United States and Canada.* New York: Macmillan, 1963–. Quarterly.

6.3 *World Meetings: Outside United States and Canada.* New York: Macmillan, 1968–. Quarterly.

6.4 *World Meetings: Medicine.* New York: Macmillan, 1978–. Quarterly.

6.5 *Mind: The Meetings Index.* InterDok Corporation. Available: www.interdok.com/mind.

6.6 *Scientific Meetings.* San Diego, CA: Scientific Meetings Publications, 1957–. Quarterly.

6.7 *International Congress Calendar.* Brussels, Belgium: Union of International Associations, 1960–. Quarterly.

The Journal of the American Medical Association (JAMA) publishes reference directories in various issues on a variety of topics, including information on forthcoming meetings both inside and outside the United States. The "Meetings in the United States" directory appears in the first issue of each month; "Meetings Outside the United States" is published once in January and once in July. Meetings are announced up to 1 year in advance of the scheduled date. Each entry includes enough information so that the interested individual will be able to write for more complete program information. General medical periodicals and the journals of other organizations should also be consulted for calendars of meetings.

A number of publications give future meeting information for all the sciences. These publications are useful in health sciences libraries because physicians and researchers are likely to need information about meetings in other areas of the sciences.

Through two separate journals, World Meetings' publications "provide information on meetings of international, national, regional interest in the sciences, applied sciences and engineering, social sciences, and professions" [Preface]. *World Meetings: United States and Canada and World Meetings: Outside United States and Canada* represent the most comprehensive and detailed listings available of future meetings in the sciences. They are quarterly publications and contain information that is maintained in the World Meetings Database.

The main entry section is a 2-year registry arranged into eight subsections, one for each quarter of the 2-year period following the date of issue of the journal. In addition to the minimum expected information, a considerable amount of detail may be supplied, including restrictions on attendance, availability of papers, submission of papers deadlines, and a brief description of technical sessions. Entries are updated in succeeding issues as more information becomes available. Six indexes provide access to the main entries: keyword, location, date, publication, sponsor, and deadline for submission of abstracts or papers.

World Meetings: Medicine follows the same format and brings together in one publication all the entries relating to medicine and health found in the two general publications.

Mind: The Meetings Index is available online from the InterDok Corporation. It is a complementary service to InterDok's *Directory of Published Proceedings.* The database, started in 1984, allows free access to locate future events. InterDok acknowledges that there are plans to implement an electronic database of the *Directory of Published Proceedings* and there are hopes that the Internet traffic on *Mind* will introduce new users to the *Directory of Published Proceedings* [FAQs, InterDok Web site].

Scientific Meetings is a directory to future meetings of scientific, technical, and medical organizations. Coverage is international in scope, and it announces meetings scheduled in the coming 15 months. The main section is a list of all meetings, arranged alphabetically by sponsoring agency. Each entry includes the inclusive dates, the content of the meeting, and the name of a contact person. The subject index and chronological index provide access to the entries.

The Union of International Associations provides coverage of international meetings in all disciplines through its *International Congress Calendar*. The *Calendar* contains information for meetings that will take place in the coming 12 to 15 months and for meetings planned up to 10 years in advance. The descriptions are listed in a geographical section by country and city and in a chronological section. A single index based on keywords in the organization name, conference name, or the conference theme refers to both sections.

Although the primary purpose of these tools is to identify future meetings, they are often used to establish that a meeting was scheduled to take place. In addition to these current tools, there are retrospective lists of the meetings that have been held. These lists may include information about publications resulting from the meetings.

6.8 *Congresses: Tentative Chronological and Bibliographic Reference List of National and International Meetings of Physicians, Scientists and Experts.* Washington, DC: U.S. Government Printing Office, 1938. Supplement to Index Catalogue, 4th series, 2nd supplement.

6.9 Council for International Organizations of Medical Sciences. *Bibliography of International Congresses of Medical Sciences.* Springfield, IL: Charles C. Thomas, Publisher, 1958.

6.10 *International Congresses, 1681 to 1899, Full List.* Brussels, Belgium: Union of International Associations, 1960. Documents, no.8: Publication no. 164.

6.11 *International Congresses, 1900 to 1919, Full List.* Brussels, Belgium: Union of International Associations, 1964. Publication no. 188.

A supplement to the *Index Catalogue* in 1938, *Congresses: Tentative Chronological and Bibliographic Reference List of National and International Meetings of Physicians, Scientists and Experts* provides information on 17,000 congresses which was available in the Army Medical Library (now the National Library of Medicine). For some of the congresses, there is very little available beyond the fact that the congress was held and the date. For others, there may be a detailed listing of the individual sessions and information about any resulting publications.

The list from the *Index Catalogue* includes those congresses that are of peripheral interest to researchers in the health sciences as well as those that are in direct relationship to the field. In 1958, the *Bibliography of International Congresses of Medical Sciences* was published under the auspices of the Council for International Organizations of Medical Sciences. This list includes only those congresses directly related to the medical sciences; 1,427 congresses in the field of medicine are identified. The basic arrangement is a chronological listing by subject.

The Union of International Associations has prepared two lists of international congresses covering all subject areas from 1861 to 1899 and from 1900 to 1919. Each provides a chronological approach, giving the name of the congress, its location, and the date. *International Congresses, 1900 to 1919, Full List* includes a subject index for both volumes.

Papers Presented at Meetings

The papers presented or discussed at meetings often represent the latest and most up-to-date information available on a topic. For the librarian, there is the difficulty of identifying the presenter, the title of the paper, and whether or not the paper has been published.

Cruzat [1] has identified six major forms of presentation for the proceedings of meetings.

1. A multivolume work encompassing the total proceedings of a conference or meeting.
2. A monograph or report with a specific title and editor.
3. A supplement, special number, or entire issue of an established journal (from either an official publication of the sponsoring society or agency or an unaffiliated publication that the society elects because of the subject content of the symposium or conference).
4. Selected papers or abstracts published in a journal because it is the official organ or because of subject content.

5. Reports of a meeting or conference in a journal that has a special section devoted to "congress or conference proceedings."
6. Dual publication as both an issue or part of a journal and as a monograph or report.

In addition, the individual papers may be submitted to appropriate journals for separate publication. These papers will then be included in the indexing and abstracting services that index the journals.

A problem of identification arises when the paper has been revised and published under another title. Identification is further complicated by the current practice of taping proceedings. These tapes, which may be the only record of a meeting, are neither likely to be included in the traditional bibliographic sources nor are they likely to be easily available.

6.12 *Conference Papers Index.* Bethesda, MD: Cambridge Scientific Abstracts, 1973–. Monthly. Formerly: *Current Programs.* Available: www.csa.com/csa/factsheets/cpilong.shtml.

Published since 1973, *Conference Papers Index* (*CPI*) provides a listing of all the papers presented at meetings, whether or not the paper appeared in published format. This source covers scientific meetings, including those in the health sciences, and is mainly prepared from programs or abstract publications of the conferences. Subject emphasis since 1995 has focused on the life sciences, environmental sciences, and the aquatic sciences. *Conference Papers Index* is arranged by topic. Information on publications resulting from the meeting is indicated, as is the name and address of the individual presenters. This source is particularly useful when a preprint distributed either before or at the meeting is the only known publication of a particular paper. The electronic database of *Conference Papers Index,* which is supplied through Cambridge Scientific Abstracts, covers 1982 to the present. Information is derived from final programs, abstract booklets, and published proceedings.

Current Bibliographies of Published Proceedings

The published proceedings may include either full-text or just an abstract of the papers presented at meetings. Some proceedings will include everything presented at the meetings and others will be selective.

There are several bibliographic sources, most of them covering all the sciences, that list published proceedings on a regular basis.

6.13 *Index to Scientific and Technical Proceedings.* Philadelphia, PA: Institute for Scientific Information, 1978–. Monthly, annual cumulation. Available: www.isinet.com/isi/products/citation/wos /wosproceedings.

6.14 *Directory of Published Proceedings: Series SEMT—Science/ Engineering/Medicine/Technology.* Harrison, NY: InterDok, 1965–. Ten issues per year, annual cumulation. *Cumulated Index Supplement.* Harrison, NY: InterDok. Quarterly, annual cumulation.

6.15 *Directory of Published Proceedings: Series MLS—Medical and Life Sciences.* Harrison, NY: InterDok, 1990–. Annual.

6.16 *Directory of Published Proceedings: Series PCE—Pollution Control/Ecology.* Harrison, NY: InterDok, 1974–. Annual.

6.17 *Proceedings in Print.* Halifax, MA: Proceedings in Print, Inc., 1964–. Six issues per year; annual cumulative index.

6.18 *Biological Abstracts/RRM.* Philadelphia, PA: BioSciences Information Service, 1980–. Semimonthly.

Index to Scientific and Technical Proceedings (*ISTP*) covers published proceedings in all the sciences. It is produced by the Institute for Scientific Information (ISI) and includes materials selected from ISI's various databases. Approximately 30 percent of the materials are in the life sciences. The proceedings, regardless of the format in which they appeared, must contain complete papers to be listed in the *ISTP*; proceedings that include both complete papers and abstracts are also included. Many indexing services index only proceedings volumes, but *ISTP* indexes to the individual papers. Published monthly, *ISTP* offers one of the fastest means of access to the proceedings literature.

The main section of *ISTP* provides complete bibliographic information for the published proceedings. The entry includes titles of papers, authors, and address of the first author in cases of multiple authorship. The category index and the permuterm subject index provide a subject approach. The sponsors of the meetings are found in the sponsor index. The author/editor index and the corporate index give access to the authors of the papers, editors of the proceedings, and corporate affiliations of the individual authors. The meetings location index provides country and city where the meeting was held. *ISTP* is also available on the Internet through the ISI Proceedings database and online through DIMDI (Deutsche Institut fuer Medizinische Documentation und Information [German Institute for Medical Documentation and Information]).

InterDok Corporation is responsible for three bibliographies of the proceedings of scientific meetings—*Directory of Published Proceedings: Series SEMT; Directory of Published Proceedings: Series MLS;* and *Directory of Published Proceedings: Series PCE.* They provide basic bibliographic information for proceedings that have been identified in their respective areas of responsibility. Since 1964, *Series SEMT* has provided monthly information on preprints and published proceedings of international congresses, conferences, symposia, meetings, seminars, and summer schools. Its principal arrangement for entries is chronological by date of meeting, with indexes by subject/sponsor, location, and editor. *Series MLS* (1990) and *Series PCE* (1974) are issued annually and are prepared from the entries in *Series SEMT* and a companion publication, *Series SSH—Social Sciences/Humanities.*

Proceedings in Print is broader in scope than the above titles; it covers all subject areas. Conferences can be identified through the alphabetical index, which uses headings found in the proceedings: corporate author, sponsoring agency, editor, and subject.

Biological Abstracts/RRM provides an extensive index to life science and biomedical meeting literature through print, CD, and Web formats. Approximately 165,000 references are provided every year from more than 1,500 annual meetings and symposia. The regularly updated CD and Web versions are available through EBSCO, SilverPlatter, and Ovid.

Because of the information provided, these current bibliographies of proceedings serve both as a means of verifying that a particular conference took place and as acquisitions sources. Once the publications of a meeting have been identified, it is then possible to acquire the proceedings by using either the information provided in the bibliographies or other sources to locate a library that may hold them.

6.19 *Index of Conference Proceedings.* Boston Spa, U.K.: British Library Document Supply Centre. No. 69–, June 1973–. Monthly. Index of Conference Proceedings. *Annual Cumulation.* 1988–. Continues: Index of Conference Proceedings Received. *Annual Cumulation.* 1985–1987.

6.20 *Index of Conference Proceedings 1964–1988.* London: Saur, 1989.

One of the most comprehensive collections of proceedings in the world is located at the British Library Document Supply Centre. The proceedings of more than 450,000 conferences, congresses, symposia, workshops, and seminars are in the collection. *Index of Conference Proceedings* includes proceedings published in monographs or parts of reports and in journals. The monthly publication is arranged alphabetically by subject keywords taken from the titles and organizers of the proceedings. Under each of the keywords there is a chronological listing of all the appropriate conferences and the published proceedings. The collection includes all subject areas, but emphasis is on the sciences. The *Index* is available online and on CD-ROM.

The *Index of Conference Proceedings 1964–1988* is a cumulation of the proceedings acquired during the 25-year period.

In addition to these titles that are specifically concerned with proceedings of meetings, the librarian must consult indexing and abstracting services for periodical coverage of proceedings and individual papers given at meetings. Sources for monographs, such as the *National Library of Medicine Current Catalog* and the *National Union Catalog*, will provide coverage of separately published proceedings.

Reviews

In an era of interdisciplinary research that requires the synthesis of information from a variety of sources, reviews of research in the health sciences are vital forms of scientific communication. The review brings together information about previously published research and provides the reader with an overview of work that has been carried out in a particular area. It brings to the researcher's attention an expert's evaluation of the most significant published research in a given field. Through reviews, the primary literature may be reduced to a more manageable state.

For the student, the review may serve as an introduction to a topic; for the practicing scientist, it may function as a guide to a field that is only of peripheral interest. The researcher in the field will find the review useful to identify items that may have previously been overlooked or to update knowledge.

A review usually cites a large number of references and is confined to examining the literature already published rather than presenting new information. Often, the title will include an identifier such as "review of," "progress in," "advances in," or "yearbook of." The review article, at the very least, will provide bibliographic information. Usually, it will also provide selection and synthesis, evaluation, and an overview of the extant research.

Typically, reviews are found in two formats. One is the serial publication devoted to review-type articles (e.g., *Annual Review of Medicine, Biological Reviews, Progress in Clinical Pathology*, and *Year Book of Surgery*). The other is in the form of individual articles found in the primary sources of information, such as books, periodicals, and technical report literature. A review may also appear in the form of a literature search that is performed by a scientist in preparation of a research study. However, it is usually more difficult to gain access to this type of review.

Bibliographic control of reviews in the health sciences has generally surpassed that in the other sciences, due in large part to the efforts of the National Library of Medicine. Other agencies have routinely included and identified review publications in indexing and abstracting activities as well.

6.21　*Bibliography of Medical Reviews.* Bethesda, MD: National Library of Medicine, 1955–. Annual, 1955–1967. Monthly, 1968–1977, separately and in *Index Medicus.* Monthly, 1978–, only in *Index Medicus.*

6.22 *Index to Scientific Reviews.* Philadelphia, PA: Institute for Scientific Information, 1974–. Semiannual.

The primary purpose of these two publications is to identify reviews. The first source deals with the health sciences and the second includes all branches of science.

The *Bibliography of Medical Reviews* (*BMR*) is a continuing feature of *Index Medicus* (*IM*). *Bibliography of Medical Reviews* first appeared in 1955 as an annual publication; a 6-year cumulation in 1961 represents review articles from the *1955–59 Current List of Medical Literature* and the *1960 Cumulated Index Medicus* (*CIM*). It continued as an annual publication through 1967; since January 1968, it has been published as a part of the monthly *IM* with an annual cumulation in *CIM*. It was also published as a separate monthly publication from 1968 through 1977. Since January 1978, *BMR* has appeared in print only as a separate section of the paper *Index Medicus*.

Bibliography of Medical Reviews follows the same format as *IM* and provides subject access to citations of reviews. In 1988, NLM expanded its definition of medical reviews to include categories of materials that were previously excluded from *BMR*. The definition now includes articles such as academic reviews, subject reviews, epidemiologic reviews, and state-of-the-art reviews. Online access to reviews found in the print *BMR* is provided through PubMed and other vendors offering access to the MEDLINE database.

Since 1974, the Institute for Scientific Information (ISI) has published the *Index to Scientific Reviews* (*ISR*) to provide separate bibliographic coverage of the world's scientific review literature. *Index to Scientific Reviews* is a semiannual publication that draws from the databases used to produce other ISI publications. It represents the most comprehensive coverage of the review literature for all of the sciences and covers the same disciplines as *Science Citation Index* (*SCI*).

Index to Scientific Reviews serves both as a source of bibliographic information for the reviews currently being published and as a citation index to these articles. The main section of *ISR* is the research front

119

specialty index, which provides bibliographies of current reviews in identified areas of intense research activity. This section is accessed using the source index and permuterm subject index. The corporate index is arranged by authors' geographic location and organizational affiliations. *Index to Scientific Reviews* can be searched in print and on the SCI and SciSearch CD-ROMs and online as a part of the SCISEARCH database.

6.23 *Biological Abstracts/RRM (Reports/Reviews/Meetings)* (see 6.18).

In 1980, *Biological Abstracts/RRM* (*BA/RRM*) succeeded the BioSciences Information Service (BIOSIS) publication *BioResearch Index*. *Biological Abstracts/RRM* covers the nontraditional forms of literature in the life sciences with particular attention to reports, reviews, and meetings. The monthly publication contains citations to a wide variety of formats that are not normally found in indexing and abstracting services or that have had limited coverage in the past. *Biological Abstracts/RRM* can be searched on regularly updated CD-ROMs and Internet versions available through EBSCO, SilverPlatter, and Ovid.

In addition to these three sources, which are designed specifically for the bibliographic control of reviews, other tools should be consulted. Citations to reviews are included in many indexing and abstracting services, some of which provide an indicator that the item cited is a review.

Translations

The promotion and stimulation of scientific progress and development depend on effective communication among the world's scientists. Frequently, this communication is hindered by the language barrier. Significant research results published in a language unfamiliar to a scientist have limited value. This situation exists with the biomedical literature as well as with that of other subject areas.

There are several options available when a research article has been published in a foreign language. On an informal level, the researcher may have someone either partially or completely translate the article to determine if a formal translation is worthwhile. On a more formal level there are three primary methods available: translation clearinghouses, cover-to-cover translations, and translation agencies or freelance translators.

The beginning source in the quest for translators or translation agencies is the American Translators Association (Available: www.atanet .org). The Web site provides two online directories: the Online Directory of Translation and Interpreting Services and the Online Directory of Languages Services Companies.

Dealing with the bibliographic control of translations is a relatively recent development. No centralized translation service existed in the United States prior to World War II. Consequently, it was necessary for the scientist either to read foreign-language articles in the original language or personally to secure translations. With the advent of more global awareness in the scientific community, there came the conviction that access to foreign scientific writing is a necessity. The end of World War II and the launching of Sputnik by the U.S.S.R. in 1957 greatly heightened this conviction. With so much of the world's scientific and technical information published in languages other than English, the need for access continues.

It is unlikely that scientists will develop greater fluency in foreign languages; as a result, their dependence on translations is likely to continue and even to increase. Cost is an important factor in the production of translation, and there have been attempts to share this expense in various ways, usually through publication of the translations or providing bibliographic access to a collection of translations.

Translation Centers

Translation centers serve as a central collecting point for translations that have been made for individuals and organizations. Translations are deposited with the center, which then provides bibliographic access to the information and may also offer reference service. Unfortunately, two of the three major centers are no longer in operation.

United States

The National Translations Center (NTC) was the primary national resource for English-language translations in the natural, physical, medical, and social sciences. Last located at the Library of Congress, the program was unable to attain cost recovery; consequently, the decision was made to discontinue the service, and the NTC closed on September 30, 1993.

The National Translations Center began after World War II as an effort of the Science-Technology Division of the Special Libraries Association (SLA). Members of the division collected unpublished translations and maintained a union catalog. In 1953, NTC was formally organized at the John Crerar Library. It continued its association with the SLA until it became an independent department of the John Crerar Library in 1970. As a part of a merger in 1984, NTC moved to the University of Chicago. In 1989, the center's materials were transferred to the Library of Congress (LC), where it was a unit of the Cataloging Distribution Service.

Information on the location of nearly 1 million translations—approximately 400,000 are held at LC—is contained in the NTC files. This collection comprises translations of journal articles, patents, conference papers, and other forms of technical literature. Translations were received from scientific and professional societies, government agencies, special libraries, corporations, universities, and other institutions.

6.24 *Translations Register-Index.* Chicago, IL: National Translations Center, John Crerar Library, 1967–1986. Continued by: *World Translations Index,* 1987–1988.

6.25 National Translations Center. *Consolidated Index of Translations into English.* New York: Special Libraries Association, 1969.

6.26 *Consolidated Index of Translations into English II: 1967–1984.* Chicago, IL: National Translations Center, 1986. 3 vols.

The *Translations Register-Index* is the bibliographic source for translations acquired by NTC from 1967 through 1986. The register section lists translations according to subject categories. The index section comprises journal and patent citations. Journals are listed alphabetically by title, followed by the year, volume, issue, and pages that are available in translation. Patents are arranged by country, and the directory is used to determine from which source the patent is available. The cumulated index includes NTC acquisitions that have been announced in the register section. The National Translations Center ceased publication of the *Translations Register-Index* and joined with the International Translation Centre for 1987 and 1988 to publish its holdings in *World Translations Index* (see 6.29).

For information on translations made available from 1953 through 1966, the *Consolidated Index of Translations into English* (*CITE I*) should be consulted. More than 142,000 translations are included. This publication is a cumulation of previously published lists from the Library of Congress, the Special Libraries Association, NTC, and a number of specialized sources.

The *Consolidated Index of Translations into English II* (*CITE II*) cumulates citation information on an additional 250,000 translations of scientific and technical journals previously listed in *Translations Register-Index.*

The translations announced in these three indexes are located at the Library of Congress.

United Kingdom

The British Library Document Supply Centre (BLDSC) is the largest depository of translations in the United Kingdom and one of the largest in the world. In addition to collecting translations, BLDSC has actively promoted cover-to-cover translations of Russian-language periodicals.

Currently, the collections include more than half a million journal articles translated into English from a wide variety of languages, particularly Japanese, Russian, German, and French, ranging in date from the 1800s to the present.

6.27 *British Reports, Translations, and Theses Received by the British Library Document Supply Centre.* Boston Spa, UK: British Library Document Supply Centre, 1986–1997. Monthly. Formerly: *British Reports, Translations, and Theses, 1981–1985; BLLD Announcement Bulletin, 1975–1980; BLL Announcement Bulletin,* June 1973–December 1974; *NLL Announcement Bulletin,* 1971–May 1973; *British Research and Development Reports,* 1966–1971. Available: www.bl.uk/services/document/translations.html.

British Reports, Translations, and Theses is a monthly listing of both technical report literature and translations acquired by the British Library. All items are held at BLDSC and photocopies may be obtained if copyright allows or the item will be loaned out. The British Library Document Supply Centre staff provide a pre-checking service that will inform the requestor if an existing English version or an English abstract exists of the requested item.

International

The International Translations Centre, located at Delft in The Netherlands, functioned from 1961 to 1976 as the European Translations Centre. The name was changed to reflect better the scope of the organization. It was dissolved at the end of 1997.

6.28 *World Transindex.* Delft, The Netherlands: International Translations Centre, 1978–1986.

6.29 *World Translations Index.* Delft, The Netherlands: International Translations Centre, 1987–1997. 10 issues per year. Continued *Translations Register-Index,* 1987–1988; and *World Transindex.*

In 1978, *World Transindex* succeeded *World Index of Scientific Translations and List of Translations Notified to the International Translation Centre, Transatom Bulletin,* and *Bulletin de Tranductions.* It is a subject listing with author and source indexes; all subject areas and languages are represented.

World Translations Index announced "translations of literature related to all fields of science and technology, from all languages into Western languages" [Introduction]. The reference section lists bibliographic details of the translation and of the original article, location where the translation may be obtained, journals containing the translation, or translations commercially issued as monographs. This section is accessed by an author index and a subject index, which cites the bibliographic information of the original publications. The indexes cumulated annually and were published in a separate volume. Many of the translations available through the International Translations Centre may be obtained/ordered through Delft Technical University.

Cover-to-Cover Translations

These publications, usually serial in nature, may enter into the normal channels of bibliography and may be indexed as a matter of course in the major indexing and abstracting services. For the librarian, it may be difficult to determine the availability of a journal that is translated on a regular basis. *Ulrich's Periodicals Directory*, *New Serial Titles*, *Chemical Abstracts Service Source Index*, and *World Translations Index* will be useful tools in identifying the journals that are or have been regularly translated. Once this is determined, the next step is to find our which indexing and abstracting services include the translated journal.

6.30 Himmelsbach CJ, Brociner GE. *A Guide to Scientific and Technical Journals in Translation*, 2nd ed. New York: Special Libraries Association, 1972.

A Guide to Scientific and Technical Journals in Translation provides a listing of those journals completely or partially translated up to 1972. There is also a guide to the volumes that have appeared in translation. Although long out of date, it is still useful in retrospective searching.

6.31 *Journals in Translation*, 5th ed. Boston Spa, U.K.: British Library Document Supply Centre; Delft, The Netherlands: International Translations Centre, 1991.

The International Translations Centre and the British Library Document Supply Centre jointly published *Journals in Translation*, which is a bibliography of periodicals that are completely or partially translated. Most of the translations are into English. The scope of this publication includes all subject areas, but emphasis is on the sciences. It is now available through the BLDSC.

References

1. Cruzat GS. Keeping up with biomedical meetings. RQ 1967 Fall; 7:12–20.

Readings

Conferences

1. Kelly JA. Scientific meeting abstracts: significance, access, and trends. *Bull Med Libr Assoc* 1998 Jan.; 86:68–76.

Reviews

1. Grogan D. Reviews of progress. In: *Science and technology: an introduction to the literature*, 4th ed. London: Clive Bingley, 1982:249–61.
2. Virgo JA. The review article: its characteristics and problems. *Lib Q* 1971 Oct.; 41:275–91.

Translations

1. Grogan D. Translations. In: *Science and technology: an introduction to the literature*, 4th ed. London: Clive Bingley, 1982:324–37.

PART III

CHAPTER 7

———

TERMINOLOGY

Fred W. Roper

To understand the literature of the health sciences, it is important to know the specialized terminology that characterizes it. This vocabulary is accessed through a variety of reference works, each one designed to answer a particular type of question, teach a particular part of the vocabulary, or provide a specific piece of information. Terminology reference tools may be grouped by type: comprehensive dictionaries of the health sciences; specialized dictionaries, such as those for abbreviations or etymology; specialized subject dictionaries; foreign-language dictionaries; and compilations of syndromes and eponyms.

General Dictionaries

An unabridged medical dictionary is first and foremost a record of the use of medical terminology. In a world where new diseases, new operations, new procedures, and new syndromes are continuously being discovered and named, dictionaries must regularly be updated. A dictionary should reflect the terminology that is currently in use in the medical professions. To serve this need, there are two unabridged medical dictionaries that are extensively used in the United States.

7.1   *Dorland's Illustrated Medical Dictionary*, 30th ed. St. Louis, MO: Harcourt Health Sciences Group, 2003. Also available on CD-ROM.

7.2   *Stedman's Medical Dictionary*, 27th ed. Baltimore, MD: Lippincott Williams & Wilkins, 2000.

Now in its 30th edition, *Dorland's Illustrated Medical Dictionary* is considered by many to be the "dean of medical dictionaries." It is comprehensive, authoritative, and has been a standby for many years. *Dorland's* contains more than 1,850 pages of definitions and many special features, foremost of which is the "Fundamentals of Medical Etymology" section. This brief introduction to the formation of medical terms includes lists of the most used prefixes, suffixes, and root words. In addition to the usual dictionary illustrations, there are 29 tables and 53 plates, all of which appear in alphabetical order.

The main section of the book contains the vocabulary with more than 121,000 terms, including over 8,100 new terms and 7,600 new entries. There are 820 illustrations including 566 new illustrations. The anatomic entries reflect the 1998 Terminologia Anatomica. Entries for *MeSH* headings are included. *Dorland's* is used by the National Library of Medicine in establishing *MeSH* headings. An electronic format is also available.

In an effort to avoid printing the same definition many times, the editors of *Dorland's* have made extensive use of cross references for words that are synonyms. The preferred term is defined and synonyms are referenced to that term. Also, anatomical terms are defined only under their official names, with cross references from common names. A major feature of word arrangement is the use of subentries. Definitions of the variations of the main entry are found in the same paragraph as the main entry. Each subentry appears in boldface type in the body of the paragraph headed by the main entry. The dictionary uses letter-by-letter alphabetization of words and abbreviations.

Stedman's Medical Dictionary is similar to *Dorland's* and is accepted by many as equal in authority and content. The 27th edition has been completely revised by many consultants and contributors. A useful feature of *Stedman's* is the opening section describing how to use the dictionary, including guides to pronunciation, derivations, abbreviations, and spelling of medical terms. It is also available in an electronic format.

The 27th edition includes more than 100,000 entries and features a genus finder. New diagnostic plates reflecting current imaging methods have been added.

The alphabetization of terms and the main entry/subentry arrangement are very similar to *Dorland's*. The subentry locator, which precedes section A of the vocabulary, lists all of the subentries used in the text of the dictionary. The subentry is followed by the main entries under which it can be found. *Stedman's* also makes frequent use of cross references to avoid duplicating definitions. Furthermore, there are many "see" references that direct the reader to related information. Eponyms and anatomical, chemical, biochemical, and pharmacological terms are included as main entries.

Stedman's is well illustrated, including tables placed throughout the textbook and color plates grouped in the center. It also includes a guide to medical etymology that contains lists of roots. The contrasting typefaces make it easy to locate and read entries.

A great deal of information not usually found in a dictionary is provided in the five appendices: a summary of blood groups, temperature equivalents, comparative temperature scales, weights and measures, and laboratory reference values.

Dorland's and *Stedman's* are very similar in size, authority, and comprehensiveness. Each is revised on a regular basis. Today's computer technology allows for faster updating of dictionaries and reduced time between revision and publication. However, even with regular revisions, no editorial board will arrive at a completely comprehensive list of medical terms. Determining which terms to delete because they are obsolete, imprecise, or no longer commonly used, and which new terms to include because they are now widely used, is a subjective editorial decision. Consequently, each dictionary contains definitions that the other excludes. All but perhaps the very smallest libraries should have both of these dictionaries in their collections to ensure the broadest coverage of vocabulary and special features.

7.3   *Blakiston's Gould Medical Dictionary*, 4th ed. New York: McGraw-Hill, 1979.

Blakiston's Gould Medical Dictionary has not been updated since the 4th edition was published in 1979. Although not as well-known as either *Dorland's* or *Stedman's*, it is nevertheless an important unabridged dictionary. The major difference between it and the previously discussed dictionaries is in terms of format. *Blakiston's* contains no subentries, but rather alphabetizes all terms and their subparts letter by letter. Synonyms are defined by the preferred term, and the preferred term is defined in full. There are no entry illustrations, but there are plates grouped together in the middle of the textbook. Like the other unabridged dictionaries, *Blakiston's* includes a brief guide to medical etymology. Also, like *Stedman's*, *Blakiston's* includes a number of very useful appendices.

Just as there are unabridged and abridged English-language dictionaries, there are both types of medical dictionaries. There are four abridged medical dictionaries of particular importance.

7.4   *Taber's Cyclopedic Medical Dictionary*, 19th ed. Philadelphia, PA: F.A. Davis Co., 2001. Available: www.tabers.com.

7.5   *Black's Medical Dictionary*, 39th ed. Lanham, MD: Madison Books Incorporated, 1999.

7.6   *The Bantam Medical Dictionary*, 3rd ed. Revised and illustrated. New York: Bantam Books, 2000. Previously published as: Urdang Dictionary of Current Medical Terms.

7.7   Dox I, Melloni BJ, Melloni JL, Eisner G, eds. *Melloni's Illustrated Medical Dictionary*, 4th ed. Boca Raton, FL: CRC Press LLC, 2001.

Taber's Cyclopedic Medical Dictionary states that it is "an abridged dictionary intended for all persons in nursing and allied health fields" [Introduction]. It includes all the standard features of an unabridged dictionary but defines fewer words. However, it provides much information not found in an unabridged dictionary, and most definitions are encyclopedic in scope. For example, the entry "cerebrospinal fluid" includes paragraphs on the formation and characteristics of the fluid.

The 19th edition includes terminology relating to alternative approaches for standard Western medical care.

A unique feature of *Taber's* is the "interpreter," which is a list of questions and statements that might be used in patient examination translated into five languages. In addition, there is a fact-finding index that lists terms that have the following subheadings: diagnosis, etiology, first aid, nursing implications, poisoning, prognosis, treatment, caution, and signs/symptoms. There are appendices that include tables, charts, and supplementary information on units of measurement, abbreviations, nomenclature, anatomy, drug interactions, and medical emergencies. *Taber's* also provides directories of burn centers and poison control centers.

Taber's is a good dictionary for paramedical personnel, health care clinicians, students, and others who need a medical dictionary but do not need the complexity and expense of one of the unabridged dictionaries.

The purpose of *Black's Medical Dictionary* ". . . is to provide a concise and understandable text in the medicine's many aspects" [Preface]. *Black's* is written for the nonprofessional who must have some basic knowledge of medicine to interact intelligently with the physician. It contains main entries in boldface type, usually followed by long articles on the subject. Broad topics, such as "Insects in relation to disease." "Injured, removal of," and "Drowning, recovery from," are discussed at length.

Although "see" references are used to link various topics, there is still considerable duplication of definitions. For example, there is a discussion of the thyroid gland under "endocrine glands" as well as under the main entry. *Black's* is distinctly different from the other dictionaries discussed because the format and style are designed to be easily accessible to the layperson.

The Bantam Medical Dictionary provides full definitions for terms in the basic sciences as well as the major specialties such as community medicine, psychology, and surgery. Special features within the definitions include subentries; "see" cross references; and starred words, which are entered and defined in their own alphabetical places. The dictionary contains about 150 fully labeled illustrations.

Melloni's Illustrated Medical Dictionary is written for the general public and students in the health sciences. It includes brief definitions of more than 30,000 terms and uses 3,000 illustrations to supplement the text. The illustrations and terms illustrated appear on the same page. It is the most heavily illustrated dictionary available. Terms are taken from the "common core of vocabulary used in medicine today" [Introduction]. Other helpful features include charts that provide conversions of measures and weights, incubation periods for various diseases, common allergic reactions to certain drugs, and an extensive section of medical abbreviations.

Medical Etymology

Etymology is important to anyone using medical terminology because it explains how words were formed. Today's medical vocabulary is based on Greek and Latin prefixes, roots, and suffixes; therefore, the definition of a medical word is a combination of the definitions of its prefix, root or roots, and suffix. If one knows the definitions of these parts, one can define the word. The importance of understanding a word's parts is demonstrated by the fact that a section on medical etymology is included in each of the major medical dictionaries discussed earlier.

7.8   Skinner HA. *Origin of Medical Terms*. Reprint. New York: Hafner, 1970.

7.9   Haubrich WS. *Medical Meanings: A Glossary of Word Origins*. Revised and expanded ed. Philadelphia, PA: American College of Physicians, 1997.

7.10   Jaeger EC. *A Source-Book of Biological Names and Terms*, 3rd ed. Springfield, IL: Charles C. Thomas, 1955.

Origin of Medical Terms is a general reference work of medical terms directed primarily at the beginning medical student. It is strongest in the basic sciences vocabulary. The book has a readable format and provides references to books or articles introducing new terms. Skinner explains some eponyms but discourages their use. One slight drawback for Americans is that the book generally uses British spellings.

Skinner's work is no longer in print, but *Medical Meanings: A Glossary of Word Origins* is intended to fill this gap in medical source material. The meanings of terms have been updated, new terms are described, and origins other than those more commonly associated with the terms are explored. *Medical Meanings* is an alphabetical list of principal words and important prefixes and suffixes. The index contains terms that are subentries, principal words that appear in more than one entry, and categories of words (e.g., colors, phobias) that are grouped together. More than 3,000 medical and related terms are included.

Jaeger's *Source-Book* is more complex than the works by Skinner and Haubrich and covers a wider range of words; hence the word "biological" rather than "medical" in the title. The 3rd edition includes a textbook and a supplement that is fully cross-referenced to the main volume. The textbook's opening section includes information about how words are formed, types of words, and an abbreviation guide. Both volumes are alphabetically arranged. Each entry defines the word parts and makes reference to the supplement if necessary. Numerous examples are given and some geographical and personal names are included.

Medical Abbreviations

The use of abbreviations and acronyms has proliferated in the health sciences, and one recurrent problem is that a single abbreviation may have a number of different meanings. For example, PPV may stand for "positive-pressure ventilation" or "progressive pneumonia virus." Conversely, multiple abbreviations may exist for a single term. It is essential for the reference collection to have up-to-date sources that list the possible meanings of acronyms and abbreviations.

7.11 Jablonski S, ed. *Dictionary of Medical Acronyms and Abbreviations*, 4th ed. Philadelphia, PA: Hanley & Belfus, 2001.

7.12 *Stedman's Abbreviations, Acronyms, and Symbols*, 3rd ed.. Baltimore, MD: Lippincott Williams & Wilkins, 2003.

7.13 Mitchell-Hatton SL. *The Davis Book of Medical Abbreviations: A Deciphering Guide.* Philadelphia, PA: Davis, 1991.

7.14 Melloni BJ, Melloni JL. *Melloni's Illustrated Dictionary of Medical Abbreviations.* Boca Raton, FL: CRC Press LLC, 1998.

7.15 Davis N. *Medical Abbreviations: 24,000 Conveniences at the Expense of Communications and Safety,* 11th ed. Huntingdon Valley, PA: Neil M. Davis Associates, 2003.

7.16 Kerr AH. *Medical Hieroglyphs.* Downey, CA: Enterprise Publications, 1970.

Jablonski's *Dictionary of Medical Acronyms and Abbreviations* lists the most frequently used acronyms and abbreviations that were identified by a systematic screening of the National Library of Medicine's (NLM) collection of books and periodicals. No definitions are given, only the full entry of possible meanings for the terms. The new edition includes more than 10,000 new entries to reflect recent advances in fields such as medical informatics, computers in biomedicine, outcomes research, and evidence-based medicine. The intent is to provide a list of frequently used acronyms and abbreviations in medicine and health care

The *Stedman's* compilation was produced by reviewing dictionaries, "approved lists" from teaching hospitals, and other compendia. Although more than 20,000 clinically relevant terms are listed, there is less overlapping than might be expected between this source and Jablonski's *Dictionary*. A comparison of the terms listed between LD and LH indicates considerable differences in the number of terms and the number of possible meanings.

The Davis Book of Medial Abbreviations: A Deciphering Guide is a useful tool because it contains obsolete, profane, slang, and nonmedical abbreviations. It includes pronunciations of acronyms and words that have been crafted from abbreviations (e.g., "trick" for Trichomonas), enabling the user to identify an unknown term. It deciphers medical codes by the use of medical specialty listings that appear after the full entry (e.g., Trichomonas [lab]).

Melloni's Illustrated Dictionary of Medical Abbreviations contains more than 17,000 medical abbreviations compiled from the latest medical books and journals to ensure their currency and accuracy. The excellent illustrations aid comprehension of the abbreviations and enhance their meanings—a unique feature for an abbreviations dictionary.

In *Medical Abbreviations: 24,000 Conveniences at the Expense of Communications and Safety*, Neil Davis has compiled 24,000 meanings for medical, nursing, and pharmaceutical abbreviations and acronyms. It contains a list of dangerous abbreviations and suggests alternatives. Included in the book price, at no extra cost, is a single user access license for the Internet version of the 11th edition of the book; a PDA version is also available.

Medical Hieroglyphs contains abbreviations taken directly from medical records, hence, it contains abbreviations that are standard or universally accepted. This book also includes a section on symbols used by physicians.

Word Finders and Concept Dictionaries

Most dictionaries consist of alphabetical lists of words followed by definitions. This arrangement is adequate if one knows the word. When only a definition or concept is known however, a dictionary that uses words as the access point is useless. In this situation, an inverted dictionary, or word finder, is necessary.

7.17 Stanaszek MJ, et al. *The Inverted Medical Dictionary,* 2nd ed. Lancaster, PA: Technomic, 1991.

7.18 Hamilton B, Guidos B. *The Medical Word Finder: A Reverse Medical Dictionary.* New York: Neal-Shuman, 1987.

7.19 Willeford G, Jr., comp. *Webster's New World Medical Word Finder,* 4th ed. New York: Prentice-Hall, 1987.

7.20 Lorenzini JA, Lorenzini-Kley L. *Medical Phrase Index: A One-Step Reference to the Terminology of Medicine,* 3rd ed. Los Angeles, CA: Practice Management Information Corporation, 1994.

Both *The Inverted Medical Dictionary* and *The Medical Word Finder* contain an alphabetical list of single words and extended phrases that are likely to be the most obvious to users. Under each heading in *The Inverted Medical Dictionary*, the proper medical term(s) is provided, and in some instances a brief definition is included as well. In addition to the main alphabetical list, this dictionary has sections on eponyms, terms used in prescription writing, drug and chemical abbreviations, and common medical abbreviations. In *The Medical Word Finder*, the entry information for the headings includes technical terminology, synonyms, and, where appropriate, commonly used prefixes and suffixes.

Webster's New World Medical Word Finder was compiled to show health professionals how to spell, syllabicate, divide, and accentuate frequently used medical terms. The book is arranged into ten sections that include a list of prefixes and suffixes; an alphabetical list of tests, arteries, syndromes, and so forth; a list of commonly prescribed drugs; and a list of phonetic spellings for 179 problem words.

The authors of *Medical Phrase Index*, both medical transcribers, have included more than 200,000 phrases used in medicine today. It consists of medical phrases, both formal and informal, cross-referenced by each of its main words. *Medical Phrase Index* contains both formal and informal terminology (e.g., barium burger and café coronary). Included in the new edition are terms used in reference to psychiatry, gerontology, cardiac care, living wills, Alzheimer disease, infection control, and AIDS.

Subject Dictionaries

There are numerous dictionaries available that are narrow in scope but expansive in a particular area. Each of these examples has features that set it apart from a general medical dictionary.

7.21 Zwemer TJ. *Boucher's Clinical Dental Terminology*, 4th ed. St. Louis, MO: Mosby, 1993.

136

7.22 Jablonski S. *Jablonski's Dictionary of Dentistry.* Reprint edition of *Illustrated Dictionary of Dentistry.* Malabar, FL: Krieger, 1992.

7.23 Miller BF. *Miller-Keane Encyclopedia and Dictionary of Medicine, Nursing, and Allied Health,* 7th ed. Philadelphia, PA: Elsevier—Health Sciences Division, 2003.

7.24 Anderson DM, et al, eds. *Mosby's Medical, Nursing, and Allied Health Dictionary,* 6th ed. St. Louis, MO: Mosby, 2002.

Dental terminology is often confusing due to the number of specialties and subspecialties in dentistry. *Boucher's* and *Jablonski's* are two dictionaries that provide comprehensive coverage of dental terminology.

Boucher's Current Clinical Dental Terminology is designed for practicing dentists, students, and anyone associated with the delivery of dental care. Terms from all areas of dentistry are alphabetically arranged; pronunciations and numerous "see" references are included. Topics covered in the appendices include abbreviations, dental etymology, nomenclature, and the official American Dental Association codes for dental procedures.

Jablonski's Illustrated Dictionary of Dentistry attempts to define all terms in all specialties of dentistry and its allied fields. It is arranged in the style of major unabridged medical dictionaries. Definitions are descriptive, include cross references from secondary to preferred terms, and are supplemented with illustrations and tables. The book contains a guide to dental etymology and appendices that include information on the American Dental Association, the Canadian Dental Association, American and Canadian dental schools, and schools for dental hygiene and dental assisting in the United States.

The *Miller-Keane Encyclopedia and Dictionary of Medicine, Nursing, and Allied Health* serves as an excellent source for anyone in the allied medical professions because it defines the terminology of those professions. It has a multidisciplinary emphasis. As the title indicates, this book is an encyclopedia and has encyclopedic definitions of key terms. As in most dictionaries, entry words are divided by syllables and are marked for pronunciation. The book contains good anatomical tables and plates. Important features include the appendices, which include weights and measures, sources of patient education materials, laboratory reference values, and voluntary health and welfare agencies.

Mosby's Medical, Nursing, and Allied Health Dictionary is very encyclopedic in style. It provides sentence definitions and additional material when a definition alone is not sufficient. *Mosby's* is directed to nurses and other health professionals, particularly those in allied health fields. There are many illustrations and tables, a special 44-page color atlas of human anatomy, and extensive appendices. Unique features of this dictionary include abbreviations and cross references alphabetized into the text and a print style and size that looks like a textbook instead of a dictionary.

7.25 King RC, Stansfield WD. *A Dictionary of Genetics*, 6th ed. New York: Oxford University Press, 2002.

7.26 Campbell RJ. *Campbell's Psychiatric Dictionary*, 8th ed. New York: Oxford University Press, 2003.

7.27 Blauvelt CT, Nelson FRT. *A Manual of Orthopaedic Terminology*, 6th ed. St. Louis, MO: Mosby, 1998.

There are literally dozens of specialized subject dictionaries in medically related fields, from chromatography to psychology. These books by King, Campbell, and Blauvelt and Nelson illustrate the diversity that is available as well as the specialized information that may be found in subject dictionaries.

A Dictionary of Genetics includes 6,580 terms, tables, abbreviations, and molecular formulas from all fields related to genetics. Appendices include a list of periodicals cited in the literature of genetics, an expanded chronology of genetic research and discoveries, and more than 100 Web sites on genetic subjects.

Campbell's Psychiatric Dictionary is one of several in this subject area. It contains encyclopedic definitions of many words, extensive cross references, eponyms, and important names in psychiatry.

A Manual of Orthopaedic Terminology may be used as a general orthopedic dictionary. Terms are classified and arranged into chapters on topics such as the classification of fractures and dislocations, orthopedic tests, signs and maneuvers, prosthetic and surgical intervention, and musculoskeletal research. Several appendices and an extensive index complete the book.

7.28 Lawrence E, ed. *Henderson's Dictionary of Biological Terms*, 11th ed. New York: J. Wiley & Sons, Inc., 1995.

7.29 Gray P. *A Dictionary of the Biological Sciences*. Reprint. Malabar, FL: Krieger, 1982.

Dictionaries of biological terms are needed because general medical dictionaries do not provide comprehensive coverage of the terminology that is related to the health sciences. *Henderson's Dictionary of Biological Terms*, the classic reference in the field, is an alphabetical listing of biological words from all biological and basic medical sciences. A straightforward, uncomplicated, unadorned dictionary, it contains more than 23,000 terms, including transliterated Greek and Russian terms, and takes into account new disciplines, such as genetic engineering, and new terms, such as chromosome painting. Plant and animal kingdom classifications (to the order level) are included in the appendices.

A Dictionary of the Biological Sciences is more complicated to use. Major terms, such as chemical terms, are alphabetically arranged, but descriptive terms that require an extended definition are arranged as in a thesaurus. This dictionary includes vernacular terms, several thousand word roots, personal names, and taxa above the ordinal rank. Latin and Greek words are anglicized whenever possible. There is also a bibliography of works consulted by the author. Both of these dictionaries are directed at the generalist.

Foreign-Language Dictionaries

There is a need for reference tools that translate a medical term from one language to another. Some definitions of words that are obtained from general dictionaries may not be accurate in the medical context. In addition, more and more health care professionals are treating non-English-speaking patients. The sources described here are examples of foreign-language dictionaries that are available.

7.30 Dorian AF, comp. *Elsevier's Encyclopaedic Dictionary of Medicine.* New York: Elsevier, 1988–1990. 4 parts.

7.31 Rogers GT. *English-Spanish/Spanish-English Medical Dictionary.* New York: McGraw-Hill, 1997.

7.32 Unseld, DW. *Medical Dictionary of the English and German Languages: Two Parts in One Volume,* 19th ed. Revised and enlarged. Stuttgart: Wissenschaftliche Verlagsgesellschaft, 1991.

Elsevier's Encyclopaedic Dictionary of Medicine is available in four separately published parts: general medicine; anatomy; biology, genetics and biochemistry; and therapeutic substances. Each title is divided into two sections. The first section is the basic table, which lists the English entries in alphabetical order. Each entry is followed by the English definition and by its French, German, Italian, and Spanish equivalents.

The second section comprises four indexes, one for each language, where the equivalents are alphabetically listed. Each entry in this section has a number that refers to the relevant entry in the basic table.

The *English-Spanish/Spanish-English Medical Dictionary* translates more than 15,000 commonly used medical, technical, common, and slang terms in both English and Spanish. Sample conversations covering history-taking for a number of medical conditions are shown in Spanish as it is spoken in the United States with English translation immediately following.

The Medical Dictionary of the English and German Languages is divided into two sections: English-German and German-English. The dictionary offers no definitions; only the equivalent term is provided. This source is intended to be useful to not only doctors and dentists, but to pharmacists, chemists, and other medical and life sciences workers.

Syndromes, Eponyms, and Quotations

A syndrome is a constant pattern or grouping of abnormal signs or symptoms. Some syndromes have descriptive names and others are eponymic (i.e., named for the individual who first described the syndrome to the medical world). They are important to physicians because they are usually associated with diseases.

7.33 Magalini SI, Maglini SC. *Dictionary of Medical Syndromes*, 4th ed. Philadelphia, PA: Lippincott-Raven, 1997.

7.34 Durham RH. *Encyclopedia of Medical Syndromes*. New York: Hoeber, 1960.

7.35 Jablonski S. *Jablonski's Dictionary of Syndromes and Eponymic Diseases*, 2nd ed. Malabar, FL: Krieger, 1991.

In terms of information about each syndrome, the *Dictionary of Medical Syndromes* is the most comprehensive and up-to-date of the three sources. More than 2,900 syndromes are described including 200 new ones, and each explanation includes most of the following information: name of syndrome, synonyms, signs, etiology, pathology, diagnostic procedures, therapy, prognosis, and bibliography. The format is designed for quick reference and is easy to read. Although the text is not cross-referenced, the index is fully cross-referenced to the major headings.

Encyclopedia of Medical Syndromes is not so detailed, but it is useful because it covers syndromes not mentioned in *Dictionary of Medical Syndromes*. The syndromes are cross-referenced in the text and indexed by classification (type or organ system). The *Encyclopedia* contains references to literature that elaborates on or clarifies the syndromes.

A typical entry in *Jablonski's Dictionary of Syndromes and Eponymic Diseases* begins with the name of the person for whom the syndrome or condition is named, the eponym, its synonyms, and the definition. The entries include a bibliography or references to recent literature and the original report of the syndrome or disease. Synonyms are separately listed. When helpful, illustrations are used.

7.36 Strauss MB. *Familiar Medical Quotations.* Boston, MA: Little, Brown, 1968.

7.37 Daintith J, Isaacs A. *Medical Quotes: A Thematic Dictionary.* New York: Facts on File, 1989.

7.38 Kelly EC. *Encyclopedia of Medical Sources.* Baltimore, MD: Williams & Wilkins, 1948.

Important statements have been made by all types of people about medicine, disease, health care, and other health-related subjects. Strauss has brought together more than 7,000 such comments in *Familiar Medical Quotations.* The quotations are arranged alphabetically by category and chronologically within categories. The index, an alphabetical listing of keywords from the quotations, gives general access to the quotations. The book is authoritative—nearly all quotations have been verified. A secondary source is usually given if a quotation could not be verified. *Familiar Medical Quotations* is a compendium of who said what in the health sciences.

Medical Quotes: A Thematic Dictionary is a collection of remarks, writings, and sayings about medical and related subjects. Quotations are arranged under theme headings of general interest. Within each theme section, the quotations are in alphabetical order by the author's last name. Entry information includes the author's name, dates, a short biography, and a source reference for the quotation. Cross references are provided to related topics. Two indexes—keyword-key phrase and author—provide access to the quotations. The reference in the index is to the theme and to the number of the quote within that theme.

The title of Kelly's work, *Encyclopedia of Medical Sources,* is somewhat misleading. The book is a list of more than 6,000 names and the medical discoveries attributed to those individuals. It includes anatomical points of reference, operations, tests, treatments, diseases, important writings, and the source of publication of the discovery. The book is fully cross-referenced. Rather than listing individual names, the index lists the anatomical parts, tests, diseases, and so on.

CHAPTER 8

HANDBOOKS AND MANUALS

Jo Anne Boorkman

Handbooks and manuals are compendia of vast amounts of information on a variety of topics and are useful in answering the so-called factual question. These publications are of prime importance to the researcher in the health sciences. Grogan states "a library with no more than a sound collection of handbooks can answer 90 percent of quick-reference queries" [1]. The practical nature of the information contained in handbooks and manuals assists the researcher or clinician in day-to-day work. Handbooks and manuals range in format from one-volume data books to multivolume compendia that may be encyclopedic in nature. As with many reference resources, handbooks and manuals are becoming available electronically over the Internet. Some are freely available online whereas others are only available through institutional licensing to Web sites (e.g., CHEMnetBASE from Chapman & Hall/CRC Press). This chapter discusses three types of handbooks and manuals: data books; laboratory compendia; and handbooks relating to diagnosis, classification, and physiology.

Guide to the Literature

8.1 Powell RH, ed. *Handbooks of Tables in Science and Technology*, 3rd ed. Phoenix, AZ: Oryx Press, 1994.

In *Handbooks and Tables in Science and Technology*, Powell has provided a comprehensive guide that brings together resources that focus on "data tabulations or compilations of physical and chemical values whether they are in a manual, databook, handbook, sourcebook table, or guide." All areas of science and technology are covered, including biological and health sciences. The work is divided into three sections: Main Entry Section, Subject Index, and Author/Editor Index. The "enriched" keyword terms used in the Subject Index "attempt to bring the subjects together by selecting the appropriate terms that do not appear in the title or annotations" [Introduction]. Although the emphasis is on English-language materials, important works from around the world are included. The critical annotations enable users to determine whether or not the work cited contains the required information.

Data Books

Data books present basic scientific information in a concise format. Tables, such as the properties of substances, mathematical data, boiling points, or toxicities, are often used in the presentation of the data and are sometimes accompanied by text. Frequent revision is necessary to assure that the material presented is up to date. The key to successful use of a data book is an adequate and detailed index.

8.2   Altman P, Dittmer D, eds. *Biology Data Book,* 3rd ed. Bethesda, MD: Federation of American Societies for Experimental Biology, 1972–1974. 3 vols.

8.3   Altman P, Dittmer D, eds. *Growth, Including Reproduction and Morphological Development.* Washington, DC: Federation of American Societies for Experimental Biology, 1962.

8.4   Altman P, Katz D, eds. *Human Health and Disease.* Bethesda, MD: Federation of American Societies for Experimental Biology, 1977.

While these publications from the Federation of American Societies for Experimental Biology (FASEB) are not current, they are nevertheless important works that are based on contributions from a large number of research scientists.

The *Biology Data Book* is intended to serve as a basic reference in the field of biology. With broadened scope and coverage in the 3rd edition, the revised publication appears in three volumes: Volume 1, genetics and cytology, reproduction, development, and growth; Volume 2, biological regulators and toxins, environment and survival, and parasitism; and Volume 3, nutrition, digestion and excretion, metabolism, respiration and circulation, and blood and other body fluids. Each volume is independently indexed. An important feature is the inclusion of references for the sources of the data. Coverage is restricted "to man and the more important laboratory, domestic, commercial, and field organisms" [Preface]. Even so, many species are included.

Growth, Including Reproduction and Morphological Development is an example of the specialized handbooks that have been produced under the auspices of FASEB. Similar in format to the Biology Data Book, it is a compendium that presents data on various aspects of normal growth. The most recent title in the series of biological handbooks is *Human Health and Disease*. The seven sections of the handbook present 186 tables of quantitative and descriptive data. Contributors are identified, and the series continues to include citations to the literature.

8.5   Lentner C, ed. *Geigy Scientific Tables*, 8th revised and enlarged ed. Basle, Switzerland: Ciba-Geigy, 1981–.

The goal of *Geigy Scientific Tables* is to provide doctors and scientists with concise compendia of data on a variety of topics. The book is a continuing publication that is divided into individual volumes. This makes it possible to incorporate additional chapters and helps ensure that the information is current. Literature references to the sources of data are a part of each presentation. The six volumes published to date provide coverage of body fluids, statistical tables, physical chemistry, biochemistry, the heart, and bacteria.

8.6   Lide DR, ed. *CRC Handbook of Chemistry and Physics,* 83rd ed. Boca Raton, FL: Chapman & Hall/CRC Press, 2002/2003. Available: www.hbcpnetbase.com.

8.7   *CHEMnetBASE.* Boca Raton, FL: Chapman & Hall/CRC Press. Available: www.chemnetbase.com.

The CRC Press publishes an important group of handbooks, now numbering more than 50 titles. The series is intended to provide coverage of many subject areas in the sciences, ranging from broad areas such as chemistry and physics to specialized topics such as chemical laboratory science, hospital safety, and applied optics. The *CRC Handbook of Chemistry and Physics* first appeared in 1913. Now in its 83rd edition, it aims to provide broad coverage of all types of information frequently needed by physical scientists. References are provided to guide users to other compilations and databases if the Handbook does not have the answer. Format for the Web version is in a three-screen window that displays Table of Contents, a Menu, and Search Results and Data. Searching allows the user a variety of options including table manipulation and the ability to produce customized tables. Access to the Web version is available to multisite organizations only, with the CD-ROM electronic option available for individual purchase.

Chapman & Hall/CRC Press now offers several handbooks via the Web through CHEMnetBase. The site includes: *The Handbook of Chemistry and Physics,* 83rd edition*, Polymers: A Property Database, The Combined Chemical Dictionary, The Dictionary of Commonly Cited Compounds, Properties of Organic Compounds, Dictionary of Inorganic and Organometallic Compounds, Dictionary of Natural Products, Dictionary of Organic Compounds,* and *Dictionary of Drugs.* This Web site is available on a site-license basis to multiuser organizations through IP recognition. Subscriptions can be for individual titles or the entire site. It is not available by individual subscription; however, most titles are also available in CD-ROM.

8.8   International Commission on Radiological Protection. *Report of the Task Group on Reference Man.* Reprint. Report No. 23. New York: Pergamon, 1992.

Although the report was prepared to assist in studies on the effects of radiation on humans, the data that have been included cause it to have broad application. The compilers limited their attention to those characteristics of humans "which are known to be important or which are likely to be significant for estimation of dose from sources of radiation within or outside the body" [Introduction]. Even with this limitation, the book serves as an important complement to the handbooks discussed above.

Laboratory Compendia

These materials serve both as encyclopedias and as textbooks. They generally consist of essays relating to techniques, methodology, interpretation, and analysis used in diagnosis. Representative examples include:

8.9   Henry JB, ed. *Clinical Diagnosis and Management by Laboratory Methods*, 20th ed. Philadelphia, PA: Saunders, 2001.

8.10 Jacobs DS, Oxley DK, DeMott WR, eds. *Jacobs & DeMott Laboratory Test Handbook, with Key Word Index*, 5th ed. Hudson (Cleveland), OH: Lexi-Comp, Inc., 2001.

8.11 Jacobs DS, Oxley DK, DeMott WR, eds. *Laboratory Test Handbook Concise with Diseases Index*, 2nd ed. Hudson (Cleveland), OH: Lexi-Comp, Inc., 2002.

8.12 *Methods in Enzymology*. New York: Academic Press, 1955–. Volume 1–. Annual.

8.13 *Current Protocols Series*. Indianapolis, IN: John Wiley & Sons, Inc., 1990–2002. Available: http://www3.interscience.wiley.com /c_p/cppub.htm.

Clinical Diagnosis and Management by Laboratory Methods is a comprehensive textbook that emphasizes molecular and clinical pathology. Information is presented through a series of 68 chapters that are arranged under seven parts: Clinical Pathology/Laboratory Medicine; Clinical Chemistry; Urine and Other Body Fluids; Hematology Coagulation and Transfusion Medicine; Immunology and Immunopathology; Medical Microbiology; and Molecular Pathology. Illustrations, tables, and color plates supplement the material presented along with additional reading for the student in the field.

Jacobs & DeMott Laboratory Test Handbook with Key Word Index arranges topics alphabetically by major clinical laboratory disciplines. The Key Word Index "provides a reference to text names based on a diagnostic property, disease entity, organ system, or syndrome for which the test may be useful" [p. 13]. Symbols within the index indicate tests essential for the diagnosis of a disease and/or the diagnosis or management of a disease. *International Classification of Disease—Ninth Revision—Clinical Modification (ICD-9-CM)* codes are also included. An Acronyms and Abbreviations Glossary and Alphabetic Index complete the volume. Tests are presented in a standardized format followed by footnotes and references and in some cases Internet Web sites. The *Laboratory Test Handbook Concise with Diseases Index* is a compact abridged version of the 5th edition which provides quick reference to 960 tests, with 200 new or revised tables and graphs. Cross references are available to Web sites.

Specialized works in laboratory analysis abound, and *Methods in Enzymology* represents this type of publication. Each volume (or group of volumes) in the series concentrates on a particular topic, with an editor and a group of contributors providing essays on a state-of-the-art approach. Since 1994, the publisher has provided an index to the series on CD-ROM as well as in print.

The *Current Protocols* series is available by subscription in looseleaf, on CD-ROM (for single or networked up to 40 users), and by license on the Web for most of the publications in the series. *Current Protocols* in the life sciences include Molecular Biology, Immunology, Human Genetics, Protein Science, Cytometry, Neuroscience, Pharmacology, Cell Biology, Toxicology, and Nucleic Acid Chemistry. Other disciplines include: Bioinformatics and Magnetic Resonance Imaging. These laboratory manuals are regularly updated and represent the latest research methods in their respective areas. Online searching can be done using a thesaurus, proximity searching, or browsing the table of contents. These are primarily used as laboratory bench tools; however, they can be useful reference resources to answer questions about particular methods.

Handbooks Related to Diagnosis and Classification

Nomenclature is defined by *Webster's Third New International Dictionary* as "a system or set of names or designations used in a particular science, discipline, or art and formally adopted or sanctioned by the usage of its practitioners." In medicine and its related fields, there are a number of works that set out a systematic terminology for a particular purpose.

8.14 *Current Procedural Terminology: CPT 2003*, 4th ed. Chicago, IL: American Medical Association, 2002.

8.15 International Union of Biochemistry and Molecular Biology. Nomenclature Committee. *Enzyme Nomenclature 1992: Recommendations of the Nomenclature Committee of the International Union of Biochemistry and Molecular Biology.* San Diego, CA: Published for the International Union of Biochemistry and Molecular Biology by Academic Press, 1992. Five Supplements published in: *Eur. J. Biochem.* 1994, 223, 1–5; *Eur. J. Biochem.* 1995, 232, 1–6; *Eur. J. Biochem.* 1996, 237, 1–5; *Eur. J. Biochem.* 1997, 250; 1–6; and *Eur. J. Biochem.* 1999, 264, 610–650; respectively [Copyright IUBMB]. Available: www.chem.qmw.ac.uk/iubmb/enzyme.

8.16 Purich DL, Allison RD. *The Enzyme Reference: A Comprehensive Guidebook to Enzyme Nomenclature, Reactions, and Methods.* San Diego, CA: Academic Press, 2002.

8.17 *Manual of the International Statistical Classification of Diseases, Injuries, and Causes of Death*, 9th revised ed. Geneva, Switzerland: World Health Organization, 1977. 2 vols.

8.18 *The International Classification of Diseases, 9th Revision, Clinical Modification: ICD-9-CM,* 4th ed. Washington, DC: U.S. Department of Health and Human Services, Public Health Service, Health Care Financing Administration, 1991. 2 vols. Available: http://online.statref.com.

8.19 *Diagnostic and Statistical Manual of Mental Disorders: DSM-IV,* 4th ed. Washington, DC: American Psychiatric Association, 1994. *Diagnostic and Statistical Manual of Mental Disorders: DSM-IV-TR,* 4th ed. Washington, DC: American Psychiatric Association, 2000.

8.20 Beers MH and Berkow R, eds. *The Merck Manual of Diagnosis and Therapy,* 17th ed. "Centennial Edition." Rahway, NJ: Merck, 1999. Available: http://online.statref.com.

The purpose of *Current Procedural Terminology: CPT 2003* is to provide a standardized listing of terms and codes for reporting medical services and procedures performed by physicians. In 2000 the U.S. Department of Health and Human Services designated the CPT Code Set as the "national coding standard for physician and other health care professional services and procedures under the Health Insurance Portability Accountability Act (HIPAA)" [Forward]. Arranged in six sections, Evaluation and Management, Anesthesiology, Surgery, Radiology (including Nuclear Medicine and Diagnostic Ultrasound), Pathology and Laboratory, and Medicine (except Anesthesiology), there are also five Appendixes and an Alphabetical Index to codes with main entries for 1) procedure or service, 2) organ or other anatomic site, 3) condition, and 4) synonyms, eponyms, and abbreviations.

Enzyme Nomenclature 1992 is an example of a standardized terminology created to bring order to a particular field. This book is based on the recommendations of the nomenclature committee of the International Union of Biochemistry and Molecular Biology (IUBMB). It was created to organize the chaos that existed in the 1950s when many new enzymes were being discovered and haphazardly named. *Enzyme Nomenclature 1992* includes the names of more than 3,196 enzymes and a detailed mechanism that is used in naming new enzymes. The first five supplements were published in the *European Journal of Biochemistry*. Subsequent supplements, 6 through 8, are only available on the Web. The IUBMB Nomenclature Committee maintains the freely available Web site as cited above. The Web version of *Enzyme Nomenclature* provides the complete text of the 1992 edition, all supplements, as well as information on "How to suggest new entries and correct existing entries" and "Rules for the Classification and Nomenclature of Enzymes."

As the subtitle suggests, *The Enzyme Reference: A Comprehensive Guidebook to Enzyme Nomenclature, Reactions, and Methods* is not limited to enzyme nomenclature. The alphabetical listing of enzymes includes the EC (Enzyme Commission) number, a description of where the enzyme was isolated, references to the literature, and brief citations to *Methods in Enzymology* articles used in kinetic investigations. Some listings include the molecular structure.

The *Manual of the International Statistical Classification of Diseases, Injuries, and Causes of Death* represents "a system of categories to which morbid entities are assigned according to some established criteria" [Introduction]. These categories make standardization of the collection of data related to diseases, injuries, and causes of death possible. To facilitate the study of disease, the scheme has been arranged so that each specific disease entity has "a separate title in the classification only when its separation is warranted because the frequency of its occurrence, or its importance as a morbid condition, justifies its isolation as a separate category" [Introduction]. This element of grouping represents the difference between a classification for statistical purposes and a nomenclature that must be as detailed as possible to provide for all possible names.

The *International Classification of Diseases (ICD-9)* is a decimal classification system. The three digits preceding the decimal represent the chosen categories in 17 broad areas: digits following the decimal represent the specific diseases found in each category. Although volume 1 (Tabular List) of *ICD-10* was published in 1992, volume 2 (Instructional Manual) and volume 3 (Alphabetical Index) are not yet available. A clinical modification, *ICD-10-CM*, is expected in 2004.

ICD-9-CM is the U.S. adaptation of *ICD-9*. The clinical modification provides a common classification of diseases and related entities to be used by all agencies and institutions. The intent of *ICD-9-CM* is "to serve as a useful tool in the area of classification of morbidity data for indexing of medical records, medical care review, and ambulatory and other medical care programs, as well as for basic health statistics" [Forward]. The modification provides the greater precision that is required for the maintenance of clinical records. STAT!Ref provides access to the Ingenix ICD-9-CM volumes 1 (Tabular List) and 3 (Alphabetical Index) and CPT with RVUs Data File version.

A complementary publication, *Diagnostic and Statistical Manual of Mental Disorders: DSM-IV,* is based on the mental disorders section in *The International Classification of Diseases.* The *DSM-IV* was prepared to coordinate with the development of *ICD-10* so that the codes and terms are fully compatible with both *ICD-9-CM* and *ICD-10.*

The *Merck Manual of Diagnosis and Therapy* contains discussions of factors related to rational diagnostic reasoning and effective therapy, including discussions of symptoms and signs. The 23 sections are subdivided into chapters that go into considerable detail. The work attempts to serve as a reference guide for the whole range of medical disorders. The 17th "Centennial Edition" is available online from Stat!Ref, which provides for keyword searching and browsing of the table of contents.

Handbooks and manuals are likely to be used heavily in ready reference because of the diverse information they contain. The titles presented in this chapter are just a few of the possible sources that could have been included. Many are standard titles that should be found in all health sciences libraries; others are here to represent the variety that is available.

References

1. Grogan D. *Science and technology: an introduction to the literature,* 4th ed., rev. London: Clive Bingley, 1982:73.

CHAPTER 9

DRUG INFORMATION SOURCES

Amy Butros and Susan McGuinness

Drug information encompasses the fields of pharmacology (the study of the physiological actions of drugs), pharmacy (the compounding, manufacture, and dispensing of drugs), and toxicology (the study of hazardous effects of chemicals). Additionally, the Human Genome Project has led to the study of pharmacogenomics (the genetic basis of drug action), adding complexity to all aspects of drug information. The volume of new information generated in the field of pharmacogenomics is almost unmanageable, requiring unprecedented computer power for data analysis and storage. In the twenty-first century, the impact of pharmacogenomics on pharmaceutical research, education, practice, and therefore on drug information, is projected to be astronomical. From drug design and discovery to the point of care, questions of individual genetic variations persist. What is the protein target for a particular drug therapy? What molecular properties can be manipulated to increase beneficial drug effects and reduce adverse effects? How does a particular genetic variation affect drug metabolism? How do these differences translate to dosing calculations? These questions represent a broader scope of information needs and reflect the increasingly multidisciplinary nature of drug information in the post—genome project era.

Change is a hallmark of drug information and is driven by technology and the evolving roles of health care professionals. The Internet has transformed scientific investigation and discovery as well as information management in health care. In this changing environment, librarians may be called on to access information not traditionally included in the category of drug information. For example, the emergence of computational modeling of drug action requires the interlacing of a wide range of chemical and physical properties, creating a multiplicity of new pharmaceutical research questions. Clinical questions are also expanding, congruent with the changing roles of health care professionals. Today's pharmacists function as integral members of health care teams, partnering with physicians to customize drug regimens for individuals. As high-level practitioners who are qualified to advise patients and physicians about drug therapies, they require timely and accurate drug information to support clinical decision making. With their professional responsibility for patient care, therapeutic outcomes, and medical standards of care requiring evidence-based practice, pharmacists play a major role in providing drug information to other health care professionals and therefore rely heavily on accurate and current resources. Librarians serving this population are challenged to participate efficiently and effectively with pharmacists to access timely and relevant drug information in a highly dynamic field.

Drug information questions are directed to librarians from a number of sources. A physician may want to know all adverse effects previously associated with the administration of a particular drug or if the drug interacts with other drugs under physiological conditions. An occupational health specialist may ask if there is a relationship between a clinical symptom and daily exposure to a chemical in a work environment. A pharmacist may need the American equivalent of a drug prescribed in another country. A nurse may want more information about a drug being administered to a patient to assist in monitoring the patient's response. Increasingly complex drug information questions are also directed to librarians from patients. The Internet provides many sources of consumer health information, some more authoritative than others, and patrons often need help evaluating Web sites. Another factor affecting the scope of information needs is direct-to-consumer drug advertising. Armed with information from the Internet and drug advertising, consumers may question the recommendations of their physicians. As a result, patients may use the library to investigate questions about drugs they are taking or about additives in the food they eat.

Physicians and pharmacists may need drug information written in lay language to optimize their communications with patients.

The number of drugs (both prescription and nonprescription) available on the market has increased substantially. In recent years, the use of herbal products and other alternative therapies has also expanded, due in large part to the empowerment of consumers with increased access to health information. With the increase in the number of drugs in use, there exists a proportional increase in the potential for adverse effects and an exponential increase in the number of possible interactions between these drugs. As a result, iatrogenic (physician-induced) pathology continues to play a significant role in medicine today.

Drug Regulation and Approval Process

Information about drugs is complex due to government regulation. The Food and Drug Administration (FDA) regulates all drugs in interstate commerce and is responsible for overseeing the labeling of drugs and ensuring that they are both safe and effective. These regulations are published in the *Code of Federal Regulations, Title 21: Food and Drugs* (available electronically through the National Archives and Records Administration, Code of Federal Regulations Web site at www.access.gpo.gov/nara/cfr). The FDA requires the pharmaceutical company to notify prescribing physicians of contraindications (i.e., when not to use a drug), warnings, and adverse effects of drugs. In December 2000, the FDA proposed new requirements for drug packaging information to make it more user-friendly for physicians and patients (21 CFR part 201; FR 81081, December 2000.) Also known as the "Daily Med" initiative, the project involves reorganization of information to include tables of contents and sections of "highlights," the most important facts about the drug. Without these highlights, it can be difficult to extract the most relevant information because pharmaceutical companies are required to list all precautions and contraindications regardless of their probability. In the industrial setting, the Occupational Safety and Health Administration (OSHA) of the U.S. Department of Labor creates and enforces safety standards in the workplace. The Occupational Safety and Health Administration often works

155

together with the National Institute for Occupational Safety and Health (NIOSH) of the U.S. Department of Health and Human Services which is responsible for conducting research and making recommendations for occupational therapy. This chapter describes sources of government regulations, standards, and practices as well as drug packaging information.

There are many stages of development before a drug is put on the market [1], with investigators at each stage creating and accessing different kinds of information. In the drug discovery stage, approaches to chemical synthesis are optimized and several candidates or analogues are usually developed. Molecular modeling techniques are used to determine drug/target interactions. Next, in vitro and animal studies are conducted. In vitro tests usually involve the determination of drug concentrations that kill or inhibit the growth of various types of human cells in culture. Animal models are used to mimic human disease states for testing drug efficacy and to determine appropriate therapeutic drug concentrations. In the next stage, routes of administration are chosen, prototype drugs are formulated, and formulations are evaluated for purity, stability, and toxicity in animal models. When a pharmaceutical company has a chemical entity that it believes has significant therapeutic value, it files an Investigational New Drug (IND) Application with the FDA. The drug company must then conduct documented studies to demonstrate the therapeutic value and safety of the drug. After substantial testing in animals, the IND testing begins in very small groups (20–200) of human volunteers (Phase 1 studies) to determine safety. Phase 1 studies may be conducted in patients or in healthy volunteers and are designed to generate information on drug metabolism, pharmacology, and side effects associated with high doses. They sometimes also provide evidence on effectiveness. Phase 2 studies evaluate safety and dose range as well as efficacy in patients (up to several hundred) with the disease the drug is intended to treat. If these trials are satisfactory, the study moves into Phase 3, where the drug is given to a larger (several hundred to several thousand) and more diverse population. When sufficient data have been collected, the pharmaceutical company submits another application to the FDA, a New Drug Application (NDA), with its data on the safety and effectiveness of the drug. Approval of the NDA means that the drug is approved for marketing and can be prescribed by licensed practitioners. Prior to this approval, the drug may be used only by certain physicians who have been approved to handle investigational drugs. As the drug is made available to potentially millions of patients, additional side effects may appear. For instance, some effects are idiosyncratic, occurring in a very small percentage of the population and often missed in the preclinical phases. Phase 4 studies, sometimes called marketing studies, investigate differences between drugs of the same type or intended to treat the same condition to determine advantages and disadvantages of one drug over another.

Information on the drug in its preclinical stages, especially before it is patented, may be difficult to obtain. Clinical trials can be found through the PubMed version of MEDLINE (Available: www.pubmed.gov) and also through the Clinical Trials Web site, ClinicalTrials.gov (Available: http://clinicaltrials.gov), maintained by the National Library of Medicine (NLM). Many studies also appear in the chemical literature (or the biological literature if it is a naturally derived substance). The biological literature is also a good place to search for early toxicity or carcinogenicity animal studies performed before the IND is submitted. Unfortunately, the NDA with its documented evidence never becomes a part of the public domain. It is considered to be proprietary information available only to the company and the FDA. However researchers often publish their experiences with the drug during clinical trials. This material is retrievable through the journal and report literature.

After the patent on a drug expires, other companies may wish to market a generic equivalent. These companies must submit an Abbreviated New Drug Application (ANDA) to show that the generic drug has the same indications for use, active ingredients, route of administration, dosage form, strength, bioavailability, and labeling. Information on therapeutic equivalence of generic drugs is listed in the FDA publication, "Approved Drug Products with Therapeutic Equivalence."

This chapter describes many Web-based resources, reflecting the influence of the Internet on drug information organization and delivery, as well as essential print resources used in education and practice. Some of the information in this chapter articulates "universal truths" from earlier editions and that information has not changed, so we would like to extend our appreciation to Julie Kuenzel Kwan and Diane L. Fishman for their work. Other areas and newer resources are the contributions of the current authors.

Guides to the Literature

Librarians and information professionals new to the drug information field should be able to rely on guides to the literature to put drug information in perspective. Current drug information bibliographies and comprehensive guides to the literature are scarce and hard to locate. There is one comprehensive and in-depth guide that stands out as essential to any collection. It is Bonnie Snow's *Drug Information* compilation. A more specialized list of resources is available from the American Association of Colleges of Pharmacy, and it can be consulted to complement Snow's work.

9.1   Snow B. *Drug Information: A Guide to Current Resources,* 2nd ed. Latham, MD: Medical Library Association and Scarecrow Press, Inc., 1999.

9.2   *Basic Resources for Pharmaceutical Education.* Alexandria, VA: American Association of Colleges of Pharmacy, 2001. Available: www.aacp.org.

9.3   Sewell W. *Guide to Drug Information.* Hamilton, IL: Drug Intelligence Publications, 1976.

Snow's *Drug Information* provides good background and descriptive information supported by many resources in several areas. It covers drug nomenclature and identification, laws and regulations, adverse drug reactions and interactions, industrial pharmacy, sources for statistical information, plus online and Internet resources. Practicum exercises, a glossary, and a detailed index add to this guide's value. The American Association of Colleges of Pharmacy (AACP) provides a detailed and lengthy list of resources for any collection involved with educating pharmacists. The AACP has an alphabetical and hierarchical listing of over 800 sources; most book entries include price and electronic resource entries include URLs.

A classic source is Sewell's *Guide to Drug Information*. This book is quite dated but it contains insightful help for librarians, such as the type of information that is in drug handbooks, considered as primary sources by pharmacists, and some timeless advice on keeping up with the literature.

Drug Nomenclature

One of the major problems in using the drug literature is recognizing the multiplicity of names for a given chemical compound and understanding how reference sources must be approached depending on the type of name. A thorough understanding of these names is essential (Fig. 9-1). When a pharmaceutical company is investigating a large number of chemicals for possible therapeutic activity, it frequently assigns alphanumeric designations or code names. Often, a code name is the first designation in the primary literature.

The Chemical Abstracts Service (CAS) provides a unique registry number for each chemical compound (including drugs). One thing to remember about the registry number is that European countries commonly name the drug for the parent compound. In the United States, it is more usual to use the salt form (the compound formulated as a salt so that it will dissolve more easily in water), which will generally have a different registry number. Because indexes vary on whether the parent or salt registry number is used, the experienced searcher should try to identify both registry numbers for full retrieval.

The chemical name describes the chemical structure of a drug. There are a number of conventions for these chemical names, which are often very lengthy. Consequently, there is a need for a shorter "common" name to describe a chemical. "Aspirin" and "tetracycline" are examples of these more easily handled names. Common names are also called "generic" and "nonproprietary" names. Names used by a manufacturer to describe marketed products are called "proprietary," "brand," or "trade" names. Proprietary names are registered trademarks, as are the color, shape, and markings of each pill or capsule.

159

Two or more manufacturers may market the same generic drug, but each may also have its own trade name representing the specific product. These products may differ: although the active ingredients are the same, each manufacturer may use different ingredients in compounding the drug or in holding it together. The composition of a pill, other than amounts of active ingredients, is proprietary, or a trade secret, but the inactive ingredients for many drugs are included with drug packaging information, which can be found in the *Physicians' Desk Reference* (*PDR*) (see 9.10, below). Inactive ingredients are also sometimes listed in resources such as POISINDEX in MICROMEDEX's Healthcare Series of online databases (see 9.50, below) and *AHFS Drug Information* (see 9.15, below).

Another source of confusion is the multiplicity of generic names. Two companies working with the same drug may call it by different generic names. In the past, this practice has led to such confusion that now "official" generic names are designated. The United States Adopted Names (USAN) Commission has the authority to declare a specific generic name as the officially recognized common name, the "adopted name," in the United States. If another company wants to market a preparation of that drug, it will use this "official" generic name.

The nomenclature problem is compounded on an international scale. Other countries also have authorized bodies to establish official names; for example, Japanese Adopted Names (JAN) and British Adopted Names (BAN). The World Health Organization's International Nonproprietary Names (INN) attempts to unify official names in all participating countries, but differences still exist. These variations in nomenclature cause a range of difficulties. For instance, a patient having been prescribed a French drug travels to the United States and needs a refill of an American equivalent. A British doctor, taking an American medical licensure exam, finds "meperidine" on the examination questions rather than "pethidine," the name to which British doctors are accustomed. American researchers looking for information on the antiviral agent acyclovir will miss sources that use the INN, aciclovir.

Librarians must understand the many types of names to use literature sources effectively. Some publications, particularly those originating from commercial sources, may be arranged by proprietary or trade name. Others, especially those from professional associations, are usually arranged by nonproprietary or generic name. Books published in other countries use their own official generic names, which are sometimes different from the American form. Some sources are limited to prescription drugs whereas others include nonprescription (over-the-counter, or OTC) medications. The librarian, presented with a drug name, may not immediately know what type of name it is. The first step is to determine the type of name and then go to appropriate reference sources. Descriptions of essential sources of drug identification follow.

Figure 9-1. Drug Formula and Identification

Research code designation:	U-18,573
CAS Registry Number:	15687-27-1
Chemical names:	a-Methyl-4-(2-methylpropyl) benzeneacetic acid
	p-Isobutylhydratropic acid
	2-(4-Isobutylphenyl)propionic acid
Generic Name:	Ibuprofen
USAN, INN, BAN, JAN:	Ibuprofen
Proprietary Names:	Advil, Midol, Motrin, Nuprin
Molecular Formula:	C13H 18O 2
Structural Formula:	

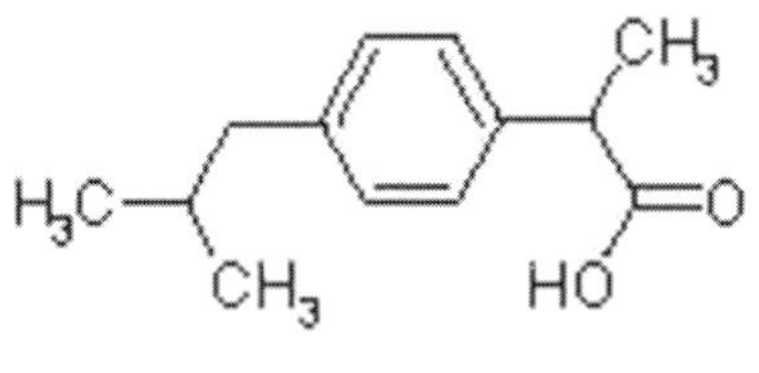

Sources of Drug Identification

For easy identification of drug names, both proprietary (trade) and nonproprietary (generic), there are a few key sources that are essential for all collections.

161

9.4   *American Drug Index.* St. Louis, MO: Facts and Comparisons, Division of Lippincott, 1956– . Annual.

9.5   *USP Dictionary of USAN and International Drug Names.* Rockville, MD: U.S. Pharmacopeia. Annual.

9.6   *The Merck Index: An Encyclopedia of Chemicals, Drugs, and Biologicals,* 13th ed. Whitehouse Station, NJ: Merck & Co., Inc., 2001.

The *American Drug Index* is an ideal source to consult first when starting your search for drug information. This source has a comprehensive alphabetical listing of proprietary and nonproprietary names for both prescription and over-the-counter drugs. The entries for proprietary names include the manufacturer's name, the nonproprietary (generic or chemical) name, composition, strength, pharmaceutical forms available, dosage, and a brief indication of use. The generic names frequently include the pronunciation, a designation of *USP*, USAN, or *NF* (*National Formulary*) to indicate where the drug name is listed, plus brief indication of use and a "see" reference to the proprietary name. Useful appendices at the back of this book include a list of medical abbreviations used in medical orders, a trademark glossary and a medical terminology glossary, a list of addresses and Web sites for drug manufacturers and distributors, plus unique information such as oral dosage forms that should not be crushed or chewed and drug names that look alike and sound alike.

The *USP Dictionary of USAN and International Drug Names* is another essential resource for basic drug information. This book is updated annually and provides a compilation of the United States Adopted Names (USAN) selected and released since June 15, 1961. This source is very useful because it is a compilation and provides entries for earlier drug names. Each USAN entry lists the year the drug name was adopted, a pronunciation guide, molecular formula, molecular weight, chemical name, CAS registry number, pharmacological or therapeutic activity, brand names under which the drug is marketed, manufacturer or distributor, and the structural formula. A detailed introduction describes the purpose and history of the USAN Council and the procedures that establish an adopted name. Several helpful appendices are included, such as a listing of brand and nonproprietary names for the USAN names, a listing of molecular formulas and CAS registry numbers, and a grouping of USAN names by category (e.g., Analgesic, Antibacterial, Food Additive, Ultraviolet Screen). Because this source also includes International Nonproprietary Names (INN), it should be noted that inclusion in this book does not necessarily mean that the drug is marketed in the United States. It only means that an official name has been designated. Frequently, U.S. drugs are named around the time that they are patented and go into clinical trials. Thus, many years may pass before the drug receives final approval for marketing.

Another brief dictionary type source is *The Merck Index*. This publication began in 1889 as a brief listing of drugs marketed by the Merck Company. It is now in its 13th edition and has grown to be a comprehensive encyclopedia of drugs, chemicals, and biological substances. *The Merck Index* should be considered as an essential part of a basic drug information collection. Although this source is alphabetically arranged by chemical name, it is easier to use the index as the entry point into the descriptive paragraphs. There are several helpful listings of tables and chemical reactions at the end of this book. The indexes that lead to the entries include registry numbers, therapeutic categories, molecular formulas, and chemical names. The entries in *The Merck Index* include registry number, chemical name, common names (in some cases), molecular formula, molecular weight, brief description of use, plus the added benefit of historical references, patent references, and preparation, synthesis, or review journal article references.

Comprehensive Treatises and Textbooks

In the medical or pharmacy library, questions frequently arise concerning the physical and chemical properties of drugs and associated mechanisms of biological activity. The librarian may begin with the sources in the previous section to obtain the necessary proprietary and generic drug names and brief information on pharmacological action. For more in-depth discussions, the following comprehensive sources are essential.

9.7   Hardman JG, Limbird LE, eds. Goodman GA, consulting editor. *Goodman & Gilman's The Pharmacological Basis of Therapeutics,* 10th ed. New York: McGraw-Hill Medical Publishing Division, 2001.

9.8   Parfitt K. *Martindale: The Complete Drug Reference,* 33rd ed. London: Pharmaceutical Press, 2002. Available: www.micromedex.com/products.

9.9   Gennaro AR. *Remington: The Science and Practice of Pharmacy,* 20th ed. Baltimore, MD: Lippincott Williams & Wilkins, 2000.

Goodman & Gilman's The Pharmacological Basis of Therapeutics, published since 1941, has been known as "the bible of pharmacology." A standard textbook on fundamental principles of drug action, it continues to be a valuable tool in medical and pharmacy schools. The book is divided into 16 sections, beginning with general principles of pharmacology and proceeding with sections organized by modes of action on physiological systems or actions related to disease states. For example, the 13 chapters of section III describe drug actions on the central nervous system, and the nine chapters of section VIII describe chemotherapy of microbial diseases. Each chapter provides in-depth discussions of pharmacological mechanisms by drug class (e.g., hypnotics and sedatives), emphasizing the comparison between individual drugs of the same class and including many useful tables of drug names and properties. The detailed index allows the user to access information by a variety of terms such as drug names, type of drug action, physiological systems, or symptoms.

Martindale: The Complete Drug Reference, provides comprehensive information similar to *Goodman & Gilman's,* but with international coverage, less emphasis on basic pharmacology, and more specific information on individual drugs. This work is divided into five parts, the first and major part being "Monographs on Drugs and Ancillary Substances." This source, and most other sources, uses the term "monographs" for the descriptive drug entries. Each chapter gives a general description of a class of drugs, followed by detailed descriptions of drugs belonging to that class, including adverse effects, drug interactions, preparations and countries of origin for each drug. Because regulations regarding new drugs are not as stringent in other countries as in the United States, Martindale's coverage includes many drugs not available in the United States and provides international equivalents of drugs marketed in this country. Drug monographs list BAN first, followed by INN and USAN where available. Also listed are chemical formulas, molecular weights, and CAS Registry numbers. References are provided at the end of each monograph. Part 2, "Supplementary Drugs and Other Substances," contains shorter monographs of similar format on herbal and other preparations. Part 3 is an index of proprietary preparations from a number of countries. Records generally include proprietary names, manufacturers or sources, and ingredients, as well as page references to the complete monographs. At the end of the book are a directory of manufacturers and a general index. The directory lists manufacturers in alphabetical order using abbreviations from Part 3. The general index includes both generic and proprietary drug names as well as synonyms and chemical names. Diseases and associated terms are also listed. *Martindale* is also available in full-text through the MICROMEDEX HealthCare Series of online databases (see 9.50, below).

Remington: The Science and Practice of Pharmacy is a standard text of pharmaceutical science used by many pharmacy schools. With an emphasis on basic science, it covers a broad range of topics including pharmaceutical chemistry, pharmaceutical manufacturing, pharmacodynamics, and the fundamentals of pharmacy practice and pharmacy law. It also provides an extensive section on therapeutic agents organized by drug class and includes brief monographs on specific drugs. These monographs generally include chemical names, formulas and molecular weights, as well as chemical structure diagrams. Brief discussions of the uses, chemical properties, and preparation are also included. The text concludes with a useful glossary of acronyms and a comprehensive subject index.

Commercial Sources of Drug Information

Numerous and varied sources exist that give information about specific drugs and pharmaceuticals that are marketed. The pharmaceutical manufacturer is responsible for providing certain basic information about their products. The FDA approves the content of this basic information. One mechanism by which the manufacturer informs the physician about a specific product is the "package insert," a brief brochure that generally includes the trade and chemical names; pharmacological action; indications and contraindications; warnings, precautions, and adverse reactions; dosage and overdosage; dosage forms; and, in most cases, references. The package insert is not necessarily complete or balanced. Although the FDA has agreed to the manufacturer's statements about the product and the manufacturer is legally responsible for the accuracy of the information included, the package insert remains a publicity and promotion mechanism for the manufacturer. A package insert does not compare or evaluate a given drug with other agents.

9.10 *Physicians' Desk Reference (PDR)*. Montvale, NJ: Thompson PDR, 1947–. Annual. Available: www.micromedex.com/products.

9.11 *Physicians' Desk Reference (PDR) for Ophthalmic Medicines*, 21st ed. Montvale, NJ: Thompson Medical Economics, 2003.

9.12 Physicians' Desk Reference (PDR) for Nonprescription Drugs and Dietary Supplements, 23rd ed. Montvale, NJ: Thompson Medical Economics, 2002.

The *Physicians' Desk Reference* (*PDR*) is an annual compilation of these package inserts. The information in the *PDR* is arranged by company name. Most of the products marketed in the United States are listed in the *PDR*, making it a handy, and frequently requested, source. The *PDR* is very useful for drug dosage, composition, contraindications, warnings, use, and adverse effects. The indexes included in the front of the *PDR* are a manufacturers' index, with addresses and contact information for most companies, a brand and generic name index, a product category index, and a product identification guide with color photographs of around 2,400 tablets, capsules, and other dosage forms. Because some omissions and inaccuracies in the color photographs have been noted, other sources to consider for visual drug identification are the *USP DI* (see 9.16, below) or Clinical Pharmacology (see 9.49, below), both available online with Web interfaces.

The *PDR* is a source of manufacturer disclaimers, cautions, precautions, and side effects, all of which are enumerated in great detail, although there is often no indication of the severity or frequency of the side effects. For example, because the manufacturing industry cannot conduct safety tests in pregnant humans, the *PDR* frequently uses the statement "safety of this drug during pregnancy is unknown."

The earliest editions of the *PDR* carried the subtitle "for the physician's desk only" and volumes are still often distributed free to physicians as a marketing tool. However, with the recent consumer movement in health care, this statement has been removed, and the PDR is now for sale throughout the country in bookstores serving the general public. Librarians should be concerned about the public's reliance on the *PDR*. First, the information is not necessarily unbiased, but represents only what the FDA has approved the manufacturer to say. Second, the coverage is selective, as drug companies are charged for inclusion. Therefore, not all drug companies participate, and those that do typically only include their more profitable drugs. Third, librarians should understand that the information included about drug use is not necessarily complete. Physicians can legally prescribe drugs for therapeutic applications that have not yet been approved by the FDA, and these unlabeled uses will not generally be addressed in the *PDR*. Finally, the information in the *PDR* is written in technical language and may be difficult for the general public to understand. Because rare side effects are included, the work may prove unnecessarily frightening to the nonprofessional. Perhaps one of the greatest challenges to the health sciences librarian is to channel members of the public from the *PDR* to more appropriate sources.

The apparent popularity and success of the *PDR* have caused a whole series of *PDR* books to appear. Some of these titles are worth listing here, but others will be covered in the following sections. *The PDR Family Guide to Prescription Drugs* and *The PDR for Herbal Medicines* will be discussed in more detail in the "Drug Information for

Patients and the Public" and the "Herbal Medicines and Natural Products" sections of this chapter. The *Physicians' Desk Reference Companion Guide* is described by the *PDR* publishers as "one of the most useful drug references in current clinical practice" and that it "provides you with a complete drug selection system" (see 9.30, below). This source does not stand alone, it really is a companion book that acts as a combined interactions index to the *PDR*, and thus will be discussed in more detail in the "Drug Interactions" section of this chapter. Two complementary *PDR* publications that librarians may consider are the *Physicians' Desk Reference for Ophthalmic Medicines* and the *Physicians' Desk Reference for Nonprescription Drugs and Dietary Supplements*. There is some overlap between these sources and the *PDR*, but there is also a lot of unique information that may be necessary in some collections.

9.13 *Drug Facts and Comparisons*, 57th ed. St. Louis, MO: Wolters Kluwer Co., 2003. Available: www.factsandcomparisons .com.

9.14 *Drug Topics Red Book*. Montvale, NJ: Thompson Medical Economics, 1896–. Annual.

Drug Facts and Comparisons is a comprehensive compendium of drug information. It is updated annually and is available as a bound volume, in loose-leaf format with monthly updates, and in an online electronic format. This source is arranged by drug therapeutic category; for example, nutritional agents, anticonvulsants, penicillins, immunologic agents, and so forth are each grouped together in distinct sections. A thorough general index lists product brand names, generic names, synonyms, and therapeutic groups, for easy page reference to each entry. Additional indexes include a Canadian Trade Name index and a Manufacturers and Distributors index. This source is worth considering for any collection; it is quite current, comprehensive, and authoritative, with an Editorial Advisory Panel and a Contributing Review Panel of physicians and pharmacists and other health care professionals from academic, private, and government institutions across the United States. Each entry or group of entries in *Drug Facts and Comparisons* includes indications, dosage, actions, contraindications, warnings, interactions, adverse reactions and patient information. Included are many useful tables that list comparisons between different brands, specific drug interactions, combinations, and supply methods.

The *Drug Topics Red Book* is well-known and trusted in the pharmaceutical marketplace. This source is in its 106th year of publication. Because it is so well-known and used by pharmacists it has become a highly requested source from any library. The *Red Book* is more of a catalog of drug products than a comprehensive drug information text. It is divided into distinct sections that can easily be accessed and browsed. Included is a brief herbal medicine guide listing descriptions of popular herbs, with a warning section under most herbs listed, plus a short herb/drug interactions section. Other sections range from pharmacy organizations, such as state boards of pharmacy, state Medicaid drug programs, and DEA offices, to manufacturer addresses, product identification with color photos, and a large section on "Rx Product Listing." This section is an alphabetical list of prescription drugs where each entry includes product names, drug class, route of administration, strength, National Drug Code, average wholesale price, and direct price. There are similar entries for the section on Over the Counter "non-drug" products. This is a good standard source for drug prices and some hard to find addresses, if you don't mind putting up with occasional advertisements.

Professional Sources of Drug Information

The sources described in this section come from professional pharmacy organizations and provide authoritative information on drugs in terms of the disorders they treat and their specific activities and formulations. The first two sources are organized in an encyclopedic format, with lengthy descriptions of drugs called "monographs."

9.15 *AHFS Drug Information.* Washington, DC: American Society of Hospital Pharmacists, 1959–. Annual. Available: www .ashp.com/ahfs/web.

9.16 *United States Pharmacopoeia Dispensing Information*, 23rd ed. Greenwood Village, CO: MICROMEDEX Thomson Healthcare, 1980–.

9.17 *Handbook of Nonprescription Drugs*, 13th ed. Washington, DC: American Pharmaceutical Association, 2002.

Formerly known as the *American Hospital Formulary Service Drug Information, AHFS Drug Information* is produced and updated annually by the American Society of Health System Pharmacists. Recommended by the National Association of Boards of Pharmacy as part of the standard reference library, it is an authoritative source of evaluative information on drugs available in the United States. *AHFS* provides drug monographs arranged by therapeutic classification, such as antineoplastic agents, diagnostic agents, and gastrointestinal drugs. It also includes a section on vitamins. This organization by class enables the user to compare easily drugs from the same family. Each section begins with a listing of the generic names of drugs described in that section, with some sections divided into subcategories. Classification numbers are assigned to major sections and subsections. For example, "Anti-Infective Agents" (section 8:00) includes subsections of amebicides (8:04), antibiotics (8:12), and more. The antibiotics subsection is further divided into nine subcategories including cephalosporins (8:12.06). The list of drugs in the cephalosporin family refers the user to page numbers, but individual drugs are not assigned classification numbers. These numeric classifications are important to pharmacists, and the International Pharmaceutical Abstracts database enables searching by these numbers. Each section includes general statements on pharmacology and basic principles of drug action for that class of compounds. The descriptions of individual drugs (monographs) emphasize the critical evaluation of clinical drug data and include information on conventional, off label, and investigational uses, preparations, dosages and administration, drug interactions and laboratory test interferences, mechanisms of action, pharmacokinetics, cautions, and contraindicatons. In cases where only the drug name is known, but not the drug classification, users may refer to the general index. The index contains both generic and proprietary names with useful cross references. *AHFS* is also available in a variety of electronic formats including stand-alone desktop, Web, and palm-based versions. The electronic database products (see Table 9-1) include bibliographies for the drug monographs not included in the print version as well as the full-text of the more specialized *Handbook of Injectable Drugs.*

The *USP DI: United States Pharmacopoeia Dispensing Information* was introduced by the *U.S. Pharmacopoeia* to provide prescribing and dispensing information not included in the official compendia (see 9.18, below), such as precautions, side effects, and dosage. In 1998 the *USP DI* was sold to MICROMEDEX, a Thomson health care company, with the agreement that an advisory council of *USP* experts would continue to participate and develop authoritative information. Volume 1 is a set of monographs written for the health care provider. This work is unique in that it describes drugs in terms of their specific areas of effect rather than therapeutic class. Drugs are described as systemic, dental, inhalation-local, ophthalmic, parenteral-local, and topical, rather than antihistamine, antineoplastic, analgesic, and so forth. Information on specific dosage forms such as tablet, injection, and ointment is also provided. Each entry lists the drug category and describes indications, pharmacology, precautions, adverse effects, overdose, patient consultation information, dosing information, and dosage forms. Single entity as well as combination drugs (drugs with more than one active ingredient) are included. To find a specific drug, the general index is the best entry point because some drugs are individually listed while others are included in sections of drug classes. For example, there is an entry for acetaminophen listed in alphabetical order before antihistamines, and the antihistamines are alphabetically listed within that section. Sections on classes of drugs include tables comparing drug characteristics as well as useful summaries of differences. The *USP DI,* Volume 1 has several useful appendices, including a listing of poison control centers in the United States and Canada and a medicine chart with color photographs of commonly used medications.

The *USP-DI,* Volume 2 was written in lay language for the patient. The first section is an alphabetical index of generic and proprietary names. Next is the same medicine chart found in Volume 1, followed by general information on the use of medications. For each drug entry,

171

the user can find information on proper usage and storage of the medication, precautions, information on pregnancy and breast-feeding, and information for different age groups. The third volume, *Approved Drug Products and Legal Requirements*, is a compilation of a variety of sources including the FDA's "Orange Book," *Approved Drug Products with Therapeutic Equivalence Evaluations*. This is an excellent source of legal information related to drug prescribing and dispensing as well as information on therapeutic equivalence (the extent to which drugs contain the same active ingredients in equal amounts, are administered by the same route, and produce the same clinical effect). Pharmacists refer to therapeutic equivalence values in determining which drugs may be substituted for others. This volume can be used to see if a prescription or nonprescription drug has been approved by the FDA and the date in which each of its forms (liquid, tablet, and so forth) was approved.

The *Handbook of Nonprescription Drugs: An Interactive Approach to Self Care,* published by the American Pharmaceutical Association, deals with over-the-counter and nonprescription drugs, including herbal remedies and dietary supplements. This information is extremely important, especially to users who may not be aware of risks associated with the use of nonprescription drugs. It is also useful to pharmacy students in developing problem-solving skills and to practitioners who interact with patients. The handbook is presented in textbook format beginning with introductory chapters on nonprescription drug therapy and followed by chapters on various disorders (mental disorders, dermatologic disorders, and so forth). There is also a chapter on home medical equipment, such as testing and monitoring devices. Many chapters describe signs and symptoms, treatment approaches, and products that can be used in treatment. Also included are useful case studies as well as treatment algorithms with assessment questions and answers. An appendix provides suggested treatment strategies for the case studies. Each chapter concludes with a bibliography of references to the literature. A general subject index is also provided.

Official Compendia

In the drug information field, an official book of legal pharmaceutical standards is known as a *pharmacopoeia*. Pharmacopoeias are published in different countries to define the accepted purity and standards of chemicals used in therapy. Many pharmacopoeias also include information on chemical tests and assay preparation.

9.18 *The United States Pharmacopeia/The National Formulary: USP NF.* Rockville, MD: United States Pharmacopeial Convention, Inc., 1979–. Annual. Available: www.usp.org and www.statref.com.

In the United States, the two official compendia are the *U.S. Pharmacopoeia* and the *National Formulary*. These two publications have been producing official standards since 1820 and 1888, respectively, although under different sponsorship. Beginning in 1979 the *U.S. Pharmacopoeia* and the *National Formulary* were published in one volume, since the *National Formulary* was acquired by the *U.S. Pharmacopoeia* after the publication of its XIV edition. This new one-volume compendium has a lengthy introduction covering the mission statement and people involved (e.g., board of trustees, executive committees, members of the U.S. Pharmacopoeia Convention). New drug admissions and revisions are also included in the introduction. Each of the drug monographs contains essential information on the drug, such as packaging and storage, identification, pH, melting range, other chemical properties, and assays. After the almost 2,000 pages of drug monographs, there are helpful chapters on general requirements for tests and assays, microbiological, biological, and chemical tests, and a large section on reagents. Also included are tables for relative solubility, atomic weights, and thermometric equivalents, and a small section on nutritional supplements. The last 200 pages comprise the *National Formulary*, containing very similar layout and information. There is a combined *USP NF* index at the end of the publication. It should be noted that the need to collect pharmacopoeias from other countries is often misinterpreted. Most drug questions relate to therapeutic use or to the general identification of a drug, rather than to official standards of purity as given in these compendia. Caution should always be exercised in evaluating any title with the word *pharmacopoeia* in it, as most sources using that term may not be pharmacopoeias in the true sense of the word because they are not listings of legal standards.

As mentioned in the previous section, the *USP DI: United States Pharmacopeia Dispensing Information* was introduced to provide prescribing and dispensing information not included in the *U.S. Pharmacopeia*. Thus, the *USP DI* should also be considered as an official compendium.

Adverse Effects, Toxicology, Poisoning

Some of the most commonly asked questions in the field of drug information deal with adverse effects of drugs and chemicals. What are the side effects of Prozac? Are there any drugs I should avoid if I am taking tamoxifen? What is the lethal dose of aspirin? Many of the sources previously described provide information on adverse effects, drug interactions, toxicity, and poisoning, but additional sources focus specifically on this area.

9.19 Dukes MNG, Aronson JK. *Meyler's Side Effects of Drugs*, 14th ed. Amsterdam, The Netherlands: Elsevier, 2002.

9.20 Aronson JK. *Side Effects of Drugs Annual 25: A Worldwide Survey of New Data and Trends in Adverse Drug Reactions*. Amsterdam, The Netherlands: Elsevier, 2002.

9.21 Leikin JB. *Poisoning & Toxicology Compendium: With Symptoms Index*, 3rd ed. Hudson, OH: Lexi-Comp, Inc., 1998.

9.22 Lee A. *Adverse Drug Reactions*. London: Pharmaceutical Press, 2001.

9.23 Shepard TH. *Catalog of Teratogenic Agents*, 10th ed. Baltimore, MD: Johns Hopkins University Press, 2001. Available: www.micromedex.com/products/reprorisk.

9.24 Friedman JM, Polifka JE. *Teratogenic Effects of Drugs: A Resource for Clinicians (TERIS)*, 2nd ed. Baltimore, MD: Johns Hopkins University Press, 2000. Available: www.micromedex .com/products/reprorisk.

9.25 Briggs GG, Freeman RK, Yaffe SJ. *Drugs in Pregnancy and Lactation: A Reference Guide to Fetal and Neonatal Risk*, 6th ed. Philadelphia, PA: Lippincott Williams & Wilkins, 2002.

9.26 Goldfrank LR. *Goldfrank's Toxicologic Emergencies*, 7th ed. New York: McGraw-Hill, Medical Publishing Division, 2002.

9.27 Lewis RJ, Sr. *Sax's Dangerous Properties of Industrial Materials (DPIM)*, 10th ed. New York: J. Wiley, 2000.

9.28 Lewis RJ, Sr. *Hazardous Chemicals Desk Reference*, 5th ed. New York: Wiley-Interscience, 2002.

9.29 Klaassen CD. *Casarett and Doull's Toxicology: The Basic Science of Poisons*, 7th ed. New York: McGraw-Hill Medical Publishing Division, 2003.

Meyler's Side Effects of Drugs includes comprehensive articles that summarize adverse drug reactions and interactions. Its presentation of data is organized by drug classification, enabling the user to easily review a family of drugs as a whole. Each chapter describes a broad class of drugs, such as central nervous system stimulants, and is divided into monographs on drug families, such as amphetamines. Each monograph provides an overview of the toxic effects and patterns of adverse reactions, specific effects on organs and systems, withdrawal effects, overdosage information, drug interactions, and brief reviews of individual drugs belonging to that family. A complementary guide to *Meyler's* is the *Side Effects of Drugs Annual,* which provides a survey of the latest developments in this field. Chapter titles correspond to those in *Meyler's,* enabling the user to combine easily the general encyclopedic information with annual updates. Libraries should maintain the full series because both sources refer to earlier editions.

The *Poisoning & Toxicology Compendium* includes six chapters on medicinal agents, nonmedicinal agents, biological agents, herbal agents, diagnostic tests/procedures, and antidotes. Each chapter lists chemicals arranged alphabetically by chemical name with entries including proprietary names, CAS registry numbers, information on dosage forms, stability, drug interactions, test interactions, mechanisms of toxicity, and more. The entries consist of brief summaries with references at the end. A symptoms index, though not comprehensive, is unique and useful for looking up entries such as "amnesia" and obtaining lists of substances known to cause that symptom. Also included are a subject index, a pregnancy risk factor index, and an index of CAS registry numbers. The subject index includes the generic and proprietary names, making it a good source for the user who does not know the generic name.

Lee's *Adverse Drug Reactions* is a useful textbook that describes drug toxicity from the viewpoint of the adverse effect, rather than the drug. The first chapter provides an overview of important concepts such as classifications of drug reactions, allergy, pharmacogenetics, and roles of the patient, prescriber, and pharmacist. Succeeding chapters describe common types of reactions, such as skin reactions and disorders of each physiological system (hepatic, renal, gastrointestinal, cardiovascular, etc.), and describe the drugs that elicit these adverse affects. Each chapter includes a case study and numerous references to the literature. A subject index is also provided.

Teratology, the study of the adverse effects of drugs on the fetus, is a widely recognized area of concern. Shepard's *Catalog of Teratogenic Agents* covers fetal exposure to over 3,000 drugs and other agents. It also includes gene mutations known to cause congenital defects. Entries are alphabetically organized by the chemical name and include synonyms, CAS registry numbers where available, descriptions of teratogenicity, and references. Author and subject indexes are also provided. This book is available in electronic format through the MICROMEDEX Healthcare Series of databases (see 9.50, below).

Teratogenic Effects of Drugs: A Resource for Clinicians (TERIS) is a useful reference for identifying teratogenic agents. Its encyclopedia format, with drugs and chemicals listed in alphabetical order by generic name, includes synonyms, a summary of teratology studies, information on the magnitude of risk, other comments, and key references. Excluded from this work are mutagens that have not been proven to be teratogenic. Information on pharmacodynamics and excretion of substances in breast milk is also excluded. This information is provided in other sources listed herein. The index includes generic and proprietary names or synonyms, with generic names in boldface type. This book is also available in electronic format through the MICROMEDEX Healthcare Series of databases (see 9.50, below).

As its name implies, *Drugs in Pregnancy and Lactation* includes not only information on possible harm to the fetus from drugs taken during pregnancy, but also on breast-feeding infants from drugs present in breast milk. Summaries of drug toxicity, in encyclopedia format, are listed alphabetically by generic drug name. Risk factors, defined in the introduction to the book, are assigned to each drug, allowing the user quickly to assess toxicity. Each entry lists the generic name, drug class, risk factor, summaries of fetal and breast-feeding risks, and references. A useful appendix of drugs, organized by category, lists drug names and risk factors. This is helpful for identifying drugs of the same class with different risk factors. The subject index lists both generic and proprietary names.

Goldfrank's Toxicologic Emergencies is a comprehensive textbook of medical toxicology covering basic principles and biochemical, molecular, and pathophysiologic foundations, with chapters on specific agents (prescription and nonprescription drugs, drugs of abuse, household toxins, heavy metals, pesticides, and other environmental and occupational toxins). Chapters on toxins describe classes of compounds, followed by specific information related to individual chemicals. Each chapter offers a case study, history and epidemiology, pharmacology, clinical manifestations, management and antidotes, summaries, and references. Answers to study questions and case studies are given at the end of the book. A subject index is also included.

An essential source of authoritative data on environmental health and safety, *Sax's Dangerous Properties of Industrial Materials* (*DPIM*) provides detailed toxicity information for over 23,000 chemicals found in the workplace, including drugs, food additives, pesticides, dyes, lubricants, soaps, plastics, and more. Each item is encoded with a unique identifier, the *DPIM* entry code, consisting of three letters followed by three numbers. Chemicals are listed in alphanumeric order by code. For example, the entry for acethion amide (AAT000) precedes the entry for acetic acid (AAT250.) The synonym cross-index of 108,000 chemical names refers to *DPIM* codes and is the best entry point for the user searching for substances by name. Each chemical listing provides the *DPIM* code, the chemical name, CAS registry number where available, and the U.S. Department of Transportation (DOT) Hazard Code. DOT codes are internationally recognized and are used in regulating shipping and labeling of hazardous materials. Also included are the molecular formula, molecular weight, and other physical properties, such as solubility and flammability data. Numeric, coded toxicity data are listed next, including skin and eye irritation, acute toxicity, mutagenic, teratogenic, carcinogenic, and other lethal or nonlethal effects. All toxicity data include literature citations. These citations consist of a journal "CODEN" character code, followed by the number of the volume, the page number of the first page of the article, and a two-digit number referring to the year of publication. Each chemical entry also lists standards and recommendations from U.S. government or expert groups, including OSHA. Safety profiles, which textually summarize toxicity and hazard data, are also provided with each entry. Consensus reports are included where applicable. The *DPIM* is a three-volume set, the first volume containing indexes needed to translate the chemical listings of toxicological information in the second and third volumes. Volume 1 provides instructions for using the *DPIM*, a key to abbreviations, a cross-index of DOT hazard codes with *DPIM* codes, a cross-index of CAS registry numbers with *DPIM* codes, the synonym cross-index, and detailed descriptions and definitions of the toxicity data found in Volumes 2 and 3. Volume 1 also includes a bibliography of cited references listed in order of CODEN and including journal titles with publishing information. A condensed version of this work is the *Hazardous Chemicals Desk Reference*. This more manageable single volume lists only the most relevant substances according to the U.S. Environmental Protection Agency Toxic Substances Control Act (TSCA) inventory. Information is provided in the same format with cross-indexes found at the end.

Casarett and Doull's Toxicology: The Basic Science of Poisons is a popular text in graduate-level pharmaceutical sciences education. It focuses mainly on mechanisms of toxicity rather than toxic effects of specific substances, though one of the seven units is devoted to classes of toxic agents, such as metals, solvents, and radioactive materials. Examples of agents are included in the discussions of toxic mechanisms. The text incorporates genetic principles underlying toxicology in descriptions of human metabolism of xenobiotics, organ specific toxicity, and carcinogenesis. Methods of toxicity measurement and risk assessment are also discussed. Each chapter includes literature references. A useful appendix lists OSHA standards and chemical substances threshold limit values (TLVs) from the American Conference of Governmental Industrial Hygienists. A comprehensive subject index is also included. This is an excellent source for the researcher interested in adverse events that can occur in the body as a result of exposure to toxic agents.

Drug Interactions

With the popularity of herbal supplements, nutritional supplements, and other over-the-counter products and with the proliferation of advertising about drugs, physicians, pharmacists, and health care providers are facing a very complex and growing problem of drug interactions. There is overwhelming evidence that the pharmacological action of a drug can be affected by the administration of other drugs, foods, alcohol, and even environmental factors, such as excessive exposure to sun or chemicals. Depending on the interaction and the chemicals involved, a drug's intended action could be minimized, increased, absorption and metabolism rate changed, toxicity levels raised, and other untoward effects could occur. For example, a person taking a monoamine oxidase inhibitor antidepressant should avoid cheese because eating tyramine-rich foods could bring about life-threatening hypertension. Similarly, a person prescribed a tetracycline or quinoline antibiotic should be warned to avoid milky foods or antacids because these will reduce or negate the effectiveness of the antibiotic.

This is a very important and challenging area of drug information. Sources of information on drug interactions are proliferating due to the new demands and popularity of the topic, so librarians need to be careful to collect well-balanced and varied sources to meet their users' needs.

9.30 *Physicians' Desk Reference (PDR) Companion Guide.* Montvale, NJ: Medical Economics Co. 1998–. Annual.

9.31 *Drug Interaction Facts.* St. Louis, MO: Wolters Kluwer Co., loose-leaf, 1998–. Available: www.factsandcomparisons .com.

9.32 *Hansten and Horn's Drug Interactions: Analysis and Management.* St. Louis, MO: Wolters Kluwer Co., loose-leaf, 2002–.

9.33 Stockley IH. *Drug Interactions: A Sourcebook of Adverse Interactions, Their Mechanisms, Clinical Importance and Management,* 6th ed. London: Pharmaceutical Press, 2002.

The main section in the *PDR Companion Guide* is an extensive interactions index. Over 1,000 pages are dedicated to interactions listed in the *PDR*, the *Physicians' Desk Reference for Ophthalmic Medicines,* and the *Physicians' Desk Reference for Nonprescription Drugs and Dietary Supplements.* The *PDR Companion Guide*'s interaction index is alphabetically arranged by brand name; each entry under the brand name contains a brief summary of the drugs this product interacts with, plus a listing of the ingredients in each of these drugs. An appropriate warning to people using this publication states "This index lists only interactions cited in official prescribing information as published by PDR. Because product labeling varies in the scope of its interaction reporting, the most prudent course is to check each product in the patient's regimen." Following the interaction index is a very brief section on food interactions, then a more lengthy side effects index. The side effects index lists the physiological effect followed by a listing of drug brand names; for example, under "Numbness, face" there is a listing for "Botox Cosmetic Purified Neurotoxin Complex." This brand name can then be looked up in the interactions index. In addition to indexes for contraindications and an international drug name index for equivalents of over 33,000 foreign pharmaceutical products, there is a very helpful "Off-Label Treatment Guide" that identifies medications routinely used for indications that they were not officially approved for. This is a very small section, unfortunately, and mentions that the information is taken from MICROMEDEX.

The *Drug Interactions Facts* has been published since 1983 by Facts and Comparisons, then a division of J. B. Lippincott, Co. and now part of the Wolters Kluwer Company. This source is in loose-leaf format due to frequent updates. The introduction states that "*Drug Interaction Facts* attempts to present all drug-drug and drug-food interactions that have been reasonably well documented to occur in humans. Simple additive or antagonistic effects that are anticipated to occur based on known pharmacological activity are not necessarily included." This is considered an authoritative source due to its reliance on current biomedical literature and a review board of physicians, pharmacologists, and clinical pharmacists. The comprehensive index lists entries by generic drug name and drug class name, with frequent cross references for product trade names. The index also notes the severity of the drug-drug interaction using a numeric code. Each entry is around one page of information with the interaction significance listed first (i.e., the onset, severity, and interaction documentation), then the effects and mechanism and management, with brief discussion and references at the end. This source is relatively easy to use and seems to be widely accepted and consulted in most health sciences libraries.

Hansten and Horn's Drug Interactions: Analysis and Management is also published by Facts and Comparisons. This source has been in publication for over 30 years, and the authors, Philip D. Hansten and John R. Horn, have been recognized as experts in the field of drug interactions for years. *Hansten and Horn's* is updated quarterly and is available in loose-leaf binder format. The format for this source has been revised to focus on management options with the goal of prevention of patient harm. Thus, each drug entry has an easy to spot boxed section for Management Options. The index is the key to using this source. Drugs are alphabetically listed by generic name, and almost all interacting drugs listed under a specific drug have a number preceding them. This number is the code to interaction severity; for example, 1 = avoid combination, 3 = minimize risk, and 5 = no interaction. In addition to the highlighted Management Options, each entry includes a brief summary, risk factors, clinical evaluation, related drugs, and references. This source is very similar to *Drug Interactions Facts*. In many cases, the clinical evaluation section (called discussion section in *Drug Interactions Facts*) lists the same clinical trial or evidence, with the same references. There are some differences in the index entries. For example, there are 112 drug entries listed under Aspirin in *Drug Interactions Facts* while there are only 50 listed under *Hansten and Horn's*, though some entries are for the same pages or drug categories, not really unique compounds. Similarly, under grapefruit juice, *Drug Interactions Facts* lists 38 drugs while *Hansten and Horn's* has 41, though some had the code for "no interaction" next to them. In general, *Drug Interactions Facts* seems to have more references after each entry while *Hansten and Horn's* "Management Options" section seems a lot more helpful for clinicians and pharmacists with headings such as "consider alternative," "circumvent/minimize," and "monitor to help in advising patients."

Stockley's *Drug Interactions* is an excellent secondary source for the circulating collection of a pharmacy school, or large health sciences, library. It contains over 2,500 monographs that briefly describe the clinical evidence, mechanism, importance, and management of proven drug interactions. Many of these monograph entries have lengthy lists of references; very few have only one or two references. After an informative introduction, there is a full chapter on alcohol interactions. This chapter is alphabetically arranged by drug categories that have interactions with alcohol; for example, benzodiazepines, CNS depressants, tricyclic antidepressants, and so forth. The rest of the entries are arranged in broad categories (e.g., analgesics, anticoagulants, beta-blockers, contraceptive, immnosuppressants, and so forth) with the drugs that cause reactions in each category. This appears to be a valuable resource, but may not be for every collection.

International Drugs

Questions about foreign drugs often are particularly challenging. For example, spelling may vary in different languages. Users often have insufficient information, and the librarian begins a search looking for the proverbial needle in a haystack. Whenever possible, the requestor should be queried for further information: Do you have the generic or chemical name and the exact spelling? For what purpose is the drug used? Do you know the manufacturer? Several sources described earlier are very useful for foreign drug names. *Martindale: The Complete Drug Reference* (see 9.8, above) is extremely valuable for its wide coverage of European drugs and extensive indexing under trade names. The *USP dictionary of USAN and international drug names with INN, JAN, and BAN* is a good place to start if the patron knows the generic or USAN name. *The Merck Index* is useful because of its broad international coverage and its inclusion of many chemical, generic, and even trade names. The DRUGDEX system, available through the MICROMEDEX Healthcare Series of databases, (see 9.50, below) is an excellent source of international drug information, providing proprietary names used worldwide, for both FDA-approved and investigational drugs. Maintaining a collection to include every country would be impractical for most libraries, and key sources will depend on geographic location and ethnicity. In the United States, Canadian and Mexican sources are often particularly useful. The following three sources are helpful for international drug identification.

9.34 Swiss Pharmaceutical Society. *Index Nominum 2000: International Drug Directory*, 17th ed. Stuttgart, Germany: Medpharm Scientific Publishers, 2000.

9.35 *Compendium of Pharmaceuticals and Specialties: The Canadian Drug Reference for Health Professionals.* Toronto, Canada: Canadian Pharmacists Association, 2002.

9.36 *Diccionario de Especialidades Farmaceuticas*, 48th ed. Mexico: Thomson PLM, 2002.

The *Index Nominum 2000* is published in English with introductory information also provided in German and French. This resource describes over 5,000 drugs and drug derivatives, arranged in alphabetical order by INN in English. Each entry, or monograph, lists German, French, Spanish, and Latin names as well as the World Health Organization's ATC (Anatomical Therapeutic Chemical) code. Also included are therapeutic classifications, such as "calcium antagonist," CAS registry numbers, chemical names, molecular formulas, chemical structure diagrams, and lists of proprietary names used in different countries. At the end of each entry is an alphabetical list of drug derivatives (e.g., salts). The book starts with an alphabetical listing of therapeutic categories, a list of ATC classification codes, a list of abbreviations and symbols, and a list of country codes. Following the drug monographs is an extensive index of proprietary names and synonyms. This index is the primary access point for patrons seeking drug information with only a proprietary foreign name to go on.

The Canadian *Compendium of Pharmaceuticals and Specialties,* a guide available on the Canadian market, is divided into seven sections. The first section is a list of new and discontinued products, including brand names, generic names, manufacturers, drug classifications, and comments. Unlike many of the resources described in this chapter, this book lists drugs in alphabetical order by proprietary name. The second section provides a useful brand and generic name index. Next is a therapeutic guide listing drugs by therapeutic classification (e.g., antidepressants and diuretics). The fourth section is a product identification table with color photographs of drug products. The fifth section is a directory of Canadian poison control centers, health organizations, and pharmaceutical manufacturers. The "Clin-Info" section contains information for clinicians on selected topics, including dosing and monitoring tools, drug use guides and summaries of therapeutic interventions, and drug interactions. This is followed by information for patients, written in lay language, on the safe and effective use of drugs. The major part of the book is devoted to product monographs, listed in alphabetical order by brand name. This information is voluntarily submitted by manufacturers and may include either the complete or abridged versions of the drug package inserts. Each entry describes pharmacology, indications for use, contraindications and other precautions, drug interactions, adverse effects, and dosing information. Appendices contain supplemental information such as medical and pharmaceutical abbreviations, nomenclature for microorganisms, and new reports of adverse drug events. The sections of this book are color-coded for convenient access.

Written entirely in Spanish, the *Diccionario de Especialidades Farmaceuticas* is similar in organization to the Canadian Compendium and the *PDR*. It contains four color-coded indexes, starting with a list of drugs having known contraindications, followed by a therapeutic index of drugs organized by classification. The third section is an index of active ingredients, which provides product names of medicines containing the ingredient either alone or in combination with other active ingredients. Fourth is an index of drugs available in Mexico, listed by brand name with therapeutic classes, generic names, and manufacturers. This is followed by a directory of manufacturers with contact information and product listings. This resource also includes a product identification table, which can be very useful in border states where patients may use medications made in Mexico. The main section is the drug monographs with information provided by manufacturers.

Drug Information for Patients and the Public

With the proliferation of Internet Web sites claiming to offer consumers the best in health care information and even attempting to sell them health care products and drugs, it is hoped that some consumers may wish to consult authoritative sources for reliable information on medications and products they are taking. To this end, librarians need to have a basic collection of easy to understand authoritative drug information sources for the average consumer. Whether librarians collect sources for consumers or not, any information given to patients should be accompanied by encouragements to consult with health care professionals for help in interpreting and evaluating the information obtained.

9.37 *The PDR Family Guide to Prescription Drugs*, 9th ed. New York: Three Rivers Press, 2002.

9.38 Rybacki JJ. *The Essential Guide to Prescription Drugs*, 2003 ed. New York: HarperCollins, 2003.

9.39 Covington TR, ed. *Nonprescription Drug Therapy: Guiding Patient Self-Care.* St. Louis, MO: Facts and Comparisons, 2002.

9.40 Griffith WH. *Complete Guide to Prescription and Nonprescription Drugs.* New York: Berkeley Publishing Group, 1983–. Annual.

In addition to the above sources, the second volume of the *USP DI* that is entitled *Advice for the Patient: Drug Information in Lay Language* is an accepted authoritative source for consumer information. This source was described previously (see 9.16, above) and is more extensive and complete than the *PDR Family Guide to Prescription Drugs.* As a patient resource it is helpful because it includes a drug information photographic section, an extensive index in front, a glossary of terms, a listing of Poison Control Centers, drug categories of use, and a pregnancy precaution listing at the back.

To complement the standard *PDR,* librarians with collections that are accessed by consumers and patients may want to consider the *PDR Family Guide to Prescription Drugs.* The publisher's note states that the information in this source is based on drug labeling that was published in the *PDR* plus "supplemented with facts from other sources the publisher believes reliable." There is an extensive "How To Use This Book" section that would be helpful to consumers and a good drug identification guide with photographs of commonly prescribed pills. The entries are one to two pages for each product and they are alphabetically arranged by brand name and include a pronunciation guide, the generic name, and sections entitled "Why Is This Drug Prescribed," "Most Important Fact About This Drug," "How Should You Take This Medication," "What Side Effects May Occur," "Special Warnings About This Medication," "Possible Food And Drug Interactions When Taking This Medication," "Special Information if You Are Pregnant or Breastfeeding," and "Recommended Dosage and Over-Dosage." Each section is written in easy to understand terms for most consumers, and advice to consult with their physicians is included in the warnings sections. In addition to the general index that contains product names, treatments, and diseases, there is a disease and disorder index and a few short chapters at the end consisting of condition overviews such as high blood pressure, osteoporosis, birth control, skin problems, kidney disease, AIDS, and aging. Format and ease of use make up for the scope and content limitations in this source.

The Essential Guide to Prescription Drugs was authored by James W. Long from 1977 to 1993, by James W. Long and James J. Rybacki from 1996 to 2000, and most recently by James J. Rybacki for the 2002 and 2003 editions. This book has been considered a well-known and trusted source for drug information for patients for over 20 years. The 2003 edition contains helpful information in the introductions, the "Points for the Patient" contains advice on the importance of medication regimens (that each patient is unique and medications need to be tailored for each patient), steps to follow when getting prescription from physician, from pharmacist, and suggestions for containing the costs of drug therapy. Introductory information is not only for the patients, but also for pharmacists and physicians in separate "Points for the Pharmacist" and "Points for the Physician" sections. An extensive "How To Use This Book" section is followed by guidelines for safe and effective drug use and a brief section on "True Breakthroughs in Medicine" with short paragraphs on medical advances, such as the AMA & JCAHO Pain Initiative, the human genome, the leukemia pill, and the NIH cholesterol guidelines. The main section of the book is the drug profiles, with two to three pages of information in each drug entry. There are around 400 drugs, over 2,000 brand names, listed in the drug profiles section. Drug entries are alphabetically listed by generic name and in some instances by broad category; easy access is by using the detailed index in the back. Many drug entries have over 40 categories of information, including pronunciations, year introduced, class, brand names, availability as a generic drug, benefits versus risks, principle uses, dosage ranges, usual duration of use, reasons to inform physicians before taking the drug, possible side effects, possible adverse effects, cautions, suggested periodic examinations, and observations to make while taking a drug. This source is revised and updated annually and is worth adding to any consumer collection due to its patient-sympathetic approach.

Nonprescription Drug Therapy: Guiding Patient Self-Care is the first edition of what promises to be a popular title. This unique source was not written for the layperson. It was intended for health professionals, to help physicians and pharmacists guide patients in their use of over-the-counter medications, but the patient-related information and advice make this book a good candidate for a consumer-oriented collection. The book is divided into sections by categories of conditions or broad topics; for example, CNS conditions, GI/GU conditions, ophthalmic conditions, home diagnostics/devices, and complementary therapies. Each of these sections has from 7 to 20 specific disorders, devices, or therapies discussed. These discussions start with a brief definition and etiology, then a few paragraphs for incidence, pathophysiology, signs/symptoms, diagnostic parameters, and treatment. The treatment section contains tables listing medications, indications, warnings, and interactions, with many helpful listings of trade names and doses of these OTC products. Informative appendices include normal laboratory values, standard abbreviations, various home administration techniques, a large section of health-related and pharmaceutical company Web sites, and, last, a detailed index of conditions, products, and devices.

Winter H. Griffith is a popular author and public speaker. His books are frequently requested in libraries, and public libraries tend to carry most of his works. His *Complete Guide to Prescription and Nonprescription Drugs* is revised annually and is described in Bowker's *Global Books in Print* as "The latest edition of the best selling reference book providing information on over 5,000 brand name drugs & over 700 generic name drugs."

Herbal Medicines and Natural Products

In these days of increased interest and usage of herbal and natural preparations, a few authoritative sources are a must. Browsing libraries for such sources in the pharmacy and pharmacology sections is not sufficient. Many of these sources are located in the complementary medicine area, so browsing both areas and consulting with large institutions for a balance in collection emphasis is recommended.

9.41 *PDR for Herbal Medicines*, 2nd ed. Montvale, NJ: Medical Economics Co., Inc., 2000.

9.42 *Herbal Companion to AHFS DI*. Bethesda, MD: American Society of Health-System Pharmacists, Inc., 2000.

9.43 *Natural Medicines Comprehensive Database*, 4th ed., Stockton, CA: Therapeutic Research Faculty, 2002. Available: www.naturaldatabase.com.

9.44 Duke JA. *Handbook of Medicinal Herbs*, 2nd ed. Boca Raton, FL: CRC Press, 2002.

9.45 DerMarderosian A. *A Guide to Popular Natural Products*, 2nd ed. St. Louis, MO: Facts and Comparisons, 2001.

As with other *PDR* publications, the *PDR for Herbal Medicines* has several helpful indexes in the front of the book. After the informative foreword, there is an in-depth alphabetical index of all the scientific, common, and brand names included in this source. There are also indexes for therapeutic categories, indications, homeopathic indications, Asian indications (to help in locating Asian botanicals used for a particular diagnosis), side effects, manufacturers, and a drug/herb interactions guide, safety guide, and a manufacturers index. There is also an extensive herb identification guide with color photographs of over 380 common medicinal plants, followed by a very brief product identification guide with only three pages of product photographs. The herbal entries include common name, genus and species, description, actions and pharmacology, indications and usage, precautions and adverse reactions, dosage, and references. While not too current or comprehensive, the *PDR for Herbal Medicines* is still a good addition to most collections.

Several herbal medicine sources state in their introductions that they base their information on the *Complete German Commission E Monographs*, which were developed by the German Federal Institute for Drugs and Medicinal Devices; Germany's equivalent to the U.S. Food and Drug Administration. The introduction to the *Herbal*

189

Companion to AHFS DI describes the German commission and states that the "accuracy of the information available within the Commission E Monographs creates a benchmark for the safety and efficacy of phytomedicine, and the monographs are regarded as *the* authoritative compendium on therapeutic medicinal herbs for healthcare professionals, representing today's highest standard in phytomedical evaluation." The *Herbal Companion to AHFS DI* is getting its information indirectly from the *German Commission E Monographs* as this publication is derived from the Integrative Medicine Communications' database, which is based on an English translation of the Commission E Monographs. The *Herbal Companion to AHFS DI* strives to offer unbiased, scientific, reference information for clinicians to assist them in integrating complementary medicine into their patients' care. A disclaimer at the beginning of this book notes that the content was not developed by the American Society of Health-Systems Pharmacists, but rather the Integrative Medicine Commission (IMC) is responsible, and that all inquires should be directed to the IMC. An Advisory Board consisting of physicians, naturopaths, pharmacists, ayurvedics, herbalists, and osteopaths was consulted. This is not a very large source, under 200 pages, but the entries are well written and organized. Each entry contains the English, botanical, and family names of the product, an overview section, usage and pharmaceutical designations, medicinal uses/indications, recommended dosage, cautions, interactions, regulatory status, and references. There are no illustrations or photographs and a brief index at the end is the only other information in this source.

The publication *Natural Medicines Comprehensive Database* is a book version of their electronic product available on the Web. The online source will be discussed further in the section on "Indexing and Abstracting Databases and Electronic Resources" (see 9.52, below). This book claims that it is recognized as "the scientific gold standard for evidence-based information on this topic." There are over 1,000 herbal and nonherbal natural products listed in this source. The products are alphabetically arranged by their most common name, with an index at the end to help provide cross references from other names. Each entry starts with a section labeled "Also Known As" to include other names and synonyms for the herbs plus scientific names; usage; safety; effectiveness; mechanism of action; adverse reactions; interactions with herbs, dietary supplements, drugs, foods, and lab tests; dosage; and comments. All references cited in various paragraphs appear at the end of the entries, arranged in numerical order by citation number. Included is a section on brand name natural products and the ingredients they contain. There are notes in several sections of the book stating that the online database contains more current and extensive information. A source worth considering if the online version's cost is prohibitive.

James A. Duke is a botanist, retired from the U.S. Department of Agriculture, and currently teaches a master's degree course in botanical healing. The first edition of this book was entitled *CRC Handbook of Medicinal Herbs,* and it was published in 1985. In the introduction, the author states that he has tried to cover most of the widely mentioned medicinal plants, including over 1,000 of the most important herbs. He also states that "Unlike Commission E and the Herbal PDR, which seem to stress European and American traditions, I include proportionately more herbs from the older African, Ayurvedic, and Chinese traditions as well, not wanting to slight any major medicinal plant from any major tradition." The herbs are listed in alphabetical order with a scientific name index and a common name index at the end of the book. Each herb entry lists the scientific name in parentheses after the common name, then a safety rating system (the safety score is explained in the introduction). Many entries include an illustration of the plant, and there are some color plates in the center of the book. The entry descriptions include many abbreviations, some of which are listed in the abbreviations section in the beginning and others in the introduction. The entries include synonyms, activities, indications, dosages, contraindications, interactions, and side effects. This source is very comprehensive and extensive, but not that easy to interpret due to the abundance of abbreviations in the descriptions.

The editor of *A Guide to Popular Natural Products* is a professor of pharmacognosy and medicinal chemistry. In his editorial work, he is assisted by an Advisory Panel and the Facts and Comparisons Editorial Advisory Panel, both of which comprise a considerable number of notable physicians, chemists, and pharmacists. This authoritative source is well written and organized for easy access to patient information and references to the literature. There are several color photographs of the herbs in the center of the book and many helpful appendices including a lengthy table of herb-drug interactions and herbal diuretics. There is a therapeutic index and primary index listing common names and scientific names. Each entry includes scientific names, common names, and a highlighted box with patient information. Following that are descriptive sections on botany, history, pharmacology, toxicology, and references. The key information is in the patient information box, which lists uses, side effects, and drug interactions when applicable. The references at the end of each entry are mainly from standard authoritative books and peer-reviewed journal articles.

Indexing and Abstracting Services and Electronic Resources

This section will focus on indexing and abstracting services, online databases, and other electronic resources, such as Internet Web sites, that are specific to drug information or that contain considerable drug information sections. For more general indexing services and sources and in-depth descriptions, please refer to Chapter 4.

Most of the databases mentioned below are available through the World Wide Web. As with all resources, licensing costs vary, and different vendors' search interfaces can also vary considerably, so librarians should be careful in selecting the most appropriate, cost-effective resource possible. Almost all vendors will allow testing of their products; requesting test accounts and inviting colleagues and users to test the systems before deciding on which to subscribe to always helps in decision making. Most libraries are noticing significant drops in the number of patrons coming in through their doors, and they are shifting their collections from mainly print-based resources to electronic resources that can be accessed remotely to respond to user needs. Thus, users are becoming more self-reliant. Selecting user-friendly search interfaces is essential for any successful collection.

The National Library of Medicine's *MeSH* (*Medical Subject Headings*) (see Chapter 4) has shown a dramatic increase in its inclusion of drug names since its inception. Earliest editions relied heavily on classes of chemical compounds. Each year, however, many drug names have been added, and today close to 40 percent of total *MeSH* descriptors belong in the "Chemicals and Drugs" section. *MeSH* entries for drugs are generic names. In a few cases, when the trade name is very common, there is a cross reference from the trade name to the generic *MeSH* term. Therefore, for the user of *Index Medicus*, tools such as the *American Drug Index* or *USAN and the USP Dictionary of Drug Names* may often be needed to convert a trade name to a generic name. Sometimes the drug name may be a minor descriptor; thus, to find information in the printed *Index Medicus*, it will be necessary to use a broader name representing a class of drugs. Because drug names have been added so frequently to *MeSH*, the user must often pay special attention to entry dates and history notes for *MeSH* terms. Often, it is useful to determine when a drug became an official USAN (or INN, if it is a foreign drug). This will give an indication of a realistic time period for a search. For example, nizatidine, an antiulcerative agent, became a USAN in 1983 and a provisional *MeSH* descriptor in 1992. To search *Index Medicus* prior to 1992, one would look under the heading "THIAZOLES" because the term nizatidine is only a provisional heading. Because other thiazoles are indexed in the same place, it would be necessary to scan for article titles that mention nizatidine or its trade name, Axid. For a MEDLINE search using subject terms (i.e., limited to *MeSH*), "NIZATIDINE" will suffice back through 1985; but for previous years, especially before 1983, when the USAN was approved, the search would have to include nizatidine as a textword, the trade name, other synonyms, and research code names. For the years before a drug is officially named, *Biological Abstracts* (see Chapter 4) and *Chemical Abstracts* or their electronic counterparts may be more useful sources.

In other cases, information may be needed about the drug therapy of a specific disease or chemicals causing a disease. In those cases, the subheadings "drug therapy" and "chemically induced" are especially useful in searching both the *Index Medicus* and MEDLINE. The librarian should be familiar with the many subheadings that would help refine and focus searches; for example, using adverse effects, poisoning, and toxicity for the untoward effects of a chemical or drug.

9.46 *ToxNet.* Besthesda, MD: National Library of Medicine. Available: http://toxnet.nlm.nih.gov.

9.47 *Registry of Toxic Effects of Chemical Substances (RTECS).* San Leandro, CA: MDL Information Systems. Available: www.cdc.gov/niosh/rtecs.html.

9.48 *International Pharmaceutical Abstracts (IPA).* Bethesda, MD: American Society of Health-System Pharmacists.

9.49 *Clinical Pharmacology.* Tampa, FL: Gold Standard Multimedia. Available: http://cp.gsm.com.

9.50 *MICROMEDEX.* Greenwood Village, CO: Thomson MICROMEDEX. Available: www.micromedex.com/products.

9.51 *Chemical Abstracts.* Columbus, OH: Chemical Abstracts Service. Available: www.cas.org.

9.52 *Natural Medicines Comprehensive Database.* Stockton, CA: Therapeutic Research Faculty. Available: www.naturaldatabase.com.

The National Library of Medicine produces ToxNet, a set of databases with information on toxicology, hazardous chemicals, and environmental health. These databases are freely available worldwide on the Web. Three categories of information are available: toxicology databanks on toxicity and additional hazards of chemicals toxicology literature, including scientific studies, reports, and other bibliographic material; toxic release information; and chemical information, with nomenclature, identification, and structures. The toxicology databanks include the Hazardous Substances Data Bank (HSDB), Integrated Risk Information System (IRIS), Chemical Carcinogenesis Research Information System (CCRIS), and GENE-TOX. The HSDB contains emergency handling procedures, human health effects, detection methods, OSHA standards, and other regulatory requirements for over 4,500 potentially harmful chemicals. Records are divided into categories including human health effects, emergency medical treatment, pharmacokinetics, and many others. This enables users to navigate quickly to specific topics. IRIS provides information from the EPA about the potential health effects of environmental pollutants, including carcinogenic and noncarcinogenic health risk information for over 500 chemicals. The CCRIS contains scientifically evaluated data from the National Cancer Institute (NCI) on carcinogenicity, mutagenicity, and tumor promotion and tumor inhibition tests for over 8,000 chemicals. GENE-TOX contains information from the EPA on over 3,000 chemicals with genotoxic potential. The literature databases include Toxline and the Developmental and Reproductive Toxicology and Environmental Teratology Information Center (DART/ETIC.) Toxline is a collection of more than 3 million bibliographic citations on drugs and other chemicals and is included in MEDLINE/PubMed as the subset, "Toxicology." The DART/ETIC covers teratology and other aspects of developmental and reproductive toxicology. It contains over 90,000 references to literature published since 1965. The Toxics Release Inventory (TRI) database provides annual estimates of toxic chemicals released to the environment. The database is searchable by chemical name, company name, or geographic region (including zip code.) ChemIDplus contains over 350,000 chemical records, of which over 114,000 include chemical structures, and is searchable by subject, chemical generic or proprietary name, CAS registry number, molecular formula, and structure. Users may search all ToxNet databases simultaneously or select individual sources.

The Registry of Toxic Effects of Chemical Substances (RTECS) emphasizes acute and chronic effects of potentially toxic chemicals. Once a part of ToxNet, RTECS was produced by NIOSH and is currently maintained by MDL Information Systems. Data on skin/eye irritation, carcinogenicity, mutagenicity, and reproductive toxicity as well as federal regulations are presented. References are available for all data. Information on availability and vendors for RTECS can be found online.

International Pharmaceutical Abstracts (IPA) is produced in print and electronic versions by the American Society of Health-System Pharmacists and covers a substantial volume of worldwide pharmacy practice literature not indexed in MEDLINE. *IPA* covers meeting abstracts of the American Society of Health-System Pharmacists

(ASHP), the Federation of International Pharmacists (FIP), and the American Association of Colleges of Pharmacy (AACP). Journals unique to *IPA* include state journals of Health System Pharmacy; natural products and alternative medicine journals such as *Integrative Cancer Therapies, Journal of Herbal Pharmacotherapy, Journal of Herbs, Spices and Medicinal Plants*; and others, like the *International Journal of Drug Policy, Journal of Pain and Palliative Care Pharmacotherapy*, and *World Health Organization Drug Information*. In addition to the typical searchable fields found in electronic bibliographic databases, *IPA* can be searched by CAS registry numbers or AHFS therapeutic drug classification. The latter is especially useful for accessing information on entire families of drugs. For example, a search of "4.00" in the therapeutic classification field retrieves articles on antihistamines. Boolean searching is also available. *IPA* is a useful supplement to MEDLINE for any library supporting pharmacy education or practice.

An excellent source of authoritative, full-text drug information is the Clinical Pharmacology database produced by Gold Standard Multimedia. Information on prescription, over-the-counter, herbal, new, and investigational drugs can be found using either generic or proprietary names. Upon entering a drug name, the system retrieves an alphabetical list of drug names and formulations from which the user can select specific products. For a given product, the user can access a broad range of information through links to a variety of sources. The Drug Information section includes monographs similar to the print sources described in this chapter, with lists of alternative names and discussions of indications, dosages, adverse effects, drug interactions, product photographs, manufacturing information, and costs. Retrieved drug monographs present highlighted keywords in context. Clinical Pharmacology also contains several useful tools for identifying and comparing drugs. The Product ID tool allows the searcher to enter any number of ingredients to build comparison tables of available drugs containing the ingredients. For example, a user could find a list of all drugs containing acetaminophen and pseudoephedrine, but no alcohol. The Clinical Reports tool generates summaries of known interactions, adverse effects, or intravenous (IV) compatibility for combinations of drugs. Patient information is available in English and Spanish.

Convenient links provide navigation between these tools from all sections of the database.

A costly but very useful resource is the MICROMEDEX suite of databases, which offers a variety of environmental health, toxicology, and drug information through its Corporate Solutions series and Healthcare series. It includes full-text electronic books such as *Martindale*, the *USP DI*, and the *PDR*, as well as sets of drug monographs, product lists, dosing calculators, drug interactions, alternative medicine, and information for patients. The drug interactions (DrugReax) tool is particularly useful, allowing the user to build a profile, adding drugs to the profile, and displaying drug interactions. MICROMEDEX resources can be purchased in various combinations or as a complete set. Examples of available resources include:

- AltMedDex (peer-reviewed information on herbal and other dietary supplements)
- DrugDex (evaluative and comparative drug information for the health care professional including investigational, non-prescription, and international drugs)
- DiseaseDex (evidence-based disease information for general and emergency medicine)
- Poisindex (product identification and toxicological information on over 1 million drugs and chemicals)
- Reprorisk (reproductive risk information for males, females, and unborn children, including the full text of Shepard's *Catalog of Teratogenic Agents*)

This system has the capability to search across all databases, by specific database, or by category. Categories include adverse reactions, contraindications, teratogenicity, treatment, and others. Search results are organized by category; each category is further divided into subcategories and grouped into sets retrieved from each resource. Each link leads to a more specific, narrower category while indicating the hierarchical path. Links are provided to return to search results, a new search, or the main menu. Links to product information are also provided if there are products associated with the search term. Considering the depth of information contained in this system, navigation is relatively simple due to the hierarchical organization.

Chemical Abstracts is also a useful source of information. Many of the biochemistry sections (e.g., pharmacodynamics, hormone pharmacology, toxicology, biochemical interactions) include drug information material. In the macromolecular chemistry sections, there are two of interest: pharmaceuticals and pharmaceuticals analysis. Many of the sections relating to industrial chemistry include references to occupational hazards. When searching *Chemical Abstracts* for a particular drug, the *Index Guide* should be consulted to find the correct index term. Specific chemicals are included in the chemical substance index. Ribavirin, for example, is indexed under 1H-1, 2, 4-triazole-3-carboxamide, -1-B-D-ribofuranosyl-. Classes of chemicals and other concepts, such as "antibiotics" and "brain neoplasms," are indexed in the general subject index. Because of its great breadth, *Chemical Abstracts* is often used to locate citations not indexed elsewhere. Patents describing the manufacture of a specific drug fall into this category. Although the emphasis is not primarily on clinical medicine, extensive research material is included, and there is substantial coverage of drugs in research. When using *Chemical Abstracts* as an electronic database, the CAS registry number for the compound may provide one of the most efficient ways of searching a drug with multiple names. SciFinder Scholar is an easy to search interface for *Chemical Abstracts* and is licensed by many large institutions for users to do their own chemical, structure, and patent searching.

Natural Medicines Comprehensive Database is available on the Web. It is more current, interactive, and comprehensive than the print product discussed in the "Herbal Medicines" section, above. The Web site allows free access to some general information, descriptions of content, and a sample record. The producers describe their site by stating: "This extremely comprehensive site is designed for medical professionals. We update this Database every business day. We analyze every important new study in this subject area, and add pertinent details to this Database. Thousands of Physicians, Pharmacists, Nurse Practitioners, PAs, Dietitians, hospitals, pharmacies, medical libraries, and clinics rely on this Database to answer their questions about natural medicines." They also have a separate Web site for patients that can be licensed separately. The patient version can search for any natural product by brand name, by ingredients, or by scientific names. In addition, there is a browsing feature so consumers can look for a product even if they do not know exactly how to spell it. The producers have a feature that enables branding locally by adding an organization's name and logo on each page. The sample record listed scientific names, a "people use this for" section, safety, effectiveness, mechanisms of actions, adverse reactions, and interactions with herbs, supplements, and drugs. This site is worth considering due to comprehensiveness and relative low cost.

These days, electronic versions of standard print sources are proliferating. These electronic resources are not just CD-ROM versions of books, databases, or Web sites of information, but also interactive online counterparts to such standard sources as the *PDR* and the *AHFS*. Since these sources abound, a comprehensive list of all of them would be out of date the minute it is written. Table 9-1 will attempt to list several of the major, more reputable, and stable Web sites and electronic resources available at this writing.

Drug Information Services

More than 100 medical centers in the United States have drug information services operated by pharmacists. They provide specialized consultation on a variety of questions related to patient care. Topics may include drug identification, prescribing, prevention and management of adverse effects, and drug interactions. Drug information services have access to specialized resources often found only in medical libraries, and pharmacists will often analyze literature and provide expert advice where conflicting information exists. It is difficult, however, to make general observations because services vary from place to place. Some may offer services only to medical and nursing staffs whereas others may extend their services to the community. Fees for service also vary. The International Drug Information Center at the Arnold and Marie Schwartz College of Pharmacy and Health Sciences, Long Island University, has published directories of drug information centers [2] since 1974. These authors periodically conduct surveys to obtain names and addresses of centers, hours of operation, and contact information. Directories are alphabetically organized by state. The most recent article cites previous articles so that updates can be found through a citation search. Librarians should be aware of nearby drug information centers and make efforts to build relationships with staff and collaborate on delivering the best possible services to users.

Table 9-1. Electronic Drug Information Resources

Resource & URL	Content	Evaluation
AHFSfirstWEB Available: www.ashp.org/ ahfs/web	Information on over 110,000 drugs and herbal products. Brings together *AHFS Drug Information* with the product summaries created by First Databank's *National Drug Data File.* Includes bibliographies and references.	Promoted heavily to pharmacy schools to help with "patient concerns." Offers the ability to create, link, and document patient records. Pricey, cost depends on institution size
Alternative Medicine Available: http://advocacynet .com/altmedicine mks.htm	4,500 links to websites on alternative and complementary medicine.	Contains advertising, huge site, gives the user an idea of the scope of information on the Internet on this topic. Free.
CenterWatch: FDA Drug Approvals Available: www.centerwatch .com	CenterWatch is a clinical trials listing service. Contains drugs in clinical trials database and drug directories for patients.	Searchable, helpful information. Subscription required for some parts, considerable amount of information available free.

Table 9.1 *continued*

Resource & URL	Content	Evaluation
Drug Info Net Available: www.druginfonet .com	Geared toward patients. Has links to hospitals, medical schools, drug manufacturers, health news, disease & drug information. Package insert information on pharmaceuticals for both health professionals and consumers provided by manufacturers and approved by U.S. FDA.	Drugs are searchable by generic name, proprietary name, therapeutic class, or manufacturer. Not as comprehensive in scope as *PDR*, also not guaranteed to have complete package info. Free, contains advertising.
Efacts Available: www.factsand comparisons.com	Produced by Facts & Comparisons, a searchable web interface to *Drug Facts & Comparisons*, *Drug Interactions Facts*, *Review of Natural Products*, and *MedFacts: Patient Information*.	Site includes brief headline and drug news items. Pricing varies, some parts free.
ePocrates Rx Available: www.epocrates.com	For handheld devices (PDAs), listing of over 2,800 drugs. Usage, administration, adverse effects, cautions, and indications included.	Popular resource for physicians and pharmacists. Updateable information in portable format with alerts and notes capabilities. Standard version available free.

Table 9.1 *continued*

Resource & URL	Content	Evaluation
FDA Web site Available: www.FDA.gov.	Information on drug safety/side effects, clinical trials, a list of all FDA approved drugs (since 1996), and searchable database of National Drug Codes. Includes searchable Approved Drug Products with Therapeutic Equivalence Evaluations/Orange Book.	Excellent site with a lot of essential relevant information. Very handy to have access to the Orange Book, which lists all FDA-approved prescription drugs, including new and generic drugs. Plus, provides therapeutic equivalence values. Free.
MedicineNet Available: www.medicinenet .com	Provided by MedicineNet, Inc. and produced by a network of board certified physicians and allied health care professionals. Provides information for patients on diseases, medications, and tests. Also has a dictionary of medical terms.	Claims to be "100% Doctor Produced." Has interesting "featured conditions" section. Medications section written in lay terms, good for patient referrals. Requires subscription, with some parts free. Contains advertising.
Medi-Lexicon Available: www.pharma -lexicon.com	A searchable dictionary of acronyms and abbreviations, plus directories of professional pharmaceutical associations, schools of pharmacy, pharmacy information services, and consultants.	Produced by Pharma-Lexicon International, based in Hastings, East Sussex, U.K. Easy to search, with several search categories. Free, with advanced search options available for a small fee.

Table 9.1 *continued*

Resource & URL	Content	Evaluation
PharmWeb Available: www.pharmweb.net	Collaborative effort of several international professional organizations, managed and operated by pharmacists and medical communications specialists. Links to authoritative information, topics such as alternative medicine, patient information, and treatment guides.	Information provided is easily accessible through the site index. Good resource for professional directories and discussion lists. Helpful patient "How to use medicines" section. Free.
Pharmacyone-source.com Available: www.pharmacy onesource.com	Drug information database produced by Multum, Inc., a reputable drug information provider. Drug searches provide navigation through therapeutic drug classes. In addition, it has news, drug alerts, employment, and other information.	It has an excellent drug information database with product names, drug interactions, adverse effects, dosing info, and allergic reactions. Has the capability to launch MEDLINE searches, as well as search the FDA Orange Book, directly from drug search results. Users must subscribe, but subscription is free.
Regsource.com Available: http://regsource .com	U.S., Canadian, and European site dedicated to regulatory information. Contains full text of *The Merck Manual*, FDA Orange Book, searchable extensive reference section.	Great source for regulatory information. Extensive comprehensive site with links to *Federal Register* and all major regulatory sites worldwide. Free, contains advertising.

Table 9.1 *continued*

Resource & URL	Content	Evaluation
SafeMedication.com Available: www.safemedication.com	Drug news, patient information and a searchable database (Medmaster) based on *ASHP's Medication Teaching Manual: The Guide to Patient Drug Information*, a publication developed for use in patient education on side effects, precautions, and more.	Authoritative source geared to consumers, developed by the American Society of Health System Pharmacists (ASHP).
STAT!Ref Available: www.statref.com.	Collection of searchable full-text medical and drug information textbooks for health care professionals.	STAT!Ref is available online, web interface, or on CD-ROM and most recently for PDAs. Can search individual textbooks, such as *USP DI*, or the whole collection. Price depends on institution size and number of books selected.
U.S. Pharmacopoeia Available: www.usp.org.	Drug information, standards, dietary supplements, veterinary medicine, and products from the *USP DI*.	Authoritative source, helpful information including conference calendar and "e-newsroom" for searchable press releases. Some sections free, pricey subscription for full *USP/NF*.

Table 9.1 *continued*

Resource & URL	Content	Evaluation
WebMD Available: www.webmd.com.	The WebMD Drug and Herb Directory, provided by Multum, contains comprehensive information on prescription drugs, over-the-counter medications, and the most popular herbal remedies.	Helpful sections in the "Drugs and Herbs" section include drug alerts, product recalls, and FAQs. Searchable drug database with extensive descriptions. Free, contains advertising.

References

1. Guarino RA, ed. *New drug approval process: the global challenge*, 3rd ed. New York: Marcel Dekker, Inc., 2000. (Drugs and the Pharmaceutical Sciences, vol. 100).
2. Rosenberg JM, Natan JP, Cicero LA. Pharmacist-operated drug information centers in the United States: A directory of centers that meet listed criteria—1999. *Hosp Pharm* 1999; 34(7):797–810.

Readings

1. Hunter TS, ed. *E-Pharmacy: a guide to the Internet care zone.* Washington, DC: American Pharmaceutical Association, 2002.
2. Keely JL. Pharmacist scope of practice. *Ann Intern Med* 2002 Jan. 1; 136(1):79–85.
3. Koo MM, Krass I, Aslani P. Factors influencing consumer use of written drug information. *Ann Pharmacother* 2003 Feb.; 37(2):259–67.
4. Uhl K, Kennedy DL, Kweder SL. Accurate information on drug effects on pregnancy is crucial. *Am Fam Physician* 2003 Feb. 15; 67(4):700–1.
5. Vogt EM. Effective communication of drug safety information to patients and the public: a new look. *Drug Saf* 2002; 25(5):313–21.

CHAPTER 10

CONSUMER HEALTH SOURCES

Mary L. Gillaspy

Overview of the Consumer Health Phenomenon

Individuals have always sought information about their health. From ancient times, shamans and other healers within cultures have provided treatments of varying efficacy to relieve disease and suffering, and the recipients of this traditional (or folk) medicine have welcomed their interventions or, at least, accepted them in the absence of any better alternative. Patients in every age have also talked with others who have shared the same or a similar experience and sought their counsel and support.

In the 1990s, the confluence of a two-decade-old fitness trend, the emergence of managed care, an aging and well-educated populace, and easy access to the Internet via the World Wide Web inspired a consumer revolution in health care. No longer willing to be passive bystanders, twenty-first-century health consumers demand active partnerships with their providers, second opinions, information about treatment options (including integrative therapies), and education so that they can better understand and manage their own health. A survey conducted in 2000 revealed that 52 million adults in the United States, equating to 55 percent of those with Internet access at that time, had used the World Wide

Web to look for health information [1]. By late 2001, when a follow-up survey was conducted, that number had jumped to 73 million [2].

Unfortunately, this trend in demand for information and education has coincided with a trend toward less physician time available per patient visit. In fact, between 1943 and 1985, the average patient visit to a physician fell from 26 minutes to 17 minutes [3]. One survey even reported that half of patients left their physicians' offices not understanding what they were told or knowing what to do to alleviate their condition [4]. Poor literacy (by some estimates, approximately one-fourth of the U.S. population is deemed functionally illiterate) undoubtedly contributes to this phenomenon [5] and is exacerbated by provider lack of time for explaining diagnoses and therapies and testing understanding of what has been communicated.

Enter the "new kid on the block" of medical libraries: consumer health information services. Although a few such services have existed for decades, hospitals, clinics, and academic health sciences centers have only quite recently begun offering reference services to the public. Today, partnerships exist between many public libraries, which have traditionally received many health information requests, and local medical libraries.

What Makes Consumer Health Information Different from Traditional Medical Reference?

Providing health information to lay people differs considerably from traditional medical reference. First, though the information may be delivered in a hospital or academic health sciences library setting, the venue may also be a storefront, public library, or community-based organization. Personnel providing the information may also be different from those in traditional settings. Most important of all, the information needs and information-seeking behaviors of a health consumer are radically different from those of a physician, researcher, nurse, or allied health professional.

Venues for Dissemination of Consumer Health Information

Consumer health information (CHI) is provided in both formal and informal settings. Informal settings include person-to-person contact, support groups, online moderated discussion lists, chat rooms, and similar venues. Discussion in this chapter will be limited to formal situations, particularly those that occur in a hospital, a public library, or an academic health sciences library that provides a special area and collection for members of the public. Libraries in community-based organizations, clinics, or storefronts may also find the references that follow are useful when making purchases.

Obviously, the venue affects the resources that are required to respond appropriately to the information needs of health care consumers. For example, some settings may offer a computer terminal, or special software, with or without personal assistance. Others may set aside a room or a corner dedicated to serving patients, families, and the general public. Still other settings may dedicate an entire facility to serving only or primarily health care consumers. The resources that are selected will vary by venue. Whether they include only print, only computer access, or a combination of the two, the information included in this chapter will help library and education professionals have references on hand that will meet many of the health information needs of consumers.

Personnel in Consumer Health Library Settings

Given the unique information needs of the lay public, information professionals play a very different role in CHI settings from the typical ones found in libraries that serve only health professionals. Their role is at least as much that of educator as of health information professional, and sometimes it is mainly educator. Health care consumers often want to discuss the information they are receiving and may require considerable assistance in locating and then understanding what they have found.

Whether the consumer health information service is located in a storefront, in a community-based organization, in an academic medical center, or in a hospital, only one medical librarian, if that, is generally available. Many of these services are operated without any information professional at all; rather, health educators, nurse educators, or other groups establish, operate, and maintain the center. In such situations, a medical librarian or staff of a nearby medical library may provide consultation services. Ideally, consumer health information services are staffed by a multidisciplinary team, the members of which may be full-time, part-time, or a combination of these. A combination of a librarian, health educator, and volunteers from varied professional backgrounds can make for a powerful team.

Volunteers are ubiquitous in these settings and generally perform useful, even essential, work for the center. From answering the telephone, to assisting with technical service tasks, to sorting mail and creating information packets, to independent projects, to helping customers directly, volunteers enhance the services that consumer health information services provide. Their training should be developed and overseen by a coordinator of volunteers, who can also act as the primary contact and screener for the program.

Volunteers who meet customers should be trained to meet and greet customers and to triage requests beyond their training to the staff on duty. When volunteers are provided with a finite group of reference resources, with clear instructions regarding when to use the tools, they can handle a great deal of the reference business. The models below can be used as a training tool for both volunteers and new, nonlibrarian staff.

Table 10-1 contains resources with which all staff are required to be familiar. These are the resources that should be exhausted first before moving on to alternatives.

Table 10-1. Baseline Resources

Order of Use	Resources
Consult first	Locally produced or approved patient education resources; locally approved database for pharmaceutical information.
Consult second	MEDLINEplus (see 10.51), Gale encyclopedias, medical dictionaries
For cancer	Cancer.gov (see 10.52), *Gale Encyclopedia of Cancer* (see 10.24), *Everyone's Guide to Cancer Therapy* (see 10.81), *Informed Decisions* (see 10.82)
Media	Locally held audiovisual resources

Table 10-2 contains more advanced references that require significantly more training time for staff. Moreover, before using these resources, staff are expected to conduct a reference interview to determine the exact information need and the level of information required to satisfy the need.

Table 10-2. Advanced Baseline Resources

Order of Use	Resources
Consult as needed	Local online public access catalog (OPAC)
Consult as indicated	Merck manuals online, Lange handbooks, *Krause's Food, Nutrition*, and *Diet Therapy* (see 10.62), *Cecil's Textbook of Medicine* (see 10.48), *Harrison's Principles of Internal Medicine* (see 10.47), *Therapeutic Guide to Herbal Medicines* (see 10.65)

Local resources will determine placement of items in these two tiers as well as resources beyond the ones indicated. For example, if the library purchases a consumer health database or electronic journals or has built a Web site with locally approved materials, these will need to be added in as nonprofessional staff increase their understanding of consumer health, their mastery of the reference interview, and their general level of comfort with the setting and the services that are provided within it.

Information Needs of Health Care Consumers

While clinicians and researchers exhibit somewhat predictable information needs, the same cannot be said for the health care consumer. Arguably, their needs are often more difficult to meet because they frequently are unsure of how to frame their questions and may be distraught from the gravity of a diagnosis, sudden financial stress, grief, or other stressors associated with negotiating the health care system. The responsibility lies with the information professional to 1) select and make available the best resources, 2) assess the consumer's level of need and willingness to learn, and 3) stage the information correctly so that the person can learn incrementally and move

211

as far along a continuum of health information need as he or she wishes, using resources appropriate to the individual's learning style. Literacy level must also be determined and taken into account when providing health information to consumers, especially that found on the Internet through the use of search engines, much of which is written at a tenth-grade level or higher [6].

Successful librarians possess finely honed interpersonal skills, and in no field are these skills more important than in consumer health. Providing health information to the public has in the past been the jealously guarded purview of physicians and nurses. This situation has begun to change, but the first and most important thing that any librarian working in consumer health in a hospital, clinic, or academic medical center must do is gain the trust of the providers in the institution. Once that hurdle has been overcome, providers are grateful for the support of a well-run consumer health information center because they no longer have the time to meet the increasing health information needs of their patients. Trust and respect for the librarian, other staff, and volunteers must be earned and carefully nurtured with all providers for the consumer health library program to prosper.

General Reference Sources for Consumer Health Information

With many excellent resources available, at different reading and usability levels, the lists below contain a variety of references, not all of which are essential except in comprehensive collections. Repetition exists among some of the resources listed in the remainder of this chapter and works covered in other parts of this book. This duplication is necessary for two reasons. First, some readers may turn to this reference and use only selected chapters. In that case, the duplication reinforces that some references are so important that they transcend the boundaries, which are artificial at best, between "professional" and "lay" literature. Second, a range of resources is essential for answering the often complicated questions that health care consumers bring to libraries and learning centers. Because people come to consumer health information venues at all levels of literacy and prior knowledge, resources that address the breadth of these needs should ideally be provided. References can be divided into the following general categories: 1) those written specifically for laypeople, including low-literacy materials; 2) midlevel resources, which encompasses works written for professionals in text that is approachable for an educated consumer or one who requires more depth of information than lay references typically provide; and 3) technical or advanced materials, like medical textbooks. The best consumer health libraries feature an array of resources (information in varied formats) at an array of levels so that the largest number of queries can be satisfied.

Guides to the Literature

10.1 Barclay DA, Halsted DD. *Consumer Health Reference Service Handbook.* New York: Neal-Schuman, 2001.

Besides providing information about how to start a reference service for consumers, this book also includes a section on common health concerns of consumers, recommended consumer health Web sites, and key print resources for collections.

10.2 Rees AM. *Consumer Health Information Source Book.* 7th ed. Westport, CN: Greenwood Publishing Group, 2003.

Now in its seventh edition, this guide has long been the most important work available for assessing and reporting the best materials available for consumer health. Recent editions have added electronic resources and Spanish language materials; the seventh edition continues this tradition and has added a chapter about consumer health libraries in North America which are models for excellence.

10.3 *Consumer and Patient Health Information Section (CAPHIS) of the Medical Library Association.* Chicago, IL: CAPHIS. Available: http://caphis.mlanet.org.

10.4 Healthnet: Connecticut Consumer Health Information Network: Lyman Maynard Stowe Library: University of Connecticut. *Recommended Books for a Consumer Health*

Reference Collection. Farmington, CT: University of Connecticut. Available: http://library.uchc.edu/departm /hnet/corelist.html.

This excellent reference includes a special section on setting up and running a small consumer health library. Several documents about collections are posted, including a core bibliography for consumer health reference from the Lyman Maynard Stowe Library at the University of Connecticut Health Center.

Directories

Many of the directories that were once essential are now marginal purchases because so much of this type of information is available on the Internet. However, some of it, such as the database from the American Board of Medical Specialties, is available only for an annual subscription fee, yet when available, it is frequently used by consumers.

10.5 *AHA Guide to the Health Care Field.* Chicago, IL: American Hospital Association. Annual. 1998. Annual. Formerly: *American Hospital Association Guide to the Health Care Field.* 1974–1997. Annual.

This annual publication lists all hospitals in the United States alphabetically by state. Helpful information such as address, telephone number, types of service provided, number of beds, and more is provided.

10.6 *The Official ABMS Directory of Board Certified Medical Specialists.* Evanston, IL: American Board of Medical Specialists, Research and Education Foundation. 1992–. Annual. See 12.2.

Published annually, this resource is an excellent one for consumers who want to know as much as they can about their physicians, particularly specialists to whom they have been referred or whom they might see only rarely.

10.7 *Medical and Health Information Directory.* Farmington Hills, MI: Gale Group, 1997–. Irregular.

Three-volume work includes 1) organizations, agencies, and institutions; 2) specific publications, libraries, and other information resources; and 3) health services, which includes such items as sleep disorder clinics, sports medicine clinics, transplant centers, and more.

10.8 *Directory of Self-Help and Mutual Aid Groups.* Chicago, IL: Mental Health Association of Illinois. 1990–. Biannual.

Self-help directories are published annually or biannually in most states. In Illinois, the Mental Health Association of Illinois publishes a biannual *Directory of Self-Help and Mutual Aid Groups.* Contents include a definition of self-help, questions to ask when looking for the "right" self-help group, and the directory itself, organized by large areas such as addiction, disability, or family issues. An alphabetical index and a concern index make the volume easy to use.

10.9 *AMA Physician Select (Doctor Finder).* Chicago, IL: American Medical Association. Available: www.ama-assn.org/ aps/amahg.htm and www.nlm.nih.gov/medlineplus/ directories.html.

More than 690,000 licensed medical doctors and osteopaths are included in this database, which can be searched by name and city or state or by medical specialty and city or state. This Internet database and several other similar ones of health professionals are also available from MEDLINEplus.

Dictionaries

Even with good online medical dictionaries available, print editions continue to be valuable and necessary in a consumer health setting. Following are the most important titles.

General Medical Dictionaries

10.10 *Dorland's Illustrated Medical Dictionary,* 30th ed. St. Louis, MO: Harcourt Health Sciences Group, 2003. Also available on CD-ROM.

Often considered the most venerable resource in its field, *Dorland's* is an optional volume for a consumer health collection. The definitions are written using sophisticated medical vocabulary, and users are directed from common names (e.g., Bell's palsy) to the name of the nerve and to the entry for *palsy.*

10.11 *Mosby's Medical, Nursing, & Allied Health Dictionary.* 6th ed. Philadephia, PA: Saunders, 2002.

Very approachable content for consumers, with copious color illustrations.

10.12 *Stedman's Medical Dictionary,* 27th ed. Baltimore, MD: Lippincott Williams & Wilkins, 2000.

Features many color illustrations and very helpful appendices, including common medical abbreviations and symbols; arteries, muscles, and nerves of the human body; and laboratory values and reference ranges.

10.13 *Taber's Cyclopedic Medical Dictionary,* 19th ed. Philadelphia, PA: F.A. Davis Co., 2001. Available: www.tabers.com.

Exceptional resource for consumer use because of its clearly written entries, many illustrations (some in color), and extensive appendices that feature multiple points of access for users.

Specialty Dictionaries

10.14 Altman R, Sarg M. *The Cancer Dictionary.* New York: Facts on File, 2000 rev. ed.

Resource written especially for the cancer patient and the general public who seeks to know more about the constellation of diseases known as *cancer.* No illustrations are included, but a well-written index and attractive format make this resource easy to use.

10.15 Jablonski S, ed. *Dictionary of Medical Acronyms and Abbreviations,* 4th ed. Philadelphia, PA: Hanley & Belfus, 2001.

Either this compendium or *Stedman's Abbreviations, Acronyms, and Symbols* (see 10.18, below) should be in every consumer health collection.

10.16 McElroy OH, Grabb LL. *Spanish-English English-Spanish Medical Dictionary.* 2nd ed. Boston, MA: Little, Brown, 1996.

Many Web-based consumer health resources are available in both English and Spanish. However, if the library is located in an area that serves a Spanish-speaking population, this is a useful resource.

10.17 Magalini SI, Maglini SC. *Dictionary of Medical Syndromes,* 4th ed. Philadelphia, PA: Lippincott-Raven, 1997.

Essential resource for consumers, many of whom suffer from rare disorders and seek information in a library. Entries include synonymous terms, symptoms and signs, etiology, pathology, diagnostic procedures, therapy, prognosis, and a brief bibliography.

10.18 *Stedman's Abbreviations, Acronyms, and Symbols,* 3rd ed. Baltimore, MD: Lippincott Williams & Wilkins, 2003.

This single volume devoted to medical abbreviations, acronyms, and symbols is an extremely helpful resource for consumers. Obviously, it is a more complete listing than can be included in a larger volume because it is a specialized resource. This volume or the Jablonski title (see 10.15, above) should be in every consumer health collection.

10.19 Sternberg MLA. *American Sign Language: Unabridged Edition.* 1st ed. New York: HarperCollins, 1998.

Excellent resource for consumers who are learning American Sign Language (ASL), for schoolchildren who are writing reports about it, and for hearing-impaired individuals and their families as well.

Encyclopedias

Gale Group's products are the best consumer health encyclopedias on the market. They are plainly written, well illustrated, updated in a timely manner, and provide introductions to most common diseases and conditions as well as some rare ones. Information is easy to find because of multiple access points within each set, and biographical and historical sidebars in all the volumes enrich understanding. A resource list is included at the end of every entry, and an index in the final volume increases ease of use. If budget and space are limited, these resources, combined with MEDLINEplus and other excellent Internet portals for consumer health, will help answer the majority of common consumer questions. Following are the titles available:

10.20 Blachford SL, ed. *The Gale Encyclopedia of Genetic Disorders.* Farmington Hills, MI: Gale Group, 2002.

In a field fraught with arcane concepts and jargon, this two-volume resource brings much of the work of the Human Genome Project to the medical consumer at the place they care about: the disorders themselves. Relatively common disorders (epilepsy, cystic fibrosis) are included as well as much rarer ones (Fahr disease, Li-Fraumeni syndrome). Articles include definitions, descriptions, genetic profile, demographics, signs and symptoms, diagnosis, treatment and management, and prognosis.

10.21 Kagan J, Gall SB. *The Gale Encyclopedia of Childhood and Adolescence.* Detroit, MI: Gale Group, 1998.

This one-volume resource is devoted to human growth and development from birth through adolescence. Illustrations and statistical charts and graphs help make the text understandable and easy to use.

10.22 Krapp K, Longe JL, eds. *The Gale Encyclopedia of Alternative Medicine.* Farmington Hills, MI: Gale Group, 2001.

This set includes four volumes. Entries in the general categories of diseases and conditions, herbs and remedies, and therapies are included. Training requirements for practitioners and lists of organizations comprise a portion of the relevant entries. The most important feature of this encyclopedia is its balance. The content is straightforward and makes no unwarranted claims.

10.23 Longe JL, ed. *The Gale Encyclopedia of Medicine.* 2nd ed. Farmington Hills, MI: Gale Group, 2002.

This set includes five volumes and was first published in 1999. Cross-references could be improved, but the content is excellent. There are entries for diseases and disorders as well as tests and treatments. In the first category, the entries typically include definitions, descriptions, causes and symptoms, diagnosis, treatments, alternative treatments (if any), prognosis, and prevention. Entries for tests and treatments include definitions, purposes, precautions, descriptions, preparation, aftercare, risks, and normal and abnormal results.

10.24 Thackery E, ed. *The Gale Encyclopedia of Cancer: A Guide to Cancer and Its Treatments.* Farmington Hills, MI: Gale Group, 2001.

Included in this two-volume set are entries on 120 different cancers, common cancer drugs, traditional and alternative treatments, and diagnostic procedures. The drug section entries are helpfully written. They appear in the encyclopedia under generic name but are indexed under both brand and generic name, with a cross-reference from the brand name to the generic. Most helpful of all, treatment acronyms such as MOPP and EVA are explained; the names of all the drugs included in the combination therapies and the types of cancer for which they are administered are also included in the entry. These articles, generally about one-and one-half pages long, are an approachable adjunct to *The Chemotherapy Sourcebook,* an excellent but technical reference. Articles on specific therapies are lengthy; for example, the "Chemotherapy" article is nine pages long while "Radiation Therapy" is four pages in length. Terms commonly used in cancer and cancer treatment, such as *adjuvant chemotherapy,* are clearly explained, and when several terms are used for the same procedure, such as *internal radiation therapy*, all of them are named and described.

10.25 Thackery E. *The Gale Encyclopedia of Mental Disorders.* Farmington Hills, MI: Gale Group, 2003.

Entries for all 150 disorders classified in the *Diagnostic and Statistical Manual of Mental Disorders*, text revision (*DSM-IV-TR*) are included in this very approachable and useful two-volume work. Medications—prescription, alternative, and over-the-counter—are discussed in detail. The large classes of drugs, such as selective serotonin reuptake inhibitors (SSRIs), do not have their own entry but are treated in the entry for each individual agent. They are grouped in the index, however, by general class. Therapies beyond pharmaceutical agents, such as electroconvulsive therapy, are also included, as are diagnostic tools such as electroencephalography.

10.26 Brickland BR, ed. *The Gale Encyclopedia of Psychology.* 2nd ed. Farmington Hills, MI: Gale Group, 2001.

First published in 1996, the nearly 700 articles of this one-volume resource provide access to important individuals, theories, and vocabulary; ground-breaking studies and experiments; applied psychology in the world around us; and psychology as a career.

10.27 *The Gale Encyclopedia of Surgery: A Guide for Patients and Caregivers.* Farmington Hills, MI: Gale Group, 2003.

Excellent supplement to online resources such as MEDLINEplus tutorials (see 10.51, below) and more current than *The Surgery Book,* an excellent reference published in 1997. A feature that consumers especially appreciate is an appendix listing the preeminent centers for specific surgical procedures.

Handbooks and Manuals

10.28 Beers MH, et al., eds. *Merck Manual of Medical Information, Second Edition: The World's Most Widely-Used Medical Reference: Now in Everyday Language,* 2nd ed. Whitehouse, NJ: Merck, 2003. Available: www.merck-homeedition.com/home.html.

10.29 Beers MH, et al., eds. *Merck Manual of Geriatrics.* 3rd ed. Whitehouse Station, NJ: Merck, 2000. Available: www.merck.com/pubs/mm_geriatrics/contents.htm.

10.30 Beers MH and Berkow R, eds. *The Merck Manual of Diagnosis and Therapy,* 17th ed. "Centennial Edition." Rahway, NJ: Merck, 1999. Available: http://online .statref.com.

The first and most important resources in the area of handbooks and manuals are these three Merck manuals, all of which should be used in their online versions because the Web sites contain corrections and changes from the original or current print editions.

10.31 Rakel RE, Bope ET. *Conn's Current Therapy.* Philadelphia, PA: Saunders, 2003. Annual.

10.32 Decherney A, Nathan L., eds. *Current Obstetric and Gynecologic Diagnosis and Treatment.* New York: Lange Medical Books/McGraw-Hill, 2003. Available: www.accessmedicine.com

10.33 Hay WW, et al., eds. *Current Pediatric Diagnosis and Treatment.* New York: Lange Medical Books/McGraw-Hill, 2002. Available: www.accessmedicine.com

10.34 Lemcke DP, et al., eds. *Current Diagnosis and Treatment of Women.* New York: Lange Medical Books/McGraw-Hill, 2003.

10.35 Skinner HB, ed. *Current Diagnosis and Treatment in Orthopedics.* New York: Lange Medical Books/McGraw-Hill, 2000.

10.36 Tierney LM, ed. *Current Medical Diagnosis and Treatment.* New York: Lange Medical Books/McGraw-Hill. Annual.

10.37 Way LW, Doherty GM, eds. *Current Surgical Diagnosis and Treatment.* New York: Lange Medical Books/McGraw-Hill, 2002.

10.38 Ahya SN, et al., eds. *The Washington Manual of Medical Therapeutics,* 30th ed. Philadelphia, PA: Lippincott Williams & Wilkins, 2001.

Conn's *Current Therapy* and the Lange series of handbooks have long been used by consumers and by reference librarians helping consumers answer questions. Before there were many quality consumer health resources available, except for pamphlets from organizations, these two series offered a gateway to medical knowledge that helped patients understand what was happening to their bodies and what to expect from treatment.

Today they are the middle ground between materials written specifically for consumers and medical textbooks. For the consumer who wants to go beyond the basic information offered by an encyclopedia article, a book from the "Mayo Clinic on" series, or printouts from a Web site, these handbooks are an excellent choice. They delve more deeply into actual disease processes than the consumer material and allow a more multifaceted understanding of the actual medical problem.

The *Washington Manual of Medical Therapeutics* is also a helpful resource in this category. Unlike *Current Therapy* and the Lange handbooks, it focuses on the seriously ill in-patient, making it a resource that might be helpful for family members.

Key Medical Book Series Written for the Consumer

Certain institutions and publishers have developed consumer health information series that, like the Gale Group encyclopedias, follow a similar format and exhibit a recognizable "look and feel." Some good choices are listed below in alphabetical order by producer or sponsoring institution. The Web site, if available, follows the name of the organization, publisher, or series. The Web site offers only online ordering; the full text of the items themselves is not available.

10.39 American Medical Association. *AMA Consumer Publications*. Chicago, IL: AMAPress. Available: www.ama assn.org/ama/pub/category/7350.html.

While few in number, these resources are well written in lay language.

10.40 American Academy of Pediatrics. *AAP Online Bookstore*. Elk Grove Village, IL: American Academy of Pediatrics. Available: www.aap.org/pubserv.

One of the best features of these resources is that they are frequently updated; moreover, many publications are available in English as well as Spanish.

10.41 *Everything You Need to Know About . . .* Springhouse, PA: Springhouse Corporation. 1996

Most of these titles are dated, but because they offer very basic information, most of it is still current and relevant. These resources are especially helpful for low-literacy customers. To find the available titles, search the Web site of an online bookseller.

10.42 *Harvard Medical School Guides.*

Search a bookseller's Web site to find the excellent resources in this series, which are published by different companies but are written under the auspices of the Harvard Medical School.

10.43 *Johns Hopkins University Press.* Available: www.press.jhu.edu/cgi-bin/bipshow.cgi?type=series &qry=jhb.

Some of the most important consumer health resources, such as *The 36-Hour Day*, *The Guide to Living with HIV Infection*, and *Dying at Home* are published by this press.

10.44 *Mayo Clinic on . . .*

Search a bookseller's Web site for "Mayo Clinic on" to retrieve a list of current titles; like the Harvard titles, they are not available from the institution itself. These are excellent references on common diseases and conditions, from arthritis to vision and eye health, and some or all of them should be available for reference in consumer health libraries.

10.45 *Omnigraphics Health Reference Series.* Detroit, MI: Omnigraphics. Available: www.omnigraphics.com.

Nearly 200 volumes are available in this series at this writing. While they are attractive on a shelf and contain accurate information, their format makes them much harder to use than the Gale encyclopedias; moreover, because of the dry presentation of material and absence of sections on school concerns for pediatric topics, they are not as useful to families as the O'Reilly guides. That being said, they can be useful for filling in areas of collections that need something beyond a brief encyclopedia article and require a work devoted to a single health topic. The series directed toward adolescents, the Teen Health Series, is well worth including in a consumer health collection that serves this age group. Unlike the original series, the format in these books is engaging, and the titles address important concerns of teenagers, such as diet, drugs, mental health, sexual health, skin health, and sports injuries.

10.46 *Patient-centered Guides: Questions Answered, Experiences Shared.* Sebastopol, CA: O'Reilly and Associates, 2001. Available: www.patientcenters.com.

Outstanding, frequently updated titles; one volume, *Your Child in the Hospital,* is also available in a Spanish-language edition. The publisher has also provided a Web site with Family Resource Centers available for eleven of the titles. These pages contain portions of the books with occasional updates. Two of the most useful features of these Family Resource Centers are sections explaining special education procedures and those for resources, with direct links into organizations that can prove helpful for specific conditions.

Category-Specific Reference Resources for Consumer Health Information

Category 1: General Health and Medical References

Libraries that serve the public cannot answer the questions asked of them without having access to a core set of medical textbooks. On a continuum of resources (an array of levels) running from materials written at a fourth- to sixth-grade reading level on up the scale, these works are the upper end of the collection. Today, they may be obtained either in print or in an electronic database or both. Moreover, materials written for the consumer complement these sophisticated, technical resources.

10.47 Braunwald EG, et al., eds. *Harrison's Principles of Internal Medicine.* 15th ed. New York: McGraw-Hill, 2001. Available: www.accessmedicine.com.

The most authoritative reference available on the diagnosis and treatment of diseases and conditions, *Harrison's* is one of the two "bibles" of internal medicine. It is, however, very technical, and only the most highly educated consumer will find it useful. If only one such advanced reference can be purchased, make it *Cecil's Textbook of Medicine* (below).

10.48 Goldman L, Bennett JC, eds. *Cecil's Textbook of Medicine.* 21st ed. Philadelphia, PA: Saunders, 2000.

With *Harrison's Principles of Internal Medicine*, this work is the other "bible" of internal medicine. It is essential in the consumer health setting for its authority and its engaging approach to its subjects. Current copies of both *Harrison's* and *Cecil's* are ideal; what one text omits, the other one explores, often in depth.

10.49 Goodman DR, Horowitz DA, ed. *American College of Physicians Complete Home Medical Guide.* 2nd American ed. New York: DK Publishing, 2003.

Excellent reference of its type. Home medical guides, by their nature, provide only cursory information about health topics. This one is beautifully produced, with well-written text, colorful illustrations, and excellent graphics. Only one such reference is required, because Web resources such as MEDLINEplus and healthfinder.gov provide so much of the same information. Examine home health guides from Harvard Medical School, Johns Hopkins, and the Mayo Clinic, as well as this one, to determine which one best meets the needs of customers.

10.50 Narins B, ed. *World of Health.* Detroit, MI: Gale Group, 2000.

Unique, one-volume reference contains 1,400 individual entries, alphabetically arranged, that explore the worlds of medical terminology, history, and biography, with an allied health encyclopedia as well. More than 300 illustrations complement the articles, and a timeline puts the items included in historical perspective.

Many excellent portals to consumer health information are available today on the Internet. The National Institute of Diabetes, Digestive, and Kidney Disorders (NIDDK) and the National Heart,

Lung, and Blood Institute (NHLBI), besides the two sites mentioned below, produce excellent information for consumers. Many private organizations (like the American Heart Association and the American Diabetes Association) have excellent information as well. The first consumer health portal from the federal government, healthfinder.gov, is continually enhanced and is particularly easy to use—because of its clean, bright format—for seniors or persons with poor vision. Medem, Virtual Hospital, KidsHealth, MayoClinic.com, and many other sites provide excellent information. However, by going to one of the two sites described below, consumers are directed to an enormous array of resources, including everything available through the federal government as well as the independent sites listed above. They truly offer one-stop shopping for consumer health reference information.

10.51 *MEDLINEplus.* Bethesda, MD: National Library of Medicine. Available: http://medlineplus.gov/.

MEDLINEplus is the premier free portal to consumer health information on the World Wide Web. Beginning with pages devoted to a mere 22 health topics in 1998, the site has grown to include more than 600 such pages. It also includes the A.D.A.M. medical encyclopedia, drug information, and more than 150 interactive health tutorials covering common diseases and conditions, diagnostic tests and procedures, surgeries and surgical procedures, and prevention and wellness information.

10.52 *Cancer.gov: Cancer Information.* Besthesda, MD: National Cancer Institute. Available: http://cancer.gov.

Cancer.gov contains comprehensive cancer treatment information from the National Cancer Institute. The site covers all aspects of cancer and should be a first stop for information about this disease. It also links out to other sources of information. Treatment documents are updated whenever new information is available.

Commercial databases of consumer health information can also be purchased; they typically include full-text periodical articles, books, and pamphlets. The best-known products are Health Source: Consumer Edition, from EBSCO Information Services, and Health Reference Center, from Gale Group. CareNotes, from MICROMEDEX, (see

10.54, below) and McKesson Clinical Reference Systems (CRS) are excellent patient education products. Clinical Reference Systems, or parts of it, is available through many other sources, including Health Source: Consumer Edition.

Category 2: Procedures, Therapies, Symptoms, and Manifestations

The organizing principle used in this section is the headings from the MEDLINEplus Web site. These terms, which are widely understood and accepted by health care consumers, serve as useful descriptors for providing access to print and audiovisual materials in a consumer health library.

Drug Information

10.53 *The United States Pharmacopoeia: USP DI.* 17th ed. Rockville, MD: United States Pharmacopoeial Convention, Inc. Annual. Vol. 1, Drug Information for the Health Care Provider; Vol 2, Advice for the Patient. Available: www.nlm.nih.gov/medlineplus/druginformation.html.

Consumers expect to see a current *Physicians' Desk Reference* in a health library, though online resources are more authoritative (because of frequent updates) and generally much easier to use because of the simplicity of search interfaces. Volume 2 of the *USP DI*, *Advice for the Patient*, is available online for free from MEDLINEplus. In most consumer health information settings, a print edition of this resource is not required, though the online version will extensively be used.

10.54 *MICROMEDEX CareNotes.* Greenwood Village, CO: Thomson MICROMEDEX. Available: www.micromedex.com /products/carenotes.

CareNotes, the patient information tool from MICROMEDEX, provides 3,000 information sheets on medications and diseases and conditions; all are available in either English or Spanish.

10.55 *Clinical Pharmacology.* Tampa, FL: Gold Standard Multimedia. Available: www.gsm.com/products_cp.htm.

Clinical Pharmacology, produced by Gold Standard Multimedia, is a very attractive product that provides technical monographs as well as patient education handouts, many of them available in Spanish as well as English. Pricing for hospitals is based on the number of beds, and the Web-based product can be accessed throughout the institution.

Diagnostic Tests

10.56 *Everything You Need to Know About Medical Tests.* Philadephia, PA: Springhouse, 1997.

Though the reference needs to be updated to include genetic testing, home tests, and other diagnostic tools, this book is so clearly and simply written that it remains an essential reference, especially helpful for use with low-literacy customers.

10.57 Fischbach FT. *Manual of Laboratory and Diagnostic Tests.* 6th ed. Philadelphia, PA: Lippincott Williams & Wilkins, 2000.

Librarians should choose one midlevel resource for the reference shelf, either this one or *Mosby's Manual of Laboratory and Diagnostic Tests* (below).

10.58 Pakana KD, Pagana TJ. *Mosby's Manual of Laboratory and Diagnostic Tests.* 2nd ed. St. Louis, MO: Mosby, 2002.

Good illustrations and current information. Very helpful if a midlevel resource is needed.

10.59 Zaret BL, ed. *The Patient's Guide to Medical Tests.* Boston, MA: Houghton Mifflin, 1997. Available: www.netlibrary.com.

Very comprehensive, clearly written, well-illustrated volume from the Yale University School of Medicine.

Symptoms and Manifestations

10.60 Margolis S. *Johns Hopkins Symptoms and Remedies: The Complete Home Medical Reference.* New York: Rebus, 2003.

Many health care consumers use a library service to "check out" symptoms prior to seeing a health care professional. This book is an authoritative answer to such an information need. The first half of the book lists symptoms, such as "swallowing difficulty," with three columns of information: associated symptoms, possible diagnosis, and distinguishing features. The possible diagnoses are listed in alphabetical order. The second half of the book is an alphabetical arrangement of disorders, with each article explaining the condition and the cause, prevention, diagnosis, treatment options, and when to call a doctor. A textbox with each article provides cross references to symptoms.

Nutrition and Diet Therapy

10.61 Duyff RL. *American Dietetic Association Complete Food and Nutrition Guide.* 2nd ed. New York: John Wiley & Sons, 2002.

Outstanding, very well written resource that provides important nutrition information for individual health issues such as fibromyalgia and hypertension, use and abuse of supplements, food-drug interactions, and much more.

10.62 Mahan LK, Escott-Stump, S, eds. *Krause's Food, Nutrition, and Diet Therapy.* 10th ed. Philadelphia, PA: Saunders, 2000.

Krause is the most authoritative resource available on diet therapy. The reference offers tables and illustrations for individual diseases and conditions and how they can be managed through diet.

10.63 Pennington JAT. *Bowes and Church's Food Values of Portions Commonly Used.* 17th ed. Philadelphia, PA: Lippincott Williams & Wilkins, 1998.

Answers many typical consumer questions regarding the specific nutrient content of certain foods and even indexes items by brand name

Alternative, Complementary, and Integrative Medicine

10.64 American Cancer Society. *Guide to Complementary and Alternative Cancer Methods.* Atlanta, GA: American Cancer Society, 2000.

Authoritative resource from the American Cancer Society provides information on what works, what might work but is unproven, and what is known to be harmful in a clear, easy-to-use format.

10.65 Blumenthal M, ed. *Therapeutic Guide to Herbal Medicines: Complete German Commission E Monographs.* Austin, TX: American Botanical Council, 1998.

This is the first English translation of the most authoritative guide to the therapeutic use of herbal medications. Originally published in Germany, where a great deal of research into the therapeutic properties of herbals has been conducted.

10.66 Blumenthal M, ed. *Herbal Medicine: Expanded Commission E Monographs.* 1st ed. Newton, MA: Integrative Medicine Communications, 2000.

Longer, more detailed articles than the original volume, with references, on the 107 most used herbals in the United States.

10.67 *Medical Advisor: The Complete Guide to Alternative and Conventional Treatments.* 2nd ed. Alexandria, VA: Time-Life Books, 2000.

Helpful format provides information for more than 300 diseases and conditions, including symptoms and warning signs that warrant medical attention. Besides giving conventional as well as alternative treatment information, home remedies are described in appropriate cases.

10.68 *PDR for Herbal Medicines.* 2nd ed. Montvale, NJ: Medical Economics Company, 2000.

This reference includes monographs based on the German Commission E Monographs. A full-color identification guide for several hundred herbs is included as well as an index to common and botanical names for each plant.

10.69 Pelletier K. *Best Alternative Medicine: What Works? What Does Not?* New York: Simon & Schuster, 2000.

Contains evidence-based reviews of alternative therapies—including homeopathy, acupuncture, naturopathy, and more—and then discusses alternative approaches to treating some ailments, such as asthma, bronchitis, headaches, sinusitis, and more.

Surgery

10.70 *Gale Encyclopedia of Surgery.* (See 10.27, above.)

10.71 Schwartz SI, ed. *Principles of Surgery.* 7th ed. New York: McGraw-Hill, 1999.

10.72 Greenfield LJ, ed. *Surgery: Scientific Principles and Practice.* 3rd ed. Philadelphia, PA: Lippincott Williams & Wilkins, 2001.

If a surgical textbook is required, choose either *Principles of Surgery*, edited by Seymour I. Schwartz, or *Surgery: Scientific Principles and Practice*, edited by Lazar J. Greenfield.

Category 3: Anatomy and Physiology

10.73 Clayman CB, ed. *The Human Body: An Illustrated Guide to Its Structure, Function, and Disorders.* 1st American ed. New York: Dorling Kindersley, 1995.

Beautiful illustrations, coupled with detailed yet lucid text, make this book an outstanding reference for laypersons.

10.74 Guyton AC, Hall JE. *Textbook of Medical Physiology.* 10th ed. Philadelphia, PA: Saunders, 2000.

Optional reference, depending on the clientele of the consumer health service. If the population includes students and professionals, then this textbook is an important work to provide in the collection.

10.75 Netter FH. *Atlas of Human Anatomy.* 2nd ed. East Hanover, NJ: Novartis, 1997.

The magnificent illustrations in this volume make it an essential purchase for any library that has a biomedical collection.

10.76 Thibodeau GA, Patton KT. *Structure and Function of the Body.* 11th ed. St. Louis, MO: Mosby, 2000.

A text written for students in allied health programs, this volume is a good choice for a midlevel resource in anatomy and physiology.

Category 4: Selected Disorders and Conditions

Bones, Joints, and Muscles

10.77 Klippel JH, et al., eds. *Primer on the Rheumatic Diseases.* 12th ed. Atlanta, GA: Arthritis Foundation, 2001.

Excellent, midlevel resource discusses individual rheumatic diseases, what is known about the role of genetics in these diseases, rehabilitation, self-management, the economic consequences of rheumatic disease, and much more. Illustrations and tables enhance the text. Appendices include criteria for the classification and diagnosis of specific rheumatic diseases, guidelines for management, drugs, and supplements.

Brain and Nervous System

10.78 Gilroy J. *Basic Neurology.* 3rd ed. New York: McGraw-Hill, 2000.

Text is divided by individual illnesses or groups of illnesses and is very helpful to consumers needing a specific, midlevel resource for the most common neurological disorders.

10.79 Victor M, Ropper AH. *Adams and Victor's Principles of Neurology.* 7th ed. New York: McGraw-Hill, 2001.

Straightforwardly written, this text can answer many complex neurology questions posed by a consumer.

10.80 Wiederholt WC. *Neurology for Non-Neurologists.* 4th ed. Philadelphia, PA: Saunders, 2000.

Excellent, midlevel resource that reviews clinical neuroanatomy and contains an especially good chapter on seizure disorders.

Cancers

10.81 Buckman R. *What You Really Need to Know About Cancer.* Baltimore, MD: Johns Hopkins University Press, 1997.

Covers some of the same ground as *Everyone's Guide to Cancer Therapy* (see 10.81, below), which is superior in its breadth and depth of coverage. *What You Really Need to Know About Cancer*, however, offers superior illustrations and graphics, which can be very helpful when explaining concepts to laypeople.

10.82 DeVita VT, Hellman S, Rosenberg SA, eds. *Cancer: Principles and Practice of Oncology.* 6th ed. Philadelphia, PA: Lippincott Williams & Wilkins, 2001.

The core medical textbook in its field, this is an essential reference for researching cancer questions.

10.83 Dollinger MA, et al. *Everyone's Guide to Cancer Therapy: How Cancer is Diagnosed, Treated, and Managed Day to Day.* 4th ed. Kansas City, MO: Andrews McMeel Publishers, 2002.

Most important of all the books about cancer written for the layperson, this resource covers all aspects of the disease, from what cancer is, to what to expect during treatments, to psychosocial factors affecting cancer patients and families, to survivorship.

10.84 Eyre H, Lange DP, Morris LB. *Informed Decisions: The Complete Book of Cancer Diagnosis, Treatment, and Recovery.* 2nd ed. New York: Viking, 2001.

In this American Cancer Society resource, much of the same ground is covered as in the Dollinger book, but the arrangement is different, with a great deal of emphasis being placed on the actual decision-making process that cancer patients face.

Diabetes

10.85 American Diabetes Association. *American Diabetes Association Complete Guide to Diabetes: The Ultimate Home Reference from the Diabetes Experts.* 3rd ed., completely revised. Alexandria, VA: American Diabetes Association, 2002.

Clearly written and well organized, this book is an essential reference because of the prevalence of Type II Diabetes. Type I Diabetes is covered as well.

10.85 Levin ME, Pfeifer MA, eds. *Uncomplicated Guide to Diabetes Complications.* 2nd ed. New York: McGraw-Hill/Contemporary Books, 2002.

Another essential reference that will answer many customer questions about peripheral neuropathy, hypoglycemia, and much more that can affect the health and quality of life of diabetic patients.

Mental Health and Behavior

10.86 *Diagnostic and Statistical Manual of Mental Disorders: DSM-IV-TR.* 4th ed. Washington, DC: American Psychiatric Association, 2000.

Essential reference for any biomedical collection.

10.87 *Gale Encyclopedia of Mental Disorders.* (See 10.25, above.)

10.88 Nicholi AM. *Harvard Guide to Psychiatry.* 3rd ed. Cambridge, MA: Belknap Press of Harvard University Press, 1999.

Useful midlevel resource for the sophisticated consumer, this work uses the *DSM-IV* definitions as an organizing principle and then briefly discusses the epidemiology, available treatments, and prevalence and etiology of each diagnosis.

Mouth and Teeth

10.89 Smith RW. *Columbia University School of Dental and Oral Surgery's Guide to Family Dental Care.* New York: Norton, 1997.

Authoritative, clearly written resource for consumers, though it needs to be updated because some sections, particularly on implants, are insufficiently covered

Skin, Hair, and Nails

10.90 Buxton PK, et al. *ABC of Dermatology.* 3rd ed. London, England: BMJ Publishing Group, 1998.

While written for practicing dermatologists, this book's excellent illustrations and format make it a good reference for consumers.

10.91 Fitzpatrick TB, et al. *Color Atlas and Synopsis of Clinical Dermatology: Common and Serious Diseases.* 4th ed. New York: McGraw-Hill, 2001.

Table of contents and excellent index make this reference easy to use. Brief articles include an illustration of the disorder, with textual content organized by description, epidemiology, pathogenesis, history, physical examination, differential diagnosis, laboratory tests, diagnosis, prognosis, and management.

Category 5: Demographic Groups

Child and Teen Health

10.92 *American Academy of Pediatrics* [some Spanish]. (See 10.40, above.)

10.93 Pruitt DB, ed. *Your Adolescent: Emotional, Behavioral, and Cognitive Development from Preadolescence Through the Teen Years.* 1st ed. New York: HarperCollins, 1999.

Essential resource from the American Academy of Child and Adolescent Psychiatry covers normal development, problem behaviors, serious problems and abnormalities, and how and when to seek help.

10.94 Pruitt DB, ed. *Your Child: Emotional, Behavioral, and Cognitive Development from Birth Through Preadolescence.* New York: HarperResource, 2000.

Essential resource from the American Academy of Child and Adolescent Psychiatry covers the same areas as the reference above, but for a younger age group.

Seniors' Health

10.95 *Merck Manual of Geriatrics.* (See 10.29, above.)

10.96 Wei J, Levkoff S. *Aging Well: The Complete Guide to Physical and Emotional Health.* New York: John Wiley & Sons, 2001.

Besides covering the basics about aging body systems, this reference includes a chapter that discusses various housing options for the elderly; risks, abuse, and legal rights; and how to assist aging parents or other family members.

10.97 Williams ME. *American Geriatric Society's Complete Guide to Aging and Health.* 1st ed. New York: Harmony Books, 1995.

Helpful topics include making health care decisions; legal, ethical, and financial considerations in health care; and a lengthy section on conditions that affect older people, such as memory disorders, digestive disorders, and much more. A list of organizations for seniors, as well as an overview of the aging process, is included.

Women's Health

10.98 Brody JE. *New York Times Book of Women's Health: Living Longer and Better in the New Millenium.* New York: Lebhar-Friedman Books, 2000.

Outstanding reference that includes 13 sections, from nutrition to violence to menopause, and much more. Attractive layout, helpful graphics and illustrations, and a special section on raising healthy daughters make this a good reference resource for consumers.

10.99 Carlson KJ, Eisentat SA, Ziporyn TD. *Harvard Guide to Women's Health*. Cambridge, MA: Harvard University Press, 1996.

Organized alphabetically by topic, this book remains a relevant and important general reference.

References

1. Fox S, Rainie L. *The online health care revolution: how the Web helps Americans take better care of themselves*. Washington, DC: The Pew Internet & American Life Project, 2000. Available: www.pewinternet.org/reports/toc.asp?Report=26.

2. Horrigan JB, Rainie L. *Counting on the Internet: most expect to find key information online, most find the information they seek, many now turn to the Internet first*. Washington, DC: The Pew Internet & American Life Project, 2002. Available: www.pewinternet.org/reports/toc.asp?Report=80.

3. Bodenheimer T. The American health care system—physicians and the changing medical marketplace. *New Engl J of Med* 1999 Feb. 18; 340(7):584–8.

4. DiMatteo MR. The role of the physician in the emerging health care environment. *West J Med* 1998 May; 168(5):328–33.

5. Ad Hoc Committee on Health Literacy for the Council on Scientific Affairs, American Medical Association. Health literacy: report of the Council on Scientific Affairs. *JAMA* 1999 Feb. 10; 281(6):552–7.

6. Berland GK, et al. Health information on the Internet: accessibility, quality, and readability in English and Spanish. *JAMA* 2001 May 23/30; 285(20):2612–21.

Readings

Besides the items in the Reference List, the articles below provide useful insights and some historical perspective on consumer health reference services.

1. The librarian's role in the provision of consumer health information and patient education. *Bull Med Libr Assoc* 1996 Apr.; 84(2):239–9.
2. Baker LM, Pettigrew KE. Theories for practitioners: two frameworks for studying consumer health information-seeking behavior. *Bull Med Libr Assoc* 1999 Oct.; 87(4):444–50.
3. Calabretta N. The hospital library as provider of consumer health information. *Med Ref Serv Q* 1996 Fall; 15(3):13–22.
4. Calvano M, Needham G. Public empowerment through accessible health information. *Bull Med Libr Assoc* 1996 Apr.; 84(2):253–6.
5. Cosgrove TL. PlaneTree Health Information Services: public access to the health information people want. *Bull Med Libr Assoc* 1994 Jan.; 82(1):57–63.
6. Fitzpatrick RB, Hendler G. What every medical librarian should know about MEDLINEplus. *Med Ref Serv Q* 1999 Winter; 18(4):11–17.
7. Goodchild EY, Furman JA, Addison BL, Umbarger HN. The CHIPS Project: a health information network to serve the consumer. *Bull Med Libr Assoc* 1978 Oct.; 66(4):432–6.
8. La Rocco A. The role of the medical school–based consumer health information service. *Bull Med Libr Assoc* 1994 Jan.; 82(1):46–51.
9. Lambremont JA. Consumer health information services in the hospital setting. *Med Ref Serv Q* 1997 Summer; 16(2):61–7.
10. Leydon GM, et al. Cancer patients' information needs and information seeking behaviour: in-depth interview study. *BMJ* 2000 Apr. 1; 320(7239):909–13.
11. Pifalo V, et al. The impact of consumer health information provided by libraries: the Delaware experience. *Bull Med Libr Assoc* 1997 Jan.; 85(1):16–22.

12. Spatz MA. Providing consumer health information in the rural setting: PlaneTree Health Resource Center's approach. *Bull Med Libr Assoc* 2000 Oct.; 88(4):382–8.
13. van der Molen B. Relating information needs to the cancer experience: 1. Information as a key coping strategy. *Eur J Cancer Care* 1999 Dec.; 8(4):238–44.
14. Van Moorsel G. Do you Mini-Med School? Leveraging library resources to improve Internet consumer health information literacy. *Med Ref Serv Q* 2001 Winter; 20(4):27–37.
15. Wood FB, et al. Public library consumer health information pilot project: results of a National Library of Medicine evaluation. *Bull Med Libr Assoc* 2000 Oct.; 88(4):314–22.

CHAPTER 11

MEDICAL AND HEALTH STATISTICS

Jocelyn A. Rankin and Mary L. Burgess

Reference staff in health sciences libraries will encounter health care statistics questions on a regular basis. However, finding the precise statistic that answers a reference question is usually a challenge, even for the most experienced reference librarian. More health care statistics are being published than ever before, both on the Internet and in print, yet it is often difficult to locate the perfect match to the reference inquiry. The successful reference librarian must not only be able to track down the requisite statistic, but also must be able to understand it and evaluate its credibility. It is also important to recognize that in spite of the ever-increasing quantities of statistical data being produced, sometimes the statistical factors being requested by a library patron are either not collected at all or possibly not analyzed in a way that serves the patron's inquiry.

So, what to do when faced with:

- How many HMOs are there in the United States and how many enrollees?
- What is the extent of alcohol consumption in the United States?
- What is the number of health care workers in Iraq?

(For answers, see page 267)

Challenges clearly abound with medical and health statistics. However, there is a logical strategy [1] to locating answers to questions about statistics.

1. Determine what type and category of statistic is being requested. For example, is the question about disease occurrence, vital statistics, or demographics?
2. Understand what variables are being asked for. Is the library patron asking for data about a specific population group, a certain time period, a certain geographic location?
3. Consider which Web sites or print resources will provide credible, timely data in the subject area. Which government and/or private organizations collect these data?
4. If there is no logical primary resource, search secondary or related resources such as journal literature, agency reports, and so forth.
5. After a reasonable search, confer with the patron, recognizing that not all statistics are collected or analyzed in a way that satisfies every inquiry.

Why Are Health Statistics So Important?

Despite the fact that statistics may frustrate, confound, and challenge the health sciences reference librarian, they are a fact of life in today's health care environment. At the national level, particularly during the last decade, efforts are underway to monitor systematically the health status of our country in order to promote healthy people and healthy lifestyles. *Healthy People 2010* [2], the ten-year road map for America's public health system, identified two overarching public health goals: to increase the quality and years of healthy life and to eliminate health disparities. Ten "Leading Health Indicators" addressing mental health, behavioral, lifestyle, and health access issues support these goals and also correlate with many specific health objectives for national, state, and local communities. Health statistics provide the tools to measure our progress as a nation in meeting these goals and objectives and also to identify the priorities for the coming decades.

Health statistics can describe health conditions and also the factors that affect health, including economic, environmental, behavioral, and lifestyle characteristics of populations. These statistics guide health care planning, health care delivery, and health care evaluation. They influence decisions and priorities about health policy, health care services, provider training, and resource and funding allocations. As the health care industry refines its business models related to accountability, managed care, and cost containment, statistics may also inform health care and financial decisions at many levels, including in government, in health care organizations and facilities, and in health sciences universities, affecting the full range of health care from general policies to day-to-day operations.

Improving health outcomes is a goal for public health and also for individual case management. The recent emphasis on evidence-based medicine (EBM), "the conscientious, explicit and judicious use of current best evidence in making decisions about the care of individual patients" [3] has given health sciences librarians the opportunity to serve as valuable members of educational and clinical care teams. EBM formalizes the process of incorporating the best relevant research evidence with clinical expertise in the practice of medicine. While statistical data do not alone provide complete information about disease etiologies, diagnoses, therapies, and outcomes, the use of data from clinical trials and reports of best practices can advise health care providers on the efficacy and safety of proposed approaches to patient care. There is often great difficulty in conducting EBM searches and identifying the best evidence. Roles for librarians include assisting in formulating the clinical questions, teaching students and clinicians effective search skills, and searching for and identifying the best resources. The critical appraisal skills of librarians help in recognizing clinical studies with strong methodologies, appropriate statistical analyses, and valid conclusions.

New Approaches in Health Statistics

Health sciences librarians should also be aware of emerging resources for health statistics that are resulting from new approaches to discovering, tracking, and understanding health data. Among these are powerful new data mining tools that are being developed to maximize the benefits of recent technological advances in large-scale data collection, data access, and data warehousing. These tools, which are essentially a new generation of statistics, can be applied to massive databases in order to search for previously unrecognized patterns, data clusters, and data models. Data mining may also yield predictive information relating to future trends and behaviors. In the health care sector, data mining and knowledge discovery tools are being applied to support both clinical care and improved business management.

11.1 *Public Health Information Network (PHIN)*. Atlanta, GA: U.S. Department of Health and Human Services, Centers for Disease Control and Prevention. Available: www.cdc.gov/phin.

11.2 *National Electronic Disease Surveillance System (NEDSS)*. Atlanta, GA: U.S. Department of Health and Human Services, Centers for Disease Control and Prevention. Available: www.cdc.gov/nedss.

While compiling health data continues to be a complex process and fraught with variability, the tracking and collection of health data is moving toward greater standardization. The National Health Information Infrastructure (NHII) [4] initiative aims to develop an overarching network, supported by technologies, data standards, and systems, that will enable health information sharing at national, state, and local levels. The Centers for Disease Control and Prevention is guiding a national approach to disease surveillance through projects such as the Public Health Information Network (PHIN) and the National Electronic Disease Surveillance System (NEDSS). Surveillance, which is the ongoing, systematic collection and analysis of health data, is fundamental to detecting epidemics, emerging or reemerging infectious diseases, and bioterrorist events.

A leading new method for understanding health data is Geographic Information Systems (GIS). Geographic Information Systems technologies are introducing an added dimension to medicine and public health by enabling the graphical display of datasets. For example, GIS can support epidemiological research by allowing for visualization of patterns of disease incidence, chemical spills, or other health-related incidents. More complex analyses through layering of datasets can illustrate additional factors, such as associated health and social impacts.

Biostatistics Basics

An introductory class in statistics at the local college campus or a continuing education course at a conference are both good approaches to gaining an overview of statistical measures and values. A basic knowledge of statistics is useful when answering reference questions and also in managing the library reference department or conducting information science research. The following are helpful resources:

11.3 Le, CT. *Health and Numbers: A Problems-based Introduction to Biostatistics.* 2nd ed. New York: Wiley-Liss, 2001.

11.4 Essex-Sorlie, D. *Medical Biostatistics and Epidemiology: Examination and Board Review.* Norwalk, CT: Appleton & Lange, 1995.

These two books are good examples of readily understandable introductions to biostatistics. Both resources are useful for health sciences library patrons as well as for reference staff members wanting to acquire a basic knowledge of statistical concepts and methods. Both are easy to read and provide clear explanations with many health sciences examples.

Health and Numbers is an introductory textbook for health sciences students with an emphasis on concepts of data analysis rather than the mathematics. *Medical Biostatistics and Epidemiology* is part of the Medical Board Review series. While intended for medical students, its approach is widely applicable. Features include clinical examples, highlighting of major points and concepts, and self-study questions with detailed answers. The final chapter on "Reading and Evaluating the Medical Literature" gives a good overview of critical appraisal of the literature and includes a checklist on how to evaluate published journal articles.

11.5   Sackett, D. L., et al. *Evidence-Based Medicine: How to Practice and Teach EBM.* 2nd ed. Edinburgh and New York: Churchill Livingstone, 2000.

The classic resource for evidence-based medicine, this handbook is intended for the busy physician and all others interested in applying the principles of EBM to the practice of clinical medicine. The chapter on searching for the best evidence is a must-read for any reference librarian involved with EBM training. Separate chapters are devoted to each of the following: diagnosis, prognosis, therapy, and harm, the latter addressing studies related to causative interventions or agents. These chapters describe the types of published reports in that area and then give guidance on how to understand and evaluate the merits of published clinical reports and studies relating to the topic. The handbook includes a CD-ROM that provides clinical examples and extended descriptions.

Many medical schools have developed Web sites about EBM. The University Health Centre Network—Mt. Sinai Hospital Centre for Evidence-Based Medicine provides a variety of EBM tools as well as support for Sackett's handbook at www.cebm.utoronto.ca.

11.6   Delwiche, LD and Slaughter, SJ . *The Little SAS Book: A Primer,* 3rd ed. Cary, NC: BBU Press, 2003.

11.7   Einspruch, EL. *An Introductory Guide to SPSS for Windows.* Thousand Oaks, CA: Sage Publications, 1998.

SAS and SPSS are the two major commercially available computer software programs used for data analysis and statistics in the health sciences sector. An introductory manual keyed to the most current version of the software is useful for both the scientific researcher and the librarian. These two examples are software user guides that provide information on basic statistical concepts; how to input, modify, and manage datasets using the selected software; and how to run basic statistical tests. Both are easy to follow and include examples and screen shots to assist the software user.

11.8   *Epi Info*. Atlanta, GA: U.S. Department of Health and Human Services, Centers for Disease Control and Prevention. Available: www.cdc.gov/epiinfo.

Epi Info is a public domain statistics software package available from the U.S. Centers for Disease Control and Prevention Web site. Regularly updated to maintain compatibility with the desktop computer environment, *Epi Info* is designed to assist basic public health data collection and analysis. However, many of its functions have broader applicability for basic statistical analysis. In addition to performing basic statistical tests, *Epi Info* includes tools for developing a questionnaire or form as well as for entering and analyzing data. Epidemiologic statistics, tables, graphs, and maps are produced with simple commands. The new Epi Map feature displays geographic maps and supports data mapping.

The *Epi Info* Web site includes the software, instructions for downloading, and user manuals in several languages. There is also a tutorial for new users and a listing of *Epi Info* training classes offered by a variety groups throughout the world.

What Is a Good Statistic?

The statistics seeker expects statistics to be drawn from consistent reporting and reliable comparisons on a specific topic or combination of topics. This can be a difficult expectation to meet. Some difficulties stem from fragmented and uncoordinated data collection efforts as well as varying data collection and statistical analysis methods. Differences in terminology, data definitions, and coverage, such as geographical areas or time periods, can influence the validity of the statistical data that the librarian may retrieve to answer a specific question.

All credible statistical tables should be accompanied by technical documentation that provides detailed information on what kind of data were collected, how they were collected, the population sample used for analysis, the methods used to construct the statistical result being evaluated, and other important information. Examine these technical notes carefully, matching the patron's parameters to the documentation.

Terminology

An understanding of the terminology used in health statistics is critical to formulating a successful search. Although the jargon used in the area of health statistics is not as extensive as in many other health-related disciplines, there are some terms that searchers should keep in mind when looking for statistical health data. Table 11-1 is a list of key health statistics terms that have been drawn from a variety of sources [5–8].

Among these definitions, *rate* is a very important term in health statistics. Rate is used with terms such as natality, mortality, incidence, and prevalence. As noted in the definition, rate expresses the frequency with which an event occurs in a defined population in a specified period of time. The use of rate rather than raw numbers is essential for comparison of experience between populations at different times, different places, or among different classes of persons. For example, it is meaningless to say there were over 65,000 deaths from pneumonia and influenza in the United States without knowing the time period during which they occurred and the population in which they occurred. A rate will express this concept. Stating that the incidence rate of death from pneumonia and influenza in all races, both sexes, age 10–14 years in the United States was 0.2 per 100,000 population in the year 2000, gives an indication of the real magnitude of the problem.

The components of a rate are the numerator (the number of events in a specified period), a denominator (average population during the specified period), and a multiplier (a power of 10 to convert fractions and decimals to whole numbers).

Table 11-1. Frequently Occurring Health Statistics Terms

Acute Condition	An acute condition is a type of illness or injury that ordinarily lasts less than 3 months, was first noticed less than 3 months before the reference data of the interview, and was serious enough to have had an impact on behavior. (Pregnancy is also considered to be an acute condition despite lasting longer than 3 months).

Age Adjusted
Death Rates

Age-adjusted death rates are calculated using age-specific death rates per 100,000 population rounded to one decimal place. Adjustment is based on 11 age groups: under 1 year, 1–4 years, 5–14 years, 15–24 years, 25–34 years, 35–44 years, 45–54 years, 55–64 years, 65–74 years, 75–84 years, and 85 years and over. The exceptions to these groupings are: 1) The age-adjusted death rates for black males and black females in 1950 are based on nine age groups, with "under 1 year" and 1–4 years of age combined as one group, and 75–84 years and "85 years of age and over" combined as one group; 2) the age-adjusted death rates by educational attainment for the age group 25–64 years are based on four 10-year age groups (25–34 years, 35–44 years, 45–54 years, and 55–64 years); and 3) the age-adjusted rates for "years of potential life lost" (YPLL) before age 75 years also use the year 2000 standard population and are based on eight age groups: under 1 year, 1–14 years, 15–24 years, and 10–year age groups through 65–74 years.

Biometry

Biometry is statistics applied to the living world. Statistical methods are applied to the study of numerical data based on biological observations and phenomena. It includes demography, epidemiology, and clinical trials.

Birth Cohort

A birth cohort consists of all persons born within a given period of time, such as a calendar year.

Birth Rate

Birth rate is the number of births occurring in a stated population during a stated period of time, usually a year. The rate may be restricted to births to women of specific age, race, marital status, or geographic location (specific rate) or it may be related to the entire population (crude rate). It is calculated by dividing the number of live births in a population in a year by the mid-year resident population.

Birthweight
Birthweight is the first weight of the newborn obtained after birth.

- Low birthweight is defined as less than 2,500 grams or 5 pounds 8 ounces. *
- Very low birthweight is defined as less than 1,500 grams or 3 pounds 4 ounces. *

Cause-of-Death
Cause-of-death is also known as multiple cause-of-death. For the purpose of national mortality statistics, every death is attributed to one underlying condition, based on information reported on the death certificate and using the international rules for selecting the underlying cause-of-death from the conditions stated on the death certificate. The World Health Organization defines underlying cause-of-death as the disease or injury that initiated the train of events leading directly to death or the circumstances of the accident or violence that produced the fatal injury. Generally, more medical information is reported on death certificates than is directly reflected in the underlying cause of death. The conditions that are not selected as underlying cause of death constitute the nonunderlying cause-of-death.

Cause-of-Death Ranking
Cause-of-death ranking is when selected causes-of death, which are determined to be of public health and medical importance, are tabulated and ranked according to the number of deaths assigned to these causes. The top-ranking causes determine the leading causes of death.

Chronic Condition
A chronic condition refers to any condition lasting 3 months or more or as a condition classified as chronic regardless of its time of onset (for

* Before 1979, low birthweight was defined as 2,500 grams or less and very low birthweight as 1,500 grams or less.

example, diabetes, heart conditions, emphysema, and arthritis).

Chronic Disease
A chronic disease is a disease that has one or more of the following characteristics:

- Is permanent;
- Leaves residual disability;
- Is caused by nonreversible pathological alteration;
- Requires special training of the patient for rehabilitation; or
- May be expected to require a long period of supervision, observation, or care.

Civilian Non-institutionalized Population
Civilian non-institutionalized population is the civilian population not residing in institutions. Institutions include correctional institutions, detention homes, and training schools for juvenile delinquents; homes for the aged and dependent (e.g., nursing homes and convalescent homes); homes for dependent and neglected children; homes and schools for the mentally or physically handicapped; homes for unwed mothers; psychiatric, tuberculosis, and chronic disease hospitals; and residential treatment centers.

Clinical Trial
A clinical trial is a research activity that involves the administration of a test regimen to humans to evaluate its efficacy and safety. The term is subject to wide variation in usage, from the first use in humans without any control treatment to a rigorously designed and executed experiment involving test and control treatments and randomization. Several phases of clinical trials are distinguished:

Phase I trial – The first introduction of a candidate vaccine or a drug into a human population to determine its safety and mode of action.
Phase II trial – Initial trial to examine efficacy usually in 200 to 500 volunteers. Usually, but not

always, subjects are randomly allocated to study and control groups.

Phase III trial – Complete assessment of safety and efficacy. It involves larger numbers, perhaps thousands of volunteers, usually with random allocation to study and control groups, and may be a multicenter trial.

Phase IV trial – Includes research to explore a specific pharmacologic effect, to establish the incidence of adverse reactions, or to determine the effects of long-term use. Ethical review is required for Phase IV clinical trials.

Cohort Study
A cohort study is a longitudinal study of the same group of people over time. Usually the members of a cohort are of approximately the same age.

Communicable Disease
Communicable disease is a disease that can be communicated by infectious agent or its products from an infected person, animal, or reservoir to a susceptible host.

Comparability Ratios
Comparability ratios measure the effect of changes in classification and coding rules. About every 10–20 years the International Classification of Diseases [9] is revised to stay abreast with advances in medical science and changes in medical terminology. Each of these revisions produces breaks in the continuity of cause-of-death statistics. Discontinuities across revisions are due to changes in classification and rules for selecting underlying cause of death. Classification and rule changes impact cause-of-death trend data by shifting deaths away from some cause-of-death categories and into others.

Death Rate
A death rate is calculated by dividing the number of deaths in a population in a year by the mid-year resident population. For census years, rates are based on unrounded census counts of

the resident population, as of April 1. For the noncensus years of 1981–1989 and 1991, rates are based on national estimates of the resident population, as of July 1, rounded to 1,000s. Population estimates for 10-year age groups are generated by summing unrounded population estimates before rounding to 1,000s. Starting in 1992, rates are based on unrounded national population estimates. Rates for the Hispanic and non-Hispanic white populations in each year are based on unrounded state population estimates for states in the Hispanic reporting area. Death rates are expressed as the number of deaths per 100,000 population. The rate may be restricted to deaths in specific age, race, sex, or geographic groups or from specific causes of death (specific rate) or it may be related to the entire population (crude rate).

Demography
Demography is the study of human populations, particularly with respect to births, marriages, deaths, employment, migration, and health.

Disability
Disability is a general term that refers to any long- or short-term reduction of a person's activity as a result of an acute or chronic condition.

Disease Classification
The International Classification of Diseases (ICD) [10] provides the ground rules for disease classification. The ICD is developed collaboratively through the World Health Organization and 10 international centers, one of which is housed at National Center for Health Statistics located in Hyattsville, Maryland. The purpose of the ICD is to promote international comparability in the collection, classification, processing, and presentation of health statistics. Since the beginning of the century, the ICD has been modified about once every 10 years, except for the 20-year interval between ICD-9 and ICD-10.

Epidemic

An epidemic is the occurrence of an illness, specific health-related behavior, or other health-related event(s) that is prevalent and rapidly spreading among many individuals in a community or region at the same time and clearly in excess of normal expectancy.

Epidemiology

Epidemiology is the branch of medicine that investigates all the elements contributing to the occurrence or nonoccurrence of a disease, specific health-related behavior, or other health-related events in a population, and the application of this study to the control of health problems.

Ethnic Group

An ethnic group is a designation of a population subgroup having a common cultural heritage, as distinguished by customs, characteristics, language, and common history. Members of the group have distinctive features in their way of life, shared experiences, and often a common genetic heritage.

Ethnicity/Race

In 1977, the Office of Management and Budget issued standards for ethnicity/race for federal government statistics and administrative reporting in order to promote comparability of data among federal data systems. The 1977 standards called for the federal government's data systems to classify individuals into the following four racial groups: American Indian or Alaska Native, Asian or Pacific Islander, Black, and White. Depending on the data source, the classification by race was based on self-classification or on observation by an interviewer or other person filling out the questionnaire. In 1997, new standards were announced for classification of individuals by race within the federal government's data systems. The 1997 standards have five racial groups: American Indian or Alaska

Native, Asian, Black or African American, Native Hawaiian or other Pacific Islander, and White. These five categories are the minimum set for data on race for federal statistics. The 1997 standards also offer an opportunity for respondents to select more than one of the five groups, leading to many possible multiple race categories. As with the single race groups, data for the multiple race groups are to be reported when estimates meet agency requirements for reliability and confidentiality. The 1997 standards allow for observer or proxy identification of race but clearly state a preference for self-classification. The federal government considers race and Hispanic origin to be two separate and distinct concepts. Thus, Hispanics may be of any race. Federal data systems are required to comply with the 1997 standards by 2003.

Fertility Rate

Fertility rate is the total number of live births, regardless of age of mother, per 1,000 women of reproductive age, 15–44 years.

Fetal Death Rate

A fetal death rate is the number of fetal deaths with stated or presumed gestation of 20 weeks or more divided by the sum of live births plus fetal deaths, stated per 1,000 live births plus fetal deaths.

Geographic Regions

The 50 states and the District of Columbia are grouped for statistical purposes by the U.S. Census Bureau into four geographic regions and nine divisions. The groupings are as follows: **Northeast**: New England: Maine, New Hampshire, Vermont, Massachusetts, Rhode Island, and Connecticut.
Middle Atlantic: New York, New Jersey, and Pennsylvania.
Midwest
East North Central: Ohio, Indiana, Illinois, Michigan, and Wisconsin.

	West North Central: Minnesota, Iowa, Missouri, North Dakota, South Dakota, Nebraska, and Kansas. **South** **South Atlantic**: Delaware, Maryland, District of Columbia, Virginia, West Virginia, North Carolina, South Carolina, Georgia, and Florida. **East South Central:** Kentucky, Tennessee, Alabama, and Mississippi. **West South Central**: Arkansas, Louisiana, Oklahoma, and Texas. **West** **Mountain**: Montana, Idaho, Wyoming, Colorado, New Mexico, Arizona, Utah, and Nevada. **Pacific**: Washington, Oregon, California, Alaska, and Hawaii.
Health Facilities	Collectively, all buildings and facilities used in the provision of health services.
Health Manpower	Health manpower is the collective of all men and women working in the provision of health services whether as an individual practitioner or as employees of health institutions and programs, whether or not professionally trained, and whether or not subject to public regulation. Facilities and manpower are the principal health resources used in producing health services.
Health Resources	Health resources are the resources (human, monetary, or material) used in producing health care and services.
Health Statistics	Health statistics are the aggregated data describing and enumerating attributes, events, behaviors, services, resources, outcomes, or costs related to health, disease, and health services. The data may be derived from survey instruments, medical records, and administrative documents. Vital statistics are a subset of health statistics.

Health Status   Health status is a measure of the nature and extent of disease, disability, discomfort, attitudes, and knowledge concerning health and of the perceived need for health care. Health status measures identify groups in need of, or at risk of needing, services.

Hispanic Origin   Hispanic origin includes persons of Mexican, Puerto Rican, Cuban, Central and South American, and other or unknown Latin American or Spanish origins. Persons of Hispanic origin may be of any race.

Hospice Care   Hospice care as defined by the National Home and Hospice Care Survey is a program of palliative and supportive care services providing physical, psychological, social, and spiritual care for dying persons, their families, and other loved ones. Hospice services are available in home and in-patient settings.

Incidence   Incidence is the number of cases of disease having their onset during a prescribed period of time. It is often expressed as a rate (e.g., the incidence of measles per 1,000 children 5–15 years of age during a specified year). Incidence is a measure of morbidity or other events that occur within a specified period of time.

Incidence Rate   Incidence rate is a rate expressing the number of new events or new cases of a disease in a defined population at risk, within a specified period of time. It is usually expressed as cases per 1,000 or 100,000 per annum.

Incubation Period   The incubation period is the time interval between invasion by an infectious agent and appearance of the first sign or symptom of the disease in question.

Instrumental Activities
of Daily Living   Instrumental activities of daily living (IADL) are activities related to independent living and

257

include preparing meals, managing money, shopping for groceries or personal items, performing light or heavy housework, and using a telephone.

Leading Health Indicators

The Leading Health Indicators are used to measure the health of the nation over the next 10 years. Each of the 10 Leading Health Indicators has one or more objectives from Healthy People 2010 [11] associated with it. As a group, the Leading Health Indicators reflect the major health concerns in the United States at the beginning of the twenty-first century. The Leading Health Indicators were selected on the basis of their ability to motivate action, the availability of data to measure progress, and their importance as public health issues. The Leading Health Indicators are physical activity, overweight and obesity, tobacco use, substance abuse, responsible sexual behavior, mental health, injury and violence, environmental quality, immunization, and access to health care.

Life Expectancy

Life expectancy is the average number of years of life remaining to a person at a particular age and is based on a given set of age-specific death rates, generally the mortality conditions existing in the period mentioned. Life expectancy may be determined by race, sex, or other characteristics using age-specific death rates for the population with that characteristic.

Life Table

A life table provides a comprehensive measure of the effect of mortality on life expectancy. It is composed of sets of values showing the mortality experience of a hypothetical group of infants born at the same time and subject throughout their lifetime to the age-specific mortality rates of a particular time period, usually a given year.

Meta-analysis

Meta-analysis refers to the analysis of analyses, that is, the statistical analysis of a large collection of analysis results from individual studies for the purpose of integrating the findings.

Metropolitan
Statistical Areas

The U.S. Office of Management and Budget defines metropolitan areas according to published standards that are applied to U.S. Census Bureau data. The collective term "metropolitan area" includes metropolitan statistical areas (MSAs), consolidated metropolitan statistical areas (CMSAs), and primary metropolitan statistical areas (PMSAs). An MSA is a county or group of contiguous counties that contains at least one city with a population of 50,000 or more or a Census Bureau-defined urbanized area of at least 50,000 with a metropolitan population of at least 100,000. In addition to the county or counties that contain all or part of the main city or urbanized area, an MSA may contain other counties that are metropolitan in character and are economically and socially integrated with the main city. If an MSA has a population of 1 million or more and meets requirements specified in the standards, it is termed a CMSA, consisting of two or more major components, each of which is recognized as a PMSA. In New England, cities and towns, rather than counties, are used to define MSAs. Counties that are not within an MSA are considered to be nonmetropolitan.

Morbidity

Morbidity is any departure, subjective or objective, from a state of physiological or psychological well-being. In this sense, sickness, illness, and morbid condition are similarly defined and synonymous. Morbidity is usually stated in terms of incidence rate and prevalence rate.

259

Mortality Rate

Mortality rate is the number of deaths occurring in a population during a given period of time, usually a year, as a proportion of the number in the population. Usually the mortality rate includes deaths from all causes and is expressed as deaths per 1,000. Also referred to as death rate.

Natality Rate

The natality rate is calculated by dividing the number of live births in a population in a year by the mid-year resident population. For census years, rates are based on unrounded census counts of the resident population, as of April 1. For the noncensus years of 1981–1989 and 1991, rates are based on national estimates of the resident population, as of July 1, rounded to 1,000s. Population estimates for 5-year age groups are generated by summing unrounded population estimates before rounding to 1,000s. Starting in 1992, rates are based on unrounded national population estimates. Birth rates are expressed as the number of live births per 1,000 population. The rate may be restricted to births to women of specific age, race, marital status, or geographic location (specific rate), or it may be related to the entire population (crude rate).

National Health
Expenditures

National health expenditures estimate the amount spent for all health services and supplies and health-related research and construction activities consumed in the United States during the calendar year. Detailed estimates are available by source of expenditures (e.g., out-of-pocket payments, private health insurance, and government programs), type of expenditures (e.g., hospital care, physician services, and drugs), and are in current dollars for the year of report. Data are compiled from a variety of sources.

Notifiable Disease	A notifiable disease is one that, when diagnosed, health providers are required, usually by law, to report to state or local public health officials. Notifiable diseases are those of public interest by reason of their contagiousness, severity, or frequency.
Occupancy Rate	The American Hospital Association defines hospital occupancy rate as the average daily census divided by the average number of hospital beds during a reporting period. Average daily census is defined by the American Hospital Association as the average number of in-patients, excluding newborns, receiving care each day during a reporting period. The occupancy rate for facilities other than hospitals is calculated as the number of residents reported at the time of the interview divided by the number of beds reported. In the CMS administrative Medicare and Medicaid Online Survey Certification and Reporting database, occupancy is the total number of residents on the day of certification inspection divided by the total number of beds on the day of certification.
Over Sample	An over sample procedure is designed to give a demographic or geographic population a larger proportion of representation in the sample than the population's proportion of representation in the overall population.
Parity	Parity is defined as the total number of live births ever had by a woman.
Population	Population is the number of inhabitants of a given country or area but also, in sampling, the whole collection of units from which a sample may be drawn. A population is not necessarily composed of persons and its units may be institutions, records, or events. The sample is intended to give results that are representative of

the whole population. The U.S. Census Bureau of the Census collects and publishes data on populations in the United States according to several different definitions. Various statistical systems then use the appropriate population for calculating rates.

Prevalence/Prevalence
Rate

Prevalence/prevalence rate is the number of cases of a disease, infected persons, or persons with some other attribute present during a particular interval of time divided by the population at risk of having the attribute or disease at this point in time or midway through the period.

Randomized Control Trial

A randomized control trial is an epidemiologic experiment in which subjects in a population are randomly allocated into groups, usually called study and control groups, to receive or not to receive an experimental preventive or therapeutic procedure, maneuver, or intervention.

Rate

Rate is a measure of the frequency of occurrence of a phenomenon in a defined population in a specified period of time. All rates are ratios, calculated by dividing a numerator (the number of events in specified time) by the denominator (the average population during the period), and multiplied by 10 to remove decimals.

Getting Started on the Search for Health Statistics

11.9 *National Center for Health Statistics.* Hyattsville, MD: U.S. Department of Health and Human Services, Centers for Disease Control and Prevention, National Center for Health Statistics. Available: www.cdc.gov/nchs.

The Internet provides a burgeoning resource of health statistics and data sets. A good place to begin is the Centers for Disease Control and

Prevention's National Center for Health Statistics (NCHS) home page. As the nation's principal statistical organization, NCHS provides national leadership in health statistics and epidemiology, collecting, analyzing, and disseminating national health statistics on vital events and health activities, including the physical, mental, and physiological characteristics of the United States population. Changes in the health status of people and environmental, social, and other health hazards are noted and statistically documented. Data are also collected, analyzed, and disseminated as national health statistics on illness, injury, impairment, the supply and utilization of health facilities and manpower, health costs and expenditures, and the operation of the health services system. The National Center for Health Statistics also administers the Cooperative Health Statistics System, stimulating and conducting basic and applied research in health data systems and statistical methodology.

The National Center for Health Statistics has two major types of data systems: systems based on populations, containing data collected through personal interviews or examinations; and systems based on records, containing data collected from vital and medical records. Some are ongoing annual systems whereas others are periodically conducted. The current data systems and surveys are:

- *National Vital Statistics System* (*NVSS*): Responsible for the Nation's official vital statistics. These vital statistics are provided through State-operated registration systems recording births, deaths, marriages, divorces, and fetal deaths.
- *National Health Interview Survey* (*NHIS*): The principal source of information on the health of the civilian noninstitutionalized population of the United States.
- *National Health and Nutrition Examination Survey* (*NHANES*): Based on laboratory and examination centers that move around the United States to obtain standardized medical information from direct physical exams, diagnostic procedures, and lab tests, this survey monitors trends in the prevalence, awareness, treatment, and control of selected diseases, trends in risk behaviors and environmental

exposure, and studies the relationship between diet, nutrition, and health.

- *National Health Care Survey* (*NHCS*): Covers a family of health care provider surveys to obtain information about the facilities that supply health care, the services rendered, and the characteristics of the patients served. Each survey is based on a multistage sampling design that includes health care facilities or providers and patient records. Data are collected directly from the establishments and/or their records rather than from the patients. These data identify health care events such as hospitalizations, surgeries, and long-term stays and offer the most accurate and detailed information on diagnosis and treatment as well as on the characteristics of the institutions. To mention a few applications of this survey information, these data are used by policymakers, planners, researchers, and others in the health community to monitor changes in the use of health care resources, to monitor specific diseases, and to examine the impact of new medical technologies.

11.10 *FASTSTATS A to Z.* Hyattsville, MD: U.S. Department of Health and Human Services, Centers for Disease Control and Prevention, National Center for Health Statistics. Available: www.cdc.gov /nchs/fastats/default.htm.

11.11 *CDC Wonder.* Atlanta, GA: U.S. Department of Health and Human Services, Centers for Disease Control and Prevention. Available: http://wonder.cdc.gov/#LogonAdvantage.

11.12 *Web-based Injury Statistics Query and Reporting System (WISQARS).* Atlanta, GA: U.S. Department of Health and Human Services, Centers for Disease Control and Prevention, National Center for Injury Prevention and Control. Available: www.cdc.gov/ncipc/wisqars/default.htm.

11.13 *National Center for Health Statistics—Other Sites.* Hyattsville, MD: U.S. Department of Health and Human Services, Centers for

Disease Control and Prevention. Available: www.cdc.gov /nchs/sites.htm.

11.14 *Statistical Resources on the Web.* Ann Arbor, MI: University of Michigan Documents Center. Available: www.lib.umich.edu /govdocs/stats.html.

The NCHS Web site provides a rich source of information about America's health. Users of the NCHS Web site can choose several avenues to access data on topics such as Births (Natality), Deaths (Mortality), Health Care Availability and Access, Aging, Women's Health, Immunizations, Marriage and Divorce, Contraception and Infertility, and Home and Hospice Care. The most frequently used method to access data on the NCHS Web is through FASTATS A to Z. FASTATS is a rich source of quick statistics organized topically. Each topic page contains commonly requested statistics and links to other sites (including those outside NCHS) that contain similar statistical information on that specific topic.

In addition to its own data sources, the NCHS Web site provides access to other CDC statistical resources, for example: CDC WONDER, which serves as a single point of access to a wide variety of CDC reports, guidelines, and numeric public health data; and WISQARS, the searchable site for injury deaths and death rates. The National Center for Health Statistics also provides a page of links to other statistical sources on the Web. The links are organized by topical area and represent the major areas in which health and medical statistics are being sought. Another excellent portal to Internet resources is the University of Michigan Document Center's Statistical Resources on the Web. This mature site includes a page of health statistics links to government and private Web sites. The links are well annotated with highlights about each site's content and coverage as well as useful tips on locating and using data from these sources. Additional pages of interest at the University of Michigan Web site cover other statistical topics related to health, including demographics, economics and finances, environment, education ,and sociology.

Other helpful tools for the health sciences reference librarian are:

11.15 Weise FO, ed. *Health Statistics: An Annotated Bibliographic Guide to Information Resources*, 2nd ed. Lanham, MD: Medical Library Association and Scarecrow, 1996.

Weise's guide to health statistical resources is a comprehensive review of print publications available at that time. Eight major chapters cover the leading topical areas of health statistics in considerable detail. A glossary of health statistics terms is also provided. This is a valuable guidebook not only because print resources are essential for most historical and trend data analyses, but also because many of these publishers may now offer datasets and/or comparable publications on the Internet.

11.16 Melnick D. *Finding and Using Health Statistics: A Self-Study Course*. Bethesda, MD: National Library of Medicine, October 2000. Available: www.nlm.nih.gov/nichsr/usestats/index.htm.

This Powerpoint self-study program introduces health statistics sources to librarians and other researchers. The course covers the major health statistical resources with an emphasis on Internet availability. The resources are given context through explanations about the goals of various data collection efforts of organizations and government entities. The course also describes what library users need, how statistics are commonly used, and the limitations of standard reference tools. There is introductory material on assessing the benefits and limitations of statistics search results. Fifteen practice exercises are given at the end of the program. This independent study program is easy to use and organized to allow the student to navigate through the presentation according to interests and knowledge level.

General and Health Statistics

11.17 *Statistical Abstract of the United States*. Washington, DC: U.S. Census Bureau (for sale by the National Technical Information

Service, Springfield, VA), 2002. Annual. Available: http://purl
.access.gpo.gov/GPO/LPS2878

First published in 1878, *Statistical Abstract* is the leading, authoritative reference source for U.S. statistical information. The breadth and scope of information makes this reference tool the first place to look for many statistical questions. It is also readily available or accessible from every type of library. While primarily a compilation of federal statistics, *Statistical Abstract* does also include information from the private sector. The focus is on national data although some state and local information is provided.

The *Statistical Abstract* contains both primary and secondary statistical information. All tables have explanatory footnotes and source information, so further detail can usually be found. The statistics may be several years old but should be considered the most current available at the time of publication.

Statistical data are presented under broad subject categories, and subject access is further augmented by a good subject index. Statistics of particular interest to health sciences librarians include population data, vital statistics, national health costs by type of expenditure, health resource utilization data, and selected national nutrition information. Also related to health care are national statistics on education and income levels and environmental quality measures.

The *Statistical Abstract* is available in print, on CD-ROM, and at the U.S. Census Bureau Web site. Not all data tables from private sources are published on the Web site.

11.18 *FedStats*. Available: www.fedstats.gov.

This Web site serves as a portal to federal statistics that are published by more than 100 U.S. federal agencies. The statistical coverage is broad, including economic and population trends, education, aviation safety, foreign trade, energy, and farm production. However, considerable health statistics data can be reached through this site. Quick subject access to FedStats' Web site links is available through a Topics A-Z index. The site is also directly searchable by program or subject area, agency, and geographical area.

11.19 *Health: United States.* Washington, DC: Centers for Disease Control and Prevention, National Center for Health Statistics, 2002. Available: www.cdc.gov/nchs/hus.htm. Annual.

An annual first published in 1975–1976, *Health, United States* is one of the few sources providing trend data on the nation's health status and other health care topics. It presents national trends in health statistics. Trend table topics include Population; Fertility and Natality; Mortality Determinants and Measures of Health; Ambulatory Care; Inpatient Care, Personnel and Facilities; National Health Expenditures; Health Care Coverage and Major Federal Programs; and State Health Expenditures and Health Insurance. Each annual volume includes a chartbook that examines a current topic of interest. The 2002 volume includes a chartbook on "Trends in the Health of Americans." A copy of the printed volume is available in PDF format on the NCHS Web site. Links to updated trend tables and errata are posted with the PDF version. All volumes are available in PDF format on the NCHS Web and on CD-ROM.

11.20 Melnick D, Rouse B, eds. *Portrait of Health in the United States,* 1st ed. Lanham, MD: Bernan, 2001.

This is a good example from among the many newer secondary heath statistical reference books, which serve as compilations of health data. The editors of this *Portrait* provide statistical data and interpretative narrative on both physical and mental health as measured by a wide range of factors. The chapter introductions are very informative, explaining scope and meaning of various health categories and indicators. Many charts are included that illustrate datasets and trends, such as the leading causes of death by age group and the cancer survival rates during the last few decades by type of cancer. While the intention is to draw a national overview, regional and state data are included.

The chapters cover health care correlates, which include factors such as environment or nutrition that influence disease and wellness; health conditions; health care delivery and access; and the consequences of health status on individuals, society, and the economy. Data are presented to enable comparisons between groups. While the tables and charts may not always present the exact comparisons being sought, source information and footnotes are provided to allow further research. Sources for the statistical data are diverse and include self-perceived health status reports to more formal measures such as medical diagnosis, hospitalization, and death rates. There is a very helpful final chapter on how to find more health statistics at libraries and on the Internet.

11.21 Darnay AJ, ed. *Statistical Record of Health and Medicine*, 2nd ed. Detroit, MI: Gale Research, 1998.

Gale has a strong record of producing valuable reference tools for libraries. The *Statistical Record* is no exception. It is a well-organized and easy to use compilation of health and medical statistics from government and private sources. Topics covered are the health status and lifestyles of Americans, the health care establishment, health in the workplace, health expenditures, health care programs, the health care professions, and medical practices and procedures. There is some miscellaneous information, difficult to locate in other sources, under a section entitled "Politics, Opinions and Law." The final chapter is a summary section of international rankings and comparisons.

11.22 *Historical Statistics of the United States: Colonial Times to 1970.* 2 vols. Washington, DC: U.S. Census Bureau, 1975.

Published as part of the bicentennial celebration, this most recent edition of *Historical Statistics* serves as a supplement to the annual *Statistical Abstract of the United States. Historical Statistics* has a wealth of information and its references are a rich resource for locating primary historical data. As in *Statistical Abstract,* the statistical data are drawn primarily from U.S. government sources but also from private organizations and individuals. In general, only annual or census period data are included. Statistics are national with only occasional data shown for regions, states, and local areas.

The challenges in compiling statistical summaries are compounded when dealing with historical data. The variations over time and by resource in data availability, data collection methods, sampling approaches, concepts and/or levels of coverage, and definitions of geographic regions and categories are just a few of the changes over the years. To aid in understanding the data, each major section in *Historical*

Statistics has an introductory narrative and discussion of the data sources. This information is essential to interpreting the statistical data presented in the tables. It is also a rich resource for locating primary historical data sources. Each statistical table also includes the source(s) of the data along with explanatory footnotes, so further analysis and research is possible.

Historical Statistics includes sections on vital statistics, life expectancy and death rates, health and medical care statistics including birth and fertility rates, national health expenditures, health care providers and their educational facilities, disease rates, hospital data, and some general public health trends such as nutrition and water fluoridation. The final chapter on colonial and prefederal statistics is a fascinating review of contemporary issues, focusing primarily on population, trade, and commerce data.

Databases

Full-text databases, such as Statistical Universe and the Cochrane Library, provide access to primary and secondary resources. PubMed, a bibliographic database, leads the searcher to a wealth of statistical information published within the context of the medical and research literature.

11.23 *PubMed.* Bethesda, MD: National Library of Medicine. Available: http://pubmed.gov.

11.24 *Health Services and Sciences Research Resources (HSRR).* Bethesda, MD: National Library of Medicine. Available: www.nlm.nih.gov/nichsr/hsrr_search.

PubMed is the leading search tool for the National Library of Medicine's MEDLINE database. Citations of articles published in the major health sciences statistical journals can be obtained through a PubMed search. In addition, references to research reports published in the medical literature and containing statistical data can be retrieved through PubMed. Major *Medical Subject Headings* (*MeSH*) such as Infant Mortality or Life Expectancy retrieve general articles on these statistical topics. For more precise search results related to particular topics or diseases, the searcher should use PubMed's statistical sub-headings attached to major *MeSH* term(s). These subheadings include: economics; epidemiology; ethnology; manpower; mortality; statistics and numerical data; supply and distribution; trends; and utilization.

PubMed also provides Clinical Queries and Systematic Reviews filters to assist in retrieving statistical data from clinical trial reports and the EBM literature. These filters can be applied during a search of a broader subject heading, such as Breast Neoplasms, using one or more of the four major disease-related subheadings: etiology, diagnosis, therapy, and prognosis. The searcher can optimize these search filters for sensitivity (recall) or specificity (precision) and retrieve references to systematic reviews, meta-analysis studies, randomized controlled trials, cohort studies, and other case-controlled studies related to the topic and subheading(s) selected.

A newly developing searchable database at NLM, currently presented as a stand-alone product, is Health Services and Sciences Research Resources (HSRR). Health Services and Sciences Research Resources contains information about research datasets and instruments employed in health services research as well as the behavioral and social sciences.

11.25 *The Cochrane Library (Cochrane Database of Systematic Reviews).* The Cochrane Collaboration. Available: www.update-software.com/Cochrane/default.HTM.

While the Cochrane Library is a literature search tool and not a source for statistics per se, it is included in this chapter on statistics because it serves as the primary gateway to reports on clinical trials, systematic reviews, and meta-analyses of clinical data. It is the leading source for identifying EBM literature and thus for learning about the Cochrane Collaboration's approach to evaluating clinical outcomes and data published in the literature and their approach to performing systematic reviews.

The Cochrane Collaboration (www.cochrane.org) is an international not-for-profit organization whose purpose is to identify and make available the evidence-based literature. The primary product is a database of systematic reviews and controlled clinical trials register,

The Cochrane Database of Systematic Reviews, which is published electronically and available by subscription to the Cochrane Library. The collection of articles is relatively small, with approximately 1,500 complete reviews and 350,000 references. These resources can be searched using the same *MeSH* headings as suggested in the PubMed section, although subheadings cannot be applied.

The highly regarded Cochrane Collaboration prepares and maintains its database through a group of volunteer health care professionals worldwide who work in one of the more than 40 Collaborative Review Groups. The review groups prepare and maintain the Cochrane reviews, working in various specialty areas and collectively covering the major areas of health care. The groups compile systematic reviews of randomized controlled trials (RCTs) that have been published in the current literature. The goal is to make the evidence-based literature more widely known by highlighting the up-to-date evidence relevant to the prevention, treatment, and rehabilitation of health problems.

11.26 *Lexis-Nexis Statistical Universe.* Dayton, OH: Lexis-Nexis Group. Available: www.lexisnexis.com.

While the availability of this commercial database is usually limited to larger libraries, it is nonetheless useful for health sciences librarians to be aware that Statistical Universe offers the most comprehensive online searching of statistics. Statistical reports and abstracts from federal, state, and private sources are indexed and accessible through Statistical Universe. The service provides for a single search of three Congressional Information Services statistical indexes including American Statistics Index, which covers all federal statistical publications from 1973 forward, Statistical Reference Index, which indexes state and private statistical resources from 1980 to date, and the Index to International Statistics, whose coverage begins in 1983. Searching options include by simple keyword, Boolean operators, and by comparative data. Retrievals include tables, content within tables, and full-text material.

Demographics

11.27 *U.S. Census Bureau.* Washington, DC: U.S. Department of Commerce, U.S. Census Bureau. Available: www.census.gov.

The U.S. Census Bureau is the gold standard for U.S. demographic data. The U.S. Census is conducted every 10 years; data releases from the 2000 census are ongoing. The Census serves as the nation's official demographic record, guiding decisions in local, state, and federal governments related to changing population trends such as for funding and other federal assistance, for legislative reapportionment, and for construction projects. The Census covers major population data, demographic profiles, and generally each decennial survey includes several special topics of interest.

The Census Web site provides a wide range of data, from national and international up-to-the-minute population totals ("Population Clock") to extensive state and county level data. The site is updated almost daily with newly released reports on topics such as fathers or grandparents as caregivers, children without health care, and industry statistics. Many of the U.S. Census Bureau's classic publications, including *Statistical Abstract of the United States*, are available from the Web site, along with older editions, but currently only in PDF format. An A–Z subject index is a link off the Census Bureau home page, providing visitors with assistance in navigating the site. The Gateway to Census 2000 page provides access to the most current population data and analytical reports. Among the searchable functions at the Web site are the Census 2000 Demographic Profiles where a specific city or county can be entered to obtain a detailed report of demographic and social characteristics, such as age, race, income, major industries, and so forth. Also noteworthy for health sciences librarians is the disability statistics information (Available: www.census.gov/hhes/www/disability.html).

11.28 Heaton TB, Chadwick BA, Jacobson CK. *Statistical Handbook on Racial Groups in the United States.* Phoenix, AZ: Oryx, 2000.

There are numerous specialized resources for demographic data about minority and ethnic groups. Web sites of government agencies and advocacy groups are good sources. This handbook provides a convenient, readily available compilation of demographic data on racial groups represented in U.S. populations. Current and some historical data are included as well as growth projections. Each major section has an introductory text, which aids in interpretation of the tables. Major sections cover demographics; education; economics and employment; health, well-being, and lifestyles; family; sex, fertility, and contraception; religion; crime and delinquency; and political participation.

Health Care Facilities

11.29 American Hospital Association. *Hospital Statistics.* Chicago: Health Forum, 2003. Available: www.AHAData.com.

Under slightly varying titles for more than 50 years, the American Hospital Association (AHA) has published an annual compilation of hospital statistics. The statistics are derived from AHA's annual survey of its accredited hospitals and are presented at the aggregate level. *Hospital Statistics* is the leading source for data on trends, current marketplace issues, and comparative hospital services. The statistical tables are presented to allow comparisons at local, state, and national levels as well as by hospital bed size. Information is provided on such categories as hospital utilization rates, staffing, physician and hospital organization structures, and hospital finances. The availability of various specialized hospital services, such as hemodialysis, emergency departments, and so forth, is reported in regional and state groupings. In some categories, historical trend data are provided.

Hospital Statistics is published in print and on CD-ROM. The AHAData Web site is also available for online searching and provides for fee-based customized queries and reports. An AHAData search accesses the most recent set of *Hospital Statistics* data as well as information from AHA's Health Care Networks and Systems Research, the AHA Complimentary and Alternative Medicine Survey, the U.S. Centers for Medicare and Medicaid Services (CMS) health care provider data, and the CMS Healthcare Cost Report Information System.

Health Education Statistics

11.30 *Bureau of Health Professions.* Rockville, MD: U.S. Health Resources and Services Administration, Bureau of Health Professions. Available: http://bhpr.hrsa.gov.

Medical education statistics have been well-covered historically by several sources. However, statistics about educational programs in the nursing, dental, and allied health education programs have irregularly been produced over time by their professional societies. Currently, the most consistent resources for these data are the U.S. National Center for Health Statistics Web site (see 11.9, above) and the U.S. Health Resources and Services Administration Bureau of Health Professions Web site.

11.31 *AAMC Data Book: Statistical Information Related to Medical Schools and Teaching Hospitals.* Washington, DC: AAMC, 2002. Annual. Available: www.aamc.org.

The Association of American Medical Colleges (AAMC) publishes an annual compilation of statistics about medical education programs at accredited medical schools and teaching hospitals. The AAMC *Data Book* draws its information from the AAMC and also from other government and educational sources, all of which are noted on each table. In addition to the print version, a Web subscription is available which provides access to up-to-date information as it becomes available during the year.

The *AAMC Data Book* covers 12 topics: accredited medical schools, medical school applicants and students, faculty, financing medical schools and student financing, graduate medical education, teaching hospitals, health care financing, biomedical research, physician services, faculty and physician compensation, and general statistical information. Examples of statistics about medical students are mean admission test scores, enrollment demographics, and specialty and geographic location choices of graduating seniors. Faculty characteristics and distribution by academic department are tabulated, including for full-time, part-time, and volunteer faculty members. Medical school and student financial data is included. Teaching hospitals are profiled by size, staffing characteristics, utilization rates, and finances. There is a small amount of information about graduate medical education, biomedical research, and national health care financing that is relevant to medical education.

11.32 Medical education issue. *JAMA: Journal of the American Medical Association.* Chicago, IL: American Medical Association. Published annually in August or September. Available: www.jama.com.

Since the early 1900s, this annual *JAMA* issue has contained extensive statistical data on undergraduate and graduate medical education. Much of the undergraduate data is drawn from surveys by the joint American Medical Association–Association of American Medical Colleges medical school accrediting committee, called the Liaison Committee on Medical Education. Statistics describe medical school faculty, medical school students, applicants, and characteristics of the applicant pool. Each year, topics of special interest are also included in the survey. A recent issue, for example, included data on the frequency of students being on call at night during clinical clerkships. The graduate medical education report is a more recent addition and includes survey data from accredited graduate medical education programs. Specialty and subspecialty programs are reported, along with information about residents by ethnicity, gender, and geographic location. This issue of *JAMA* also typically includes other articles about medical education topics.

11.33 *Nursing Data Review 2002.* New York: National League for Nursing, 1985–1997, 2003–. Available: www.nln.org.

11.34 *Nursing Educators 2002.* New York: National League for Nursing, 2003. Available: www.nln.org. (Formerly part of *Nursing Data Review.*)

The National League for Nursing tracks nursing education statistics. After a hiatus in publishing, these statistics are becoming available once again. The *Nursing Data Review* analyzes bachelor and graduate degree nursing programs. Statistics and graphs show admission trends and student and graduate student data such as gender, race, ethnicity, and geographic location. The new *Nursing Educators* report is based on a faculty survey of approximately 1,500 nursing schools. Information covers number of faculty and full-time positions by program type; racial, ethnic, geographic, and gender profiles of faculty; faculty degrees and academic ranks; salaries; and recruitment and turnover data.

The NLN Web site makes some excerpts from the *Nursing Data Review* and the *Nursing Educators* report freely available. The National League for Nursing also publishes a variety of one-time reports on the nursing profession and nursing education. An example of a recent report is "Trends in Registered Nurse Education Programs: A Comparison across Three Points in Time—1994, 1999, 2004," which is available at www.nln.org/aboutnln/nursetrends.htm.

Health Manpower

As part of its mission to achieve equitable access to health care professionals across the nation, the Bureau of Health Professions (BHP) in the U.S. Health Resources and Services Administration (see 11.30, above) maintains a wide range of data on health manpower at its Web site. The Bureau of Health Professions conducts its own research studies, data collections, and analyses to assess supply and demand in the health care workforce and to analyze the effects on manpower of changes in the health care system. In addition to statistics provided at the BHP Web site, two tools are offered for more specialized health workforce analysis and forecasting. The Area Resource File (ARF) is a CD-ROM database that includes many variables for each county in the United States. There is also a computer simulation model that enables local forecasting of primary care health care providers.

The Bureau of Health Professions is responsible for designating health manpower shortage geographic areas (HPSAs), Medical Underserved Areas (MUAs), and Medically Underserved Populations (MUPs). These designations provide widely recognized evidence of need and eligibility for specialized federal programs. A Web-based query system also produces current HPSA status of states and geographic regions.

The following resources are also useful for health manpower data:

11.35 *United States Health Workforce Personnel Factbook.* Washington, DC: U.S. Department of Health and Human Services, Health Resources and Services Administration, Bureau of Health Professions, 1998–. Available: http://bhpr.hrsa.gov/healthworkforce/factbook.htm.

The *Health Workforce Personnel Factbook* maintains fairly current information about the health workforce in its publication and on its Web site. Through 71 detailed tables, information is provided about physicians, nurses, dentists, and selected allied health professionals. Data are provided about historical and current health manpower supply trends as well as future projections. Health professionals are profiled through data on current enrollees in health educational institutions, graduates, and the currently employed. Physician-to-population ratios are provided by geographic area and specialty group. Data on the public health workforce are also included along with some health economic data. This factbook is available in print and also in PDF format.

11.36 *Physician Characteristics and Distribution in the U.S.* Chicago, IL: American Medical Association, 1963–. Annual.

11.37 *Access Physician Statistics Now.* Chicago, IL: American Medical Association. Available: www.ama-assn.org/ama/pub/category/2676.htm.

The American Medical Association publishes extensive data summary on physician characteristics for annual comparisons and analyses of the physician population. The statistics are drawn from the AMA's Physician Masterfile, which is derived primarily from survey data but also includes information from other organizational and institutional sources. Each of the five chapters in *Physician Characteristics and Distribution in the U.S.* has a short introductory text with summary findings. Among the physician characteristics that are profiled are age, specialty and board certification, gender, ethnicity, geographic region, and year and school of graduation. The current edition contains new information on women physicians. The physician distribution sections show summary data by state, age, and gender, as well as specialty and activity by location and physician-to-population ratios. Trends in manpower and supply are presented, including projections on physician supply to the year 2020. The book is indexed. If physician information cannot be found in the print version, the AMA can be contacted for specialized data requests.

Access Physician Statistics Now at the AMA Web site contains a limited amount of physician statistical information. The site offers high-level specialty data and selected demographic characteristics about physicians, but has the advantage of being current.

11.38 *The Registered Nurse Population.* Rockville, MD: U.S. Health Resources and Services Administration, Bureau of Health Professions, Office of Data Analysis and Management, 2002. Available: http://purl.access.gpo.gov/GPO/LPS11936.

Beginning in 1977, the HRSA Bureau of Health Professions has conducted seven National Sample Surveys of Registered Nurses. These surveys provide the most comprehensive data about licensed nurses in the United States. Information collected includes numbers of RNs, their educational preparations, current employment status, income, geographical location, gender, race, age, and family status. The full report is available in print; the preliminary report can be accessed online.

Health Utilization and Costs

Utilization rates and costs of health care are covered in many of the general statistical resources. *Health: United States* (see 11.19, above) is particularly useful for this kind of information. Other sources include the following:

11.39 *Vital and Health Statistics.* Hyattsville, MD: U.S. Centers for Disease Control and Prevention, National Center for Health Statistics, 1963. Available: www.cdc.gov/nchs/products/pubs /pubd/series/sr13/ser13.htm.

This series presents statistics on the utilization of health manpower and facilities providing long-term care, ambulatory care, and family planning services. The highest numbers are most recent publications. All volumes of Series 13 are also available in PDF format on the NCHS Web site.

11.40 *Health Care Financing Review.* Washington, DC: U.S. Centers for Medicare and Medicaid Services, vol. 1–, 1979–. Available: http://cms.hhs.gov/review/default.asp.

The *Health Care Financing Review* is the subscription journal of the U.S. Centers for Medicare and Medicaid Services (CMS). The *Review* seeks to improve understanding of the Medicare and Medicaid programs and the U.S health care system by presenting information and analyses on a broad range of health care financing and delivery issues. The journal highlights the results of policy-relevant research and provides a forum for a broad range of viewpoints to stimulate discussion. The target audience includes policymakers, planners, administrators, insurers, researchers, and health care providers. The *Review* appears quarterly, with an additional statistical supplement issue every year, and is indexed by PubMed.

11.41 *Source Book of Health Insurance Data.* Washington, DC: Health Insurance Association of America, 2002.

Published annually, this statistical report of the private health insurance business in the United States provides the latest data on major forms of health insurance, such as hospital, surgical, major medical, disability, physicians' expense, and dental insurance. It also contains information on medical care costs, health manpower in the United States, as well as general morbidity statistics. A large number of tables on health insurance are brought together in this book. No data are supplied for individual companies. The *Source Book* has an index and contains a glossary.

11.42 American Medical Association, Center for Health Policy Research. *Physician Socioeconomic Statistics.* Chicago, IL: AMA, 1999–.

This publication provides a comprehensive overview of the physician marketplace and practice trends with a focus on financial information. The statistics come from the AMA Physician Masterfile including AMA survey data and datasets from the U.S. Centers for

Medicare and Medicaid Services (CMS, formerly HCFA). There is considerable detail given on physician workplace characteristics including practice size, employment status, hours and weeks worked, time in various tasks, hospital utilization, total expenses, professional liability premiums, physician payroll expense, total revenue, net income, Medicare involvement, and managed care involvement. Summary statistics are portrayed for the major specialties. Data on trends in practice size, type of employment (self or group), and income and revenues are helpful in guiding career selections and for benchmarking. Available in print and on CD-ROM.

11.43 American Medical Association, Center for Health Policy Research. *Practice Patterns Series.* Chicago: AMA. (Various dates.)

This series of publications provides very detailed practice and financial information for the five major medical specialty areas. A separate issue covers each of the following: family medicine, internal medicine, obstetrics and gynecology, pediatrics, and surgery. Information includes physician incomes, practice revenues and expenses by category, practice size, hospital utilization, liability premiums, and practice characteristics.

Vital Statistics

Vital statistics are records of life's major milestones. They are systematically tabulated information concerning births, marriages, divorces, separations, and deaths based on registration of these events by various local and national governments. In the United States, the U.S. National Center for Health Statistics tracks these events across the U.S. population through a series of publications, many of which are available and searchable at the NCHS Web site (see 11.9, above). Access to these reports is also possible through PubMed (see 11.23, above) and Statistical Universe (see 11.26, above).

11.44 *Vital Statistics of the United States.* Hyattsville, MD: U.S. Department of Health and Human Services, Centers for Disease Control and Prevention, National Center for Health Statistics,

1937–. Available: www.cdc.gov/nchs/products/pubs/pubd/vsus/vsus.htm.

First published in 1937, *Vital Statistics* is the official record of numbers of U.S. births, deaths, fetal deaths, marriages, and divorces. Consequently, the most current data available are always several years old. The Web site provides historical marriage and divorce data through 1988 and annual compilations of mortality and natality data, with extensive demographic and geographic detail through 1992. Beginning with 1997 mortality and natality data, users can access extensive demographic detailed tables through the NCHS Web site (see 11.9, above).

11.45 *National Vital Statistics Reports.* Hyattsville, MD: U.S. Department of Health and Human Services, Centers for Disease Control and Prevention, National Center for Health Statistics, 1952–. Available: www.cdc.gov/nchs/products/pubs/pubd/mvsr/mvsr.htm.

Formerly *Monthly Vital Statistics Report,* this series provides monthly and cumulative data on vital events (birth, death, marriage, and divorce) with brief analyses. Because each issue carries the same type of information from month to month, the current issue should be a useful tool at any reference desk where vital statistics are in demand.

11.46 *Advance Data from Vital and Health Statistics.* Hyattsville, MD: U.S. Department of Health and Human Services, Centers for Disease Control and Prevention, National Center for Health Statistics, 1976–. Available: www.cdc.gov/nchs/products/pubs/pubd/ad/ad.htm.

These are summary reports that provide the first release of data from NCHS health and demographic surveys. Topics include hospital discharge, ambulatory medical care, adoption, injury statistics, and office visits to physicians.

11.47 Vital and Health Statistics Series. Hyattsville, MD: U.S. Department of Health and Human Services, Centers for Disease Control and Prevention, National Center for Health Statistics, 1963–. Available: www.cdc.gov/nchs/products/pubs/pubd/nvsr/nvsr.htm.

Also known as the "Rainbow Series," these publications include background information, methodology, and analytical studies and presentations of findings from NCHS data collection programs. The various active subseries and areas they cover are listed in Table 11-2. Series information can be located on the NCHS Web site.

Table 11-2. Vital and Health Statistics Series

Series 1   *Programs and Collection Procedures.* Reports describing the general programs of the U.S. National Center for Health Statistics, its offices and divisions and the data collection methods used. Series 1 reports also include definitions and other material necessary for understanding the data.

Series 2   *Data Evaluation and Methods Research.* Studies of new statistical methodology including experimental tests of new survey methods, studies of vital statistics collection methods, new analytical techniques, objective evaluations of reliability of collected data, and contributions to statistical theory. Studies also include comparison of U.S. methodology with those of other countries.

Series 3   *Analytical and Epidemiological Studies.* Analytical or interpretive studies based on vital and health statistics. These reports carry the analyses further than the expository types of reports in the other series.

Series 4   *Documents and Committee Reports.* Final reports of major committees concerned with vital and health statistics and documents such as recommended model vital registration laws and revised birth and death certificates.

Series 5   *Comparative International Vital and Health Statistics Reports.* Analytical and descriptive reports comparing U.S. vital and health statistics with those of other countries.

Series 6   *Cognition and Survey Measurement.* Reports from the National Laboratory for Collaborative Research in Cognition and Survey Measurement using methods of cognitive science to design, evaluate, and test survey instruments.

Series 10   *Data from the National Health Interview Survey.* Statistics on illness, accidental injuries, disability, use of hospital, medical, dental, and other services, and other health-related topics, all based on data collection in the continuing national household survey.

Series 11   *Data from the National Health Examination Survey and the National Health and Nutrition Examination Survey.* Data from direct examination, testing, and measurement of national samples of the civilian noninstitutionalized population provide the basis for estimates of the medically defined prevalence of specific diseases in the United States and the distribution of the population with respect to physical, physiological, and psychological characteristics and analysis of relationships among the various measurements without reference to an explicit finite universe of persons.

Series 12   *Data from the Institutionalized Population Survey.* Discontinued after No. 24.: Reports from the Health Records Survey now appear in Series 13.

Series 13   *Data on Health Resources Utilization.* Statistics on the utilization of health manpower and facilities providing long-term care, ambulatory care, and family planning services.

Series 14   *Data on Health Resources: Manpower and Facilities.* Professional and facilities statistics on the number, geographic distribution, and characteristics of health professionals and facilities.

Series 15   *Data from Special Surveys.* Statistics on health and health-related topics collected in special surveys that are not a part of the continuing data systems of the National Center for Health Statistics.

Series 16   *Compilations of Advance Data from Vital and Health Statistics.* These reports provide early release of data from the health and demographic surveys of the National Center for Health Statistics. Many of these releases are followed by detailed reports in the Vital and Health Statistics series.

Series 20   *Data on Mortality.* Various statistics on mortality other than as included in regular annual or monthly reports. Special analyses by cause of death, age, and other demographic variables; geographic and time series analyses; and statistics on characteristics of death not available from the vital records based on sample surveys of those records.

Series 21   *Data on Natality, Marriage, and Divorce.* Reports of special in-depth analysis of birth, marriage, and divorce data by numerous variables.

Series 22   *Data from the National Mortality and Natality Surveys.* Discontinued after No. 15.: Reports based on sample surveys of death records now appear in Series 20, and those based on sample surveys of birth records now appear in Series 21.

Series 23   *Data from the National Survey of Family Growth.* These reports are based on data collected in periodic surveys of a nationwide probability sample of women 15–44 years of age.

Series 24   *Compilations of Data on Natality, Mortality, Marriage, Divorce, and induced Terminations of Pregnancy.* Advance reports of births, deaths, marriages, and divorces are based on final data from the National Vital Statistics System that were published as special reports to the National Vital Statistics Reports (NVSR). These reports provide highlights and summaries of detailed data subsequently published in annual volumes of Vital Statistics of the United States. Other special reports provide selected findings based on data from the National Vital Statistics System and may be followed by detailed reports in Series 20 or 21.

11.48 *Morbidity and Mortality Weekly Report (MMWR).* Atlanta, GA: Centers for Disease Control and Prevention, 1952–. Available: www.cdc.gov/mmwr//about.html.

Morbidity and Mortality Weekly Report is the leading national publication of up-to-date statistical information on vital statistics, disease outbreaks, and other health incidents occurring both nationally and internationally. It is important to remember that the data in the weekly *MMWR* are provisional, based on weekly reports to CDC by state health departments. The reporting week concludes at close of business on Friday and compiled data on a national basis are officially released to the public during the succeeding week. The full-text of *MMWR* is available electronically at the *MMWR* Web site beginning with volume 31, no. 5, February 12, 1982. An e-mail subscription and alert service is also offered.

In addition to the weekly publication, *MMWR* releases quarterly and annual *Surveillance Summaries* as well as *Recommendations and Reports.* The *Surveillance Summaries,* available at the *MMWR* Web site beginning with volume 32 in 1983, give detailed interpretation of trends and patterns based on surveillance data collected by the CDC. The *Recommendations and Reports* provide updated and in-depth guidelines on prevention and treatment in all health areas related to CDC's scope of responsibility.

State and Local Statistics

11.49 *StatePublicHealth.org.* Washington, DC: Association of State and Territorial Health Officials. Available: www.statepublichealth.org /index.php.

Measures of the public's health are first and foremost local and state data. However, the resources yielding state and local health statistics vary widely. Nearly all states have some level of health statistics on their official state Web site. In addition, the state public health departments, which can be linked to from the State Public Health Web site, often provide statistics. Medical school libraries within a state are also an excellent resource for these statistics because many specialize in collecting health data related to their own states. The U.S. National Center for Health Statistics Web site (see 11.9, above) maintains state data on vital statistics and other major health issues. Additional resources include:

11.50 *State Health Profile.* Atlanta, GA: Centers for Disease Control and Prevention, 1987–. Available: www.cdc.gov/nchs/datawh /stprofiles.htm.

The CDC has published a *State Health Profile* for each state and the District of Columbia annually since 1987. These publications, which aim to consolidate the most current data on the health of the U.S. population by state, can be ordered from the CDC. The profiles include selected information on demographics, prevention and control efforts, and CDC's health care expenditures within the states. These data are also available on the Web site.

11.51 *Health Care State Rankings,* 11th ed. Lawrence, KS: Morgan Quitno Press, 2003.

This annual publication compiles health data from all the states and displays them in rank order. Over 500 tables of state health comparisons are provided which cover the following major categories: birth and reproductive health, deaths, health care facilities, health insurance and finance, disease incidence, health care providers, and physical fitness measures. The tables are easy to use and understand; however, the content is wide-ranging under each of the major categories, requiring familiarity with the resource to anticipate its applicability in a reference inquiry. For example, tables address teen birth rates, births by Caesarian delivery, percentage of mothers not receiving prenatal care, death rate from drugs, in-patient days in community hospitals, persons not covered by insurance, average health care employee pay, and participation in selected sports. The data are drawn from both private and government sources. Based on their annual data compilations, the publishers announce a "Healthiest State" award each year.

The CD-ROM version provides the data in a searchable PDF format as well as in database formats.

11.52 *County and City Data Book,* 13th ed. Washington, DC: U.S. Census Bureau, 2000. Available: http://landview.census.gov /statab/www/ccdb.html.

11.53 *State and Metropolitan Area Data Book: 1997–98,* 5th ed. Washington, DC: U.S. Census Bureau, 1998. Available: http://purl.access.gpo.gov/GPO/LPS2647.

Published as supplements to the *Statistical Abstract of the United States,* these two references provide detailed state and local information. Both include statistics drawn from the latest national census as well as other government and private sources. Therefore, the source material is variable and documentation is provided.

The *County and City Data Book,* published irregularly since 1944, provides official population and housing data as well as other social and economic statistics. Statistics are reported for all U.S. counties, cities with populations of 25,000 or more, and incorporated places with 2,500 or more inhabitants. Health science librarians will find this a useful resource for local demographics, vital and health statistics, birth and death rates, health care practitioner statistics and rates, Medicare enrollment, education, and income and poverty levels.

First published in 1979, the *State and Metropolitan Area Data Book,* although currently somewhat out of date, contains similar information for states and metropolitan areas. Both resources are accessible in PDF format at the U.S. Census Bureau Web site.

11.54 *State Health Workforce Profiles.* Rockville, MD: Health Resources and Services Administration, Bureau of Health Professions, various dates. Available: http://bhpr.hrsa.gov/healthworkforce /profiles/default.htm.

State Health Workforce Profiles are available for all the states at the Bureau of Health Professions Web site. These reports provide current overview information on each state's health status followed by more detailed data describing the health care workforce. Tables, graphs, charts and narrative provide extensive information on more than 25 different categories of health care professionals. Data are presented on supply, demand, distribution, education and use of health personnel. The size of the state's health workforce and per capita ratios facilitate comparisons with other states and the nation. All *State Health Workforce Profiles* can be obtained in print, on CD-ROM, and in PDF format at the BHP Web site.

International Statistics

11.55 *U.S. Department of State.* Washington, DC: U.S. Department of State, Bureau of Public Affairs. Available: www.state.gov.

11.56 *Organization for Economic Cooperation and Development (OECD).* Paris: Organization for Economic Cooperation and Development. Available: www.oecd.org.

11.57 *World Agricultural Information Centre.* Rome: Food and Agricultural Organization of the United Nations. Available: www.fao.org/waicent/portal/statistics_en.asp.

11.58 *UNICEF.* New York: UNICEF. Available: www.unicef.org/statis/.

Numerous Internet sites provide international health data. The major Web sites and print resources are described below. However, the category of the statistics being sought may suggest searches of other more specialized Web sites. For example, the U.S. State Department Web site provides basic population, health, and mortality data for many countries. The Organization for Economic Cooperation and Development (OECD) offers a statistics portal linked from its home page for economic data of its member nations. The Food and Agriculture Organization (FAO) of the United Nations has a searchable statistics gateway page that retrieves reports on topics such as nutrition and pesticide use. UNICEF also has a searchable statistics Web site that provides access to country-specific child health indicators.

As with all statistical data, but particularly with international statistics, it must be emphasized to the library patron that the data sources vary widely, with the result that statistical reports may be inconsistent and incompatible for valid comparative analyses.

11.59 *WHO Statistical Information System (WHOSIS)*. Geneva: World Health Organization. Available: http://www3.who.int/whosis /menu.cfm.

The World Health Organization Web site serves as a major source for international health information and statistical data. The WHOSIS Web site serves as WHO's guide to statistical information. WHOSIS is a developing portal for international statistical and epidemiological information. Many WHO technical programs generate statistical information and these data are being made available through this Web site. Datasets relate to mortality, burden of disease, disease incidence, health personnel, immunizations, health systems performance, and selected areas about topical health issues such as AIDS and current disease outbreaks. The WHOSIS page of Links to National Health-Related Web sites (Available: http://www3.who.int/whosis/national_sites/index.cfm ?path=whosis,national_sites&language=English) leads to health information of many countries, including at their national ministries of health and health statistics offices when available.

11.60 *Weekly Epidemiology Record; Relevé épidémiologique hebdomadaire*. Geneva: World Health Organization, 1926–. Available: www.who.int/wer.

This newsletter is the international reporting mechanism for epidemiological information about disease outbreaks subject to International Health Regulations and other major communicable diseases. Published weekly in a bilingual English and French format, the

Weekly Epidemiology Record (WER) provides a method for rapid communication of newly emerging or reemerging infections and other diseases of public health importance. In addition to outbreak news, the *WER* publishes international health regulations, position statements and recommendations, and other information essential to global surveillance. For example, a recent issue published a reporting template for severe acute respiratory syndrome (SARS) with the goal of standardizing international data collection related to this outbreak.

Electronic access to volume 71, 1996 forward, of the *Weekly Epidemiology Record* is available at the Web site. Additionally, an electronic archive of *WER* issues from 1926 to 1995 is under construction. An e-mail service provides tables of contents and summary information.

11.61 *United Nations Statistics Division.* New York: United Nations. Available: http://unstats.un.org/unsd.

11.62 *Population Information Network.* New York: United Nations. Available: www.un.org/popin.

The U.N. Statistics Division maintains a Web site that provides a wide range of statistical information about U.N. countries. Information is provided about demographics, population and vital statistics, housing, and social indicators and measurements including age distributions of populations, education levels, and employment status. The Statistics Division compiles statistics from many international sources and also works to facilitate data comparability by developing specifications for compiling statistical data. The statistical databases page (Available: http://unstats.un.org/unsd/databases) offers several datasets on social indicators and populations. It also includes links to other national and international data sources. Disability statistics (Available: http://unstats.un.org/unsd/disability/dataset) show incidence of disability by country, although methods of calculating these rates vary widely. The Population Information Network provides population data for countries of the world.

11.63 Pan American Health Organization. *Health in the Americas*. Washington, DC: PAHO, 2002. 2 vols. Available: www.paho.org /English/SHA/profiles.htm.

This publication is considered the authoritative resource for health trends and health data for Central and South America. *Health in the Americas* offers an overview of the health status of the Pan American region, often emphasizing health disparities. Volume 1 includes chapters describing regional health issues, demographics, and mortality trends as well as current sociopolitical factors affecting health, including health reform efforts and environmental and political conditions. Volume 2 provides health data and information by country including an overview, demographics and mortality data, disease incidence, national health plans, policies and organizations, and expenditure information. These data are also available in summary form at the PAHO Basic Country Health Profiles Web site. The main PAHO Web site (Available: www.paho.org) is itself an excellent resource, providing information on diseases endemic to the region as well as health indicators of the various Pan American countries.

11.64 Reddy MA, ed. *Statistical Abstract of the World*, 3rd ed. Detroit, MI: Gale Research, 1997.

Another well-presented Gale reference tool, *Statistical Abstract of the World* needs updating. We hope there will be a new edition. Organized by country and equipped with an extensive keyword index, this reference source provides standard data on 185 countries. Tables are designed in a consistent fashion within each country, and sources of data are provided. Topics of particular interest to health sciences librarians are population data, vital statistics and life expectancies, health manpower and provider-population ratios, health expenditures, infant health indicators, and prevalence of malnutrition.

Health Sciences Library Statistics

It is important to remember that today's academic, hospital, and specialty health sciences libraries operate in a health care environment that emphasizes performance measures and business strategies. To effectively compete for visibility and funding within the organization, the library's contribution to the institution should be documented through both quantitative and qualitative measures. Comparative library data are effective benchmarking indicators for demonstrating a library's successes and its needs. These data can suggest best practices and can also be used to demonstrate one library's performance relative to selected libraries at peer institutions. In addition to sources for comparative statistical resources for libraries, this section includes a guide to library data analysis and library service evaluation.

11.65 *Annual Statistics of Medical School Libraries in the United States and Canada.* Seattle, WA: Association of Academic Health Sciences Libraries, 2002.Available: www.aahsl.org/default home.cfm.

Since 1978, the Association of Academic Health Science Libraries has published an annual compilation of medical school library statistics. Data on library collections, staffing, service utilization, and annual expenditures are reported by library, along with a composite medical school library profile, which suggests benchmarks for the average medical school library. Descriptive information, such as library space allocations and reporting channels, are included every five years. Performance measures and ratios and statistical trends have been included in some years. Because many medical school administrative staffs evaluate their programs by comparing themselves to other schools with comparable missions and characteristics, it is a valuable benchmarking tool. Available in print and electronically, and, for members only, in a Web-based format.

11.66 *The Composite Hospital Library: 2001 Benchmarking Aggregate Data Tables.* Chicago, IL: Medical Library Association, 2002. Available: www.mlanet.org/resources/benchmark/index.html.

The publication is the product of the Medical Library Association's initiative to support hospital library best practices by collecting descriptive and performance statistics about hospital and specialty libraries. *The Composite Hospital Library* profiles twelve typical hospital libraries with representative data on library finances, staffing, collection and resource utilization, and specialized services such as clinical medical librarian and consumer health programs. While all hospital libraries may enter data into the system and purchase the aggregate data tables, use of the Interactive Report Site that generates customized reports is limited to survey participants. Available in print, electronically, and in a Web-based searchable format.

11.67 Burroughs CM. *Measuring the Difference: Guide to Planning and Evaluating Health Information Outreach.* Seattle, WA: National Network of Libraries of Medicine, Pacific Northwest Region; Bethesda, MD: National Library of Medicine, [2000]. Available: www.nnlm.gov/evaluation/guide/frontmatter.pdf.

This manual is not a source of statistical information itself but rather is a step-by-step approach to generating credible library program performance measurements. Although focused on methods to assess the effectiveness of library outreach programs, this introduction to program evaluation provides a useful framework for all library services. Topics covered include conducting a community assessment, developing goals and measurable objectives, planning the program activities and strategies, planning the evaluation approach, gathering and analyzing data, and utilizing and reporting the results.

And, by now you know where to find the answers to these questions:

1. *How many HMO's are there in the United States and how many enrollees?*

Just go to Health Maintenance Organizations in the index of *Statistical Abstract of the United States* and you will be referred to a table on HMOs.

2. *What is the extent of alcohol consumption in the United States?*

Check out the Fast Stats A-Z at the U.S. National Center for Health Statistics at www.cdc.gov/nchs/fastats/alcohol.htm.

3. *What is the number of health care workers in Iraq?*

Under the heading of Health Personnel, WHOSIS gives numbers of physicians, nurses, midwives, dentists, and pharmacists per 100,000 population at www.who.int/whosis.

References

1. Based on Weise F., Johnson J. Medical and health statistics. In: Roper FW, Boorkman JA, eds. *Introduction to reference sources in the health sciences*, 3rd ed. Metuchen, NJ: Scarecrow Press, 1994.
2. *HealthyPeople 2010*. Washington, DC: Office of Disease Prevention and Health Promotion, U.S. Department of Health and Human Services, 2000. Available: www.health.gov/healthy-people.
3. Sackett DL, Rosenberg WM, Gray JA, Haynes RB, Richardson WS. Evidence-based medicine: what it is and what it isn't. *Br Med J* 1996 Jan.; 312(7023):71–2.
4. U.S. National Committee on Vital and Health Statistics. *Information for Health: A Strategy for Building the National Health Information Infrastructure: Report and Recommendations*. Washington, DC: U.S. Department of Health and Human Services, Office of Disease Prevention and Health Promotion, Office of Public Health and Science and National Center for Health Statistics, Centers for Disease Control and Prevention, 2001. Available: www.ncvhs.hhs.gov/nhiilayho.pdf.
5. *National Center for Health Statistics*. Atlanta, GA: United States Department of Health and Human Services, Centers for Disease Control and Prevention. Available: www.cdc.gov/nchs.
6. Upton G, Cook I. *A Dictionary of Statistics*. New York: Oxford University Press, 2002.
7. Last JM, ed. *A Dictionary of Epidemiology*, 4th ed. New York: Oxford University Press, 2001.
8. Everitt B. *Cambridge Dictionary of Statistics in the Medical Sciences*. Cambridge: Cambridge University Press, 1995.
9. *International Statistical Classification of Diseases and Related Health Problems: ICD-10*. Geneva: World Health Organization, 1992.
10. Ibid.
11. *Healthy People 2010*, op. cit.

CHAPTER 12

DIRECTORIES AND BIOGRAPHICAL SOURCES

Cheryl Dee

Directories are among the most frequently consulted ready reference tools. Directories are often used for a quick answer about people and organizations. Directories are available in printed books and in electronic format or in a combination of both formats. Many libraries purchase online access to electronic versions of directories that reside on the servers of vendors. Online directories can frequently be updated. With proper authentication, end users can consult proprietary online directories. In some cases, print directories may no longer be available. Online directories may be more current than print, but may be difficult or time consuming to use. Open-access Internet sites are quick to use, but with so many sites available, it may be hard to decide which one to use. It may be difficult to determine if an open-access site is authoritative. For directory questions, the decision between printed references and online sources is based on the librarian's perception of a quick, accurate, current, and easy to use resource. These criteria are not, however, clear-cut.

Currency is a major factor to consider because the accuracy of the information will be related to the degree that the directory contains up-to-date material. For example, editors of the *Encyclopedia of Associations* note that the 39th edition added 500 organizations and estimate that 40 percent of the respondents to the survey for information reported some change to their main contact information [Introduction] highlighting the fact that organizations constantly change, and directories must reflect the changes. Online sources are able to stay more current than the printed counterpart. The Ulrichsweb.com electronic source, for example, states that it is updated weekly compared to the annual printed *Ulrich's Periodicals Directory*.

Katz [1] tells us, however, that most reference librarians turn to print to answer the quick fact question from ready reference sources. Most print factbooks are easy to use, and the answers can be found in a few seconds. A printed directory with an easy to use index which is located close to the reference desk might be the quickest route to an answer for some librarians whereas another librarian will chose the online version of the same directory, believing it to be the most available. Perceived ease of use will also influence the selection. Like almost all information seeking, the perceived availability of the resource will often determine its usage [2].

Biographical Sources and Directories of Scientists

Some of the most frequent reference requests are for biographical information. Biographical questions may be complicated. As Boorkman points out, "while apparently straightforward and uncomplicated, the client may not always know the first name of Dr. Smith in Los Angeles, and Dr. Smith's specialty may be internal medicine, but then again it may be gastroenterology. A secretary might just have the doctor's signature, and it 'looks like' T. J. Crandell, or is that F. J. Granville? Thus, two seemingly direct requests for information are often less than clear" [3].

Print or electronic biographical sources must be based on accurate material to be authoritative. Biographical sources may rely on questionnaires supplied by the people in the directory, subsequently compiled and written by editors; or an expert in the health care field may write them; or, unfortunately, unknown and unqualified authors may write them. The unqualified are most often located on the Internet. Katz [4] states that the authoritative printed biographical titles should be listed in basic bibliographies such as *Guide to Reference Books* [5] and *Walford's* [6], or the online American Reference Books Annual. In addition, librarians can verify a source by using publishers of reliable biographies such as the Gale Group, H.W. Wilson, and recognized medical organizations.

The biographical sources and directories discussed in this chapter are examples of major sources. In addition to these sources, the librarian may refer to local, state, and regional directories as well as directories of professional associations and the telephone directory, sometimes said to be the most frequently used reference book, but also frequently overlooked. Many of these are now available on the Web, and representative examples are included in this chapter.

The following sources are primarily for physicians and scientists in the United States, with a few examples of directories to scientists in Great Britain and other countries.

United States

12.1 *American Men and Women of Science,* 21st ed. New York: Gale, 2003. 8 vols. Available: netLibrary eBooks, www.netlibrary.net.

American Men and Women of Science (*AMWS*) provides biographical sketches of 129,769 living people in the physical and biological fields as well as public health scientists, engineers, mathematicians, statisticians, and computer scientists. Information is provided from the entrants who are citizens of the United States or Canada or who have performed a significant amount of their work in North America. The alphabetical arrangement in the first seven volumes has more than 4,000 scientists. The directory includes "if available and applicable" birth date, birthplace, citizenship, spouse, children, specialty, education, honorary degrees, professional experience, present position, memberships, research addresses, fax numbers, and e-mail addresses for each entrant. The eighth volume, the discipline index, organized by field of interest, is adapted from the National Science Foundation's Taxonomy of Degree and Employment Specialties and is classified by 192 subject specialties, arranged by state or province within each subject specialty. *American Men and Women of Science* includes statistical information presenting the entrants' distribution by age and discipline and the recipients of the Nobel Prize, Crawford Prize, Charles Stark Draper Prize, National Medals of Science, the Fields Medal, the Alan T. Waterman Award, and the National Medal of Technology. *American*

Men and Women of Science in this first Gale edition states that it is comprehensive, but does not intend to include all U.S. and Canadian scientists. Entrants are meant to be limited to those who made significant contribution to their field and meet the following criteria: 1) distinguished achievement by experience, training, or accomplishment; 2) research activity of high quality; or 3) attainment of a position of substantial responsibility requiring training and experience [Introduction].

The following physicians directories provide three different approaches to biographical information.

12.2   *The Official ABMS Directory of Board Certified Medical Specialists.* Evanston, IL: American Board of Medical Specialists, Research and Education Foundation. 1992– Annual. Formed by the union of: *Directory of Medical Specialists* and *The Official American Board of Medical Specialties (ABMS) Directory of Board Certified Medical Specialists,* continuing the edition numbering of the former. *Board Certified Docs.* Available: www.boardcertified-docs.com/abms/default.asp.

12.3   *Directory of Physicians in the United States.* Chicago, IL: American Medical Association, 1992–. Irregular. Continues *American Medical Directory, 1906–1990. AMA Physician Select.* Available: www.ama-assn.org/aps/amahg.htm.

12.4   *Who's Who in Medicine and Health Care,* 3rd ed. Wilmette, IL: Marquis Who's Who, 2000–2001. Preceding title: *Who's Who in Health Care. Marquis Who's Who ON THE WEB.* Available: www.marquiswhoswho.com/ontheweb.asp.

The Official ABMS (American Board of Medical Specialists) *Directory of Board Certified Medical Specialists* is published annually in four volumes by the American Board of Medical Specialists in cooperation with Elsevier Science. The 2003 edition provides professional and biographical information on 617,000 board certified physicians in the United States and Canada and is authorized by the 24 medical specialty boards of the American Board of Medical Specialists. Biographies include medical school and year of degree, place and date of internship and residency, fellowship, academic and hospital appointments, professional associations, type of medical practice (with addresses and telephone/fax numbers), and specialty and certification by the 24 Member Boards of the ABMS. The directory also includes an alphabetical index of the specialists, a geographical distribution of diplomats by state and by specialty, a medical association resource list with addresses and telephone numbers for national and international medical associations, names and addresses for U.S. and Canadian medical schools, state licensing boards, and a necrology of all deceased specialists identified since the last edition. The directory states that it is the primary source for board certification information by the National Committee for Quality Assurance (NCQA) and the Joint Commission for Accreditation of Healthcare Organizations (JCAHO). Certification data are obtained from the certifying boards with additional data obtained from questionnaires mailed to the specialists. The electronic version of the *ABMS Directory of Board Certified Medical Specialists* is available by subscription from the American Board of Medical Specialists under the name Board Certified Docs. The electronic version is updated daily using the data from the database used to compose the *ABMS Directory*. In addition, all of the information found in the four-volume set of the *ABMS Directory* is on a single CD-ROM, *ABMS Medical Specialists Plus*, that is updated twice a year.

The *Directory of Physicians in the United States*, compiled and published by the American Medical Association, is a source of demographic and professional information on physicians located in the United States, Puerto Rico, Virgin Islands, and certain Pacific Islands and includes both members and nonmembers of the American Medical Association (AMA). The four-volume-set 38th edition includes almost 800,000 physicians and doctors of osteopathy who are members of the AMA. Volume one includes the alphabetical index and volumes two, three, and four are the geographical register, arranged alphabetically within each state and city. Information for inclusion is obtained directly from each physician and from "verified information supplied by medical schools, licensing agencies and the American Board of Medical Specialists" [Introduction]. Electronic access to *The Directory of Physicians in the United States* from the American Medical Association provides electronic access to basic professional information on licensed physicians in the United States and its possessions in AMA Physician

Select. The database includes doctors of medicine (MD) and doctors of osteopathy or osteopathic medicine (DO), which is almost every licensed physician in the United States and its possessions. Information is available to the public and includes address, phone number, education, graduation year, residency, professional organizations, and certification.

The third edition of *Who's Who in Medicine and Healthcare*, formerly *Who's Who in Health Care,* provides biographical background on over 28,000 successful medical administrators, educators, researchers, clinicians, and other health care leaders. The majority of the biographies come from the United States, but many come from more than 115 other nations, and the careers span over 100 specialties. Also included are those who support health care, such as association, governmental and industrial administration; corporate management; and legal practice. A geographical index and a classified index include name, occupation, vital statistics, parents, marriage, children, education, professional certifications, career, career-related activities, writings and creative works, civic and political activities, military, awards and fellowships, professional and association memberships, clubs and lodges, political affiliations, religion, home address, and office address. Inclusion in *Who's Who in Medicine and Healthcare* is determined by position of responsibility, contributions to the field, and accomplishments. Specifically, selection for inclusion is "judged on either of two factors: 1) the position of responsibility held, or 2) the level of achievement attained by the individual, such as deans, directors, administrators, board heads, executive officers, winners of major awards from top U.S. medical and health-related associations and all living American winners of the Nobel Prize of Physiology and Medicine" [Standards of Admission]. Marquis Who's Who ON THE WEB offers real-time access by subscription to an online database of over 1 million biographies with advanced searches of worldwide biographical databases including Who's Who in Medicine and Healthcare.

The affiliation of the physicians is different in two of the biographical directories. The *Directory of Physicians in the United* States contains 800,000 AMA physicians whereas the *ABMS Directory* contains 617,000 board certified medical specialist physicians. Clearly, there is overlap in coverage, but the amount of information on each physician is very different. The AMA *Directory* provides only brief coded information whereas the *ABMS Directory* includes a considerably more complete professional history for many physicians. Almost twice as many libraries have some edition of the annual *ABMS Directory* compared to the *Directory of Physicians in the United States* according to WorldCat. In contrast to the AMA and the ABMS directory, the *Who's Who in Medicine and Health Care* offers only selected successful physicians in their directory listings.

The following works represent directories of professional societies. Each organization has criteria for membership and lists only those individuals who have applied for or been sponsored for membership and meet the qualifications.

12.5 *Yearbook American College of Surgeons.* Chicago, IL: American College of Surgeons, 1953–. Irregular.

12.6 *AVMA Directory.* Schaumburg, IL: American Veterinary Medical Association; Division of Membership and Field Services, 1984–. Annual. Formerly: *American Veterinary Medical Association Directory*, 1943–1983.

12.7 *Who's Who in Managed Health Care Directory.* Laguna Hills, CA: HealthQuest Publishers, c1994–.

12.8 *American Dental Directory.* Chicago, IL: American Dental Association, 1947–2001. Ceased publication. Available: www.ada.org/public/directory.

The *Yearbook of the American College of Surgeons* provides biographical and geographical listings of Fellows of the American College of Surgeons. Biographical entries in the alphabetical name section include address, specialty, medical school attended, hospitals, year fellowship conferred, and memberships. Also contains historical and organizational information about the American College of Surgeons.

The *AVMA Directory* lists AVMA members in the United States, Canada, and other countries and from those nonmember veterinarians for whom data is available and who ask to be listed. The *AVMA Directory* is organized in four sections. The resource section contains tabbed sections with AVMA organizations and history, names and addresses of other related veterinary associations, federal and state government agencies, veterinary colleges, material available from the AVMA, a catalog of free loan videotapes, and AVMA forms. The auxiliary section lists information on auxiliary members including spouse's name, city, and state. The alphabetical section lists each veterinarian in alphabetical sequence and the geographic section provides a geographic listing by state and town and includes name, full address, telephone, e-mail address, school and year of graduation, professional specialty, type of employment, and employment function.

Who's Who in Managed Health Care Directory provides biographical information on leaders in the managed care industry. In addition to demographic information, the directory highlights the experience, education, credentials, significant achievements, professional affiliations, and activities of hundreds of men and women in leadership positions affecting managed care throughout the nation. The leadership profiles are also indexed by name, title, organization, and state. The directory also includes a listing of HMO CEOs with contact information.

The *American Dental Directory* ceased publication in 2001 according to WorldCat. The older editions may be of use for retrospective searching because the directory listed all dentists, not just American Dental Association members. Coded information includes a professional biography with dental education, year of graduation, and type of practice.The online American Dental Directory provides information for the dental professional and the public. The public site gives the dentist's name, address, and e-mail address. Clicking the hyperlink on a dentist's name displays a map to the dentist's office.

Other Countries

12.9   *Who's Who of British Scientists.* London: Longman, 1970–1981. Preceding title: *Directory of British Scientists.* New York: St. Martin's Press, 1963–1967.

This directory covers scientists in all fields; however, it is only useful for retrospective biographies because it is somewhat dated. *Who's Who of British Scientists* lists men and women in biological sciences in a classified arrangement by discipline. Biographical information includes name, address, phone number, current position, degrees obtained, and important writings. The earlier *Directory of British Scientists* is also arranged by discipline with an alphabetical name index.

12.10 *Medical Directory.* London: Churchill, 1845–. Vol. 1–. 2 vols. Annual.

12.11 *Medical Register.* London: General Medical Council, 1959–. Vol. 1–. 2 vols.

The *Medical Directory,* published in "official association" with the Royal Society of Medicine, is a source of information on physicians practicing in the United Kingdom. The 158th edition of the *Medical Directory* contains full biographical profiles of over 132,000 medical practitioners and the details of over 5,000 health care organizations, including an alphabetical listing of all NHS (National Health Service) trusts and hospitals.The *Medical Directory* is published in both paper and CD-ROM formats.

The *Medical Register* lists physicians in the United Kingdom. The alphabetical listing gives a physician's name, address, registration date, and degrees and includes foreign medical graduates certified to practice medicine in the United Kingdom. This directory is useful for locating practitioners in the Commonwealth, especially Australia and New Zealand, if licensed in the United Kingdom. The latest edition is 1995.

12.12 *Canadian Medical Directory.* Don Mills, ON: Business Information Group of HCN Publications Co, 1955–. Vol. 1–. Annual.

The *Canadian Medical Directory* provides brief biographical listings in alphabetical order. Section one includes "qualified doctors known to be in Canada at the time of publication" [User's Guide] and provides office address (if in private practice), university and year of graduation, medical degree, fellowships from the Royal College, specialist certification (field of practice), appointments, office telephone and fax numbers, and languages. Abbreviations used in this section are listed in the front of the directory. The geographical listing (blue tabs) includes general practitioners and family medicine physicians listed alphabetically by region. The third section (orange pages) lists certified specialists listed by specialty and geographic location Section four (purple tabs) includes all Canadian hospitals and an index of hospitals. Section five (ivory tabs) includes a resources section with the current-year graduates in medicine from Canadian universities, a list of the medical officers of the Armed Forces, and information about universities and health departments. Section six (green tabs) contains listings of Canadian health care associations arranged alphabetically by association name. Section seven includes a current year in review summarizing the major medical news items from the *Canadian Medical Association Journal* and the Canadian Medical Hall of Fame, which honors physicians, researchers, and health care builders.

The following directories help locate people outside of the English-speaking countries.

12.13 *Who's Who in Science and Engineering.* Wilmette, IL: Marquis Who's Who, 2003. *Marquis Who's Who ON THE WEB.* Available: www.marquiswhoswho.com/ontheweb.asp.

12.14 *International Who's Who in Medicine,* 2nd ed. Cambridge, U.K.: International Biographical Centre, 1995.

12.15 *Medical Sciences International Who's Who.* Harlow, U.K.: Longman; Detroit, MI: Distributed in the United States by Gale Research Co., 1987–1996. Formerly: *International Medical Who's Who.* Harlow, U.K.: Hodgson, 1980–1985.

Who's Who in Science and Engineering will provide key biographical facts on the more than 34,000 men and women leading today's scientific and technological revolution . . . who are "innovators in the medicine and healthcare fields" according to the Bowker Web site announcing the 6th edition, 2002–2003. The directory provides data on "inventors, discoverers, award winners, industry executives, educators, writers, and philosophers whose efforts are advancing human knowledge" with ". . . exclusive 'life records,' including personal data, achievements, discoveries, research findings, patents, and career histories of today's leaders from all areas of pure and applied science and engineering" such as medicine, information science, computer science, life sciences, and social sciences. Marquis Who's Who *ON THE WEB* also offers daily updates and access to *Who's Who in Science and Engineering*.

The *International Who's Who in Medicine* provides alphabetical biographical listings of health professionals worldwide but the information is old: 1995 appears to be the last publication date. The book includes "doctors in general practice, surgeons, consultants, administrators, senior teaching staff, nurses, dentists, and those concerned with public health and rehabilitation, mental health, research, laboratory science, chiropody, physiotherapy, dietetics, acupuncture and medical hypnosis from many different countries" [Foreword]. Biographical information from questionnaires includes personal data, current position, educational degrees, memberships, selected publications, awards, hobbies, and business address. The Foreword states "future editions will offer relatively few updated entries, space being given instead to additional individuals."

Medical Sciences International Who's Who ceased publication with the 7th edition (1996) according to WorldCat. The directory provides an alphabetical listing of senior medical and biomedical scientists from 90 countries and is an alphabetically arranged biographical listing with information on birth, educational information, and professional information with country and subject indexes.

Internet Directories

12.16 *MEDLINEplus: Directories.* Besthesda, MD: U.S. National Library of Medicine. Available: www.nlm.nih.gov/medlineplus/directories.html.

12.17 *Biography.com.* Arts & Entertainment Television Network. Available: www.biography.com.

12.18 *World Biographical Index.* Munich: K. G. Saur Publishing. Available: www.biblio.tu-bs.de/wbi10_en.

12.19 *AIM DocFinder.* Association of State Medical Board Executive Directors. Available: www.docboard.org/docfinder.html.

12.20 *The DocFinderPlus*. Avon, CT: National Physicians DataSource. Available: www.docfinderplus.com/begin.asp.

12.21 *Medicare Participating Physician Directory*. Baltimore, MD: Centers for Medicare and Medicaid Services. Available: www.medicare.gov/Physician/Home.asp.

MEDLINEplus, produced by the National Library of Medicine, provides links to 43 sources of directory information on general and specialist doctors and dentists with links to other health care providers.

Biography.com from the Arts & Entertainment Television Network is composed of 20,000 to 25,000 biographies of famous people including famous physicians and nurses (and annoying advertisements). Includes some medical entries.

World Biographical Index, published by K. G. Saur Publishing, provides free access to a large biographical database containing over 2 million references to persons. Search by name (or part of name) in combination with occupation, year of birth or death, year cited, and biographical archive. The Health Care section lists physicians, veterinarians, pharmacists, nurses, and others.

AIM DocFinder gives the health professional licensing listings by state, if the state is participating (17 are), and provides data from state government licensing boards and licensing background and disciplinary information of physicians and other health care practitioners. Searching is by state.

The DocFinderPlus is a product of National Physicians DataSource LLC (NPDS), publishers of *The Little Blue Book*. The Web site is searchable by doctor's name, zip code, or city. Provides only name, address, city, and state.

Medicare Participating Physician Directory contains names, addresses, and specialties of Medicare participating physicians who have agreed to accept assignment on all Medicare claims and covered services.

Proprietary databases

12.22 Biography Resource Center and The Complete Marquis Who's Who. Farmington Hills, MI: Thomson Gale. Available: www.gale-group.com/pdf/facts/brc.pdf.

Biography Resource Center is available by subscription from the Gale Group and includes full-text articles from hundreds of periodicals. The database is searchable based on one or more personal facts such as birth and death year, nationality, ethnicity, occupation, or gender, or combined criteria to create a targeted custom search. The Complete Marquis Who's Who provides quick reference information on an additional 900,000 people.

Directories of Organizations

Information requests about medical organizations, particularly hospitals, are popular. Again, addresses and telephone numbers are most often needed, although information about an organization's structure, purpose, meetings, and membership make up a great number of requests.

12.23 *Encyclopedia of Associations*, 39th ed. Detroit, MI: Gale, 1961–. 2 vols. Annual 1975–; Irregular 1961–1973. *Gale's Ready Reference Shelf.* Available: www.galegroup.com; *LexisNexis.* Available: www.lexis-nexis.com.

12.24 *Research Centers Directory*, 30th ed. Detroit, MI: Gale, 2003. 2 vols. Supplemented between editions by *New Research Centers. Gale's Ready Reference Shelf.* Available: www.galegroup.com; *LexisNexis.* Available: www.lexis-nexis.com.

12.25 Noce J, ed. *Medical and Health Information Directory*, 15th ed. Detroit, MI: Gale, 2003. Annual. 3 vols. *Gale's Health and Wellness Resource Center* Available: www.galegroup.com.

12.26 *Encyclopedia of Medical Organizations and Agencies: A Subject Guide to More Than 11,250 Associations, Foundations, Federal and State Government Agencies, Research Centers, and Medical and Allied Health Schools,* 13th ed. Detroit, MI: Gale, 2003.

12.27 Poland UH, ed. *World Directory of Biological and Medical Sciences Libraries.* Munchen: K.G. Saur, 1988. (IFLA Publication 42).

12.28 Directory of Special Libraries and Information Centers, 28th ed. Detroit, MI: Gale Research Co., 2002. Gale's Ready Reference Shelf. Available: www.galegroup.com; LexisNexis. Available: www.lexis-nexis.com.

The *Encyclopedia of Associations (EA)* is a general directory of organizations in the United States. Entries are arranged into 18 subject sections (Section 8: Health and Medical Organizations) and within each section organizations are arranged in alphabetical order according to the subject keyword. Within each keyword, entries are listed alphabetically by the organization's name. Volume One, in three parts, includes national organizations of the United States and the name and keyword index. Volume 2 includes the geographic and executive indexes. Each entry potentially provides up to 35 categories, for example: organization name; acronym; address; telephone, fax, and telex number; chief official and title; e-mails; Web site; founding date; membership dues; membership size; staff; budget; regional, state, and local groups; geographic scope; purpose of the organization; libraries; awards; computer services; affiliates; publications (including price); circulation; advertising and electronic formats; and meetings or conventions. Also see the volumes of *The Encyclopedia of Associations: Regional, State and Local Organizations* and *The Encyclopedia of Associations: International Associations.* The Gale Research Company publishes electronic formats of *The Encyclopedia of Associations: National Associations, The Encyclopedia of Associations: International Associations,* and *The Encyclopedia of Associations: Regional, State and Local Associations* in Gale's Ready Reference Shelf. The complete *Encyclopedia of Associations* including international and regional, state, and local editions is also available through the Gale Group and LexisNexis.

The *Research Centers Directory* (*RCD*) presents information on nonprofit research institutes, foundations, laboratories, bureaus, experiment stations, farms, technology transfer centers, think tanks, incubators, research parks, and more. The 30th edition lists more than 13,000 centers in North America. Entries are arranged into sections by subject, one of which is Medicine and Life Sciences. Within each section, entries are alphabetically arranged by sponsoring organization name and by center name. Four indexes assist with location including a master index arranged with all research centers in a single alphabetical index, a personal name index, a geographic index, and a subject index with cross references. Entries include 35 potential informational pieces including research center name, acronym, address, telephone number, fax number, head of organization, e-mail, Web page, founding date, membership dues, membership, staff, research budget, financial support, educational activities, databases, library holdings and specific subject specialties in the library, librarians, awards, services, publications, scholarships, meetings, and affiliated centers. *New Research Centers* provides periodic supplements to the *Directory*. *Research Centers Directory* is also available online through Gale's Ready Reference Shelf and LexisNexis.

The *Medical and Health Information Directory* is extremely useful because the directory brings together a wide range of information into a single source. The directory is a guide to more than 49,000 associations, agencies, companies, institutions, research centers, hospitals, clinics, treatment centers, educational programs, publications, audiovisuals, databases, libraries, and information services in clinical medicine, basic biomedical science, and the technological and socioeconomic aspects of health care. Volume one provides contact and descriptive information on medical and health organizations, agencies, and institutions and is organized into 20 chapters, each consisting of broad groups of organizations such as national and international, state and regional, foundations, consulting, peer review, government, and so forth with a master name and keyword index. Volume two provides contact and descriptive information on nearly 12,000 domestic and foreign medical and health-related publications, libraries, and other information resources from sources such as journals, abstracting and indexing services, newsletters, directories, publishers, electronic resources, U.S. and Canadian libraries and information centers, and Internet search engines. The volume consists of the descriptive listings organized according to type of publication or information resource and also includes an alphabetical name and keyword index that includes significant keywords appearing in names or titles. Volume three is intended for health care professionals as well as the public and includes information on clinics, treatment centers, care programs, counseling, and diagnostic services. The descriptive listings are organized into 35 chapters according to type of health service and are as diverse as headache clinics, eating disorder clinics, domestic violence programs, services for the blind, home health care agencies, and sports medicine clinics. Like the other volumes, an alphabetical name and keyword index consolidates all the listings in a single alphabetic list for easy access. The *Medical and Health Information Directory* is included in Gale's *Health and Wellness Resource Center.*

The *Encyclopedia of Medical Organizations and Agencies* (*EMOA*) is a subject guide to medical and health-related organizations and institutions, including national, international, state, and regional organizations; foundations and other funding organizations; U.S. federal and state government agencies; and research centers and medical and allied health schools. The *Encyclopedia* includes more than 18,500 entries arranged within 69 subject chapters. The subject cross-index provides an overview of all topics, and the alphabetical name and keyword index contains citations to all organizations listed in the *Encyclopedia* as well as to subject keywords appearing in the organizations' names.

The information in the *World Directory of Biological and Medical Sciences Libraries* is compiled from a questionnaire sent to all countries of the world as a project of the Working Group of the Biological and Medical Sciences Libraries Section of the Division of Special Libraries, International Federation of Library Associations and Institutions. Included in the directory are nonprofit libraries worldwide in the following subject areas: biological sciences, medical sciences (including allied health), dentistry, veterinary sciences, and pharmaceutical sciences. All libraries in developing countries have been

310

included. For developed countries, the 25 major resource libraries have been listed.

The *Directory of Special Libraries and Information Centers* is a guide to more than 34,000 special libraries, research libraries, information centers, archives, and data centers maintained by government agencies, businesses, industries, newspapers, educational institutions, nonprofit organizations, and societies in fields including science, engineering, and medicine. Volume one, in three parts, consists of descriptive listings, appendices, and the subject index. Entries within the main section are arranged in alphabetical order; libraries associated with a company, institution, agency, or association are grouped under the official name of the parent organization. Some exceptions to this organization are described in the User's Guide. Extensive cross references are interfiled and are supplied for libraries with, for example, acronyms or multiple sponsors. The *Directory* is accessible in electronic format through Lexis-Nexis and also as a part of *Gale's Ready Reference Shelf.* A *Geographic and Personnel Index,* available separately, provides a geographical rearrangement of basic contact information for libraries in volume one of the *Directory* as well as an alphabetical listing by surname of all librarians mentioned within the listings.

12.29 *World Guide to Scientific Associations and Learned Societies*, 8th ed. Munich and New York: K. G. Saur, 2002.

12.30 *Yearbook of International Organizations: Guide to Global and Civil Society Networks*, 39th ed. Brussels: Union of International Associations, 2002/2003. 3 vols. Annual. Available: www.uia.org/organizations/ybonline.php.

The *World Guide to Scientific Associations and Learned Societies* is an international directory of associations and societies representing all fields of science, culture, and technology. The text of the *World Guide* is alphabetically arranged with some 17,500 entries. Each entry includes the association name, address, year of foundation, telephone or fax, e-mail, Web page, names of officials, number of members, details of periodical publications, descriptive details on aims and activities, awards, grants, scholarships, frequency and kind of meetings, lectures, and association library and/or archives. The work is alphabetically

311

arranged by name of country and also contains an alphabetical index of association names with name variants of international associations' names, a persons' index, and a subject index.

The *Yearbook of International Organizations* states that it attempts to cover all "international organizations" according to a broad and widely interpreted range of criteria. Descriptions of organizations are from the organizations themselves and efforts are made by the editors to check this information against other sources (periodicals, official documents, media, and so forth). Entries include information such as name, address, telephone number, fax, e-mail, Web page, aims, events, founding date and place, member information, structure, staff, finances, languages, activities, and publications. The first volume of the current edition has an alphabetical arrangement with cross references; volume two is a country directory of secretariats and membership; volume three is a subject directory and index; volume four is an international organization bibliography and resource; and volume five covers statistics, visualizations, and patterns. Seven appendices include contents of organization descriptions, types of organizations, statistics, number of international organizations, editorial policy, related reference works, and the United Nations and the *Yearbook of International Organizations*. *Yearbook of International Organizations* is also accessible online by subscription.

The *Yearbook of International Organizations* provides considerably more information about each organization it lists as well as more indexes than the *World Guide*. Both directories are useful in locating information about organizations outside the United States.

Internet Directories

Frequently, information is requested about organizations. Electronic sources for organizational information are popular because these sources can be updated as frequently as the changes occur in the organization. Some examples follow.

12.31 *DIRLINE.* Bethesda, MD: U.S. National Library of Medicine. Available: dirline.nlm.nih.gov.

12.32 *Health Hotlines: Toll-free Numbers from the U.S. National Library of Medicine*. Bethesda, MD: U.S. National Library of Medicine Available: www.sis.nlm.nih.gov/hotlines.

12.33 *MEDLINEplus: Organizations*. Bethesda, MD: U.S. National Library of Medicine. Available: www.nlm.nih.gov/medlineplus /organizations.html

12.34 *Firstgov.gov*. Washington, DC: Federal Citizen Information Center, Office of Citizen Services and Communications, U.S. General Services Administration. Available: http://firstgov.gov.

12.35 *SAMHSA's National Mental Health Information Center: The Center for Mental Health Services*. Washington, DC: Substance Abuse and Mental Health Services Administration, National Mental Health Information Center. Available: www.mentalhealth.org /databases/default.asp.

12.36 "Associations on the Net" on *The Internet Public Library*. Ann Arbor, MI: University of Michigan School of Information. Available: www.ipl.org/div/aon.

12.37 *Scholarly Societies*. Waterloo, ON: University of Waterloo Library. Available: www.lib.uwaterloo.ca/society/overview.html.

12.38 *World Health Organization*. Geneva: World Health Organization. Available: www.who.int/en.

Sponsored by the NLM, DIRLINE includes location and descriptive information about a wide variety of information resources including organizations, research resources, projects, and databases concerned with health and biomedicine. Contains approximately 10,000 records and focuses primarily on health and biomedicine, with limited coverage of federal, state, and local government agencies; information and referral centers; professional societies; self-help groups and voluntary associations; academic and research institutions and their programs; and information systems and research facilities

Health Hotlines is derived from DIRLINE and provides information on health-related organizations operating toll-free telephone services with descriptions of over 14,000 biomedical information resources, including organizations, databases, research resources, and so forth. The database is searchable by keyword and by browsing the subject list. The site also includes information on services and publications available in Spanish.

MEDLINEplus: Organizations includes extensive information from the NIH from trusted sources aimed toward the consumer.

Firstgov is the U.S. government's official Web portal and provides extensive online services for citizens, business, and governments including some medical documents. Organizations can be located by using the site's search box.

SAMHSA is a specialized directory sponsored by the U.S. Department of Health and Human Services, Substance Abuse and Mental Health Services Administration for mental health statistics, resources, and services.

"Associations on the Net" is available from The Internet Public Library (IPL) at the University of Michigan School of Information and includes a guide to Web sites of prominent organizations and associations. The Health and Medical Sciences heading has hyperlinks to medical subject categories.

Scholarly Societies is sponsored by the University of Waterloo and is searchable by subject, country, language, and founding dates and many more options

World Health Organization provides topics by country, health topic, publications, research tools, and World Health Organization sites. Of particular interest is the link to Health Topics.

Proprietary Databases

12.39 *ReferenceUSA*. Omaha, NE: InfoUSA. Available: www.reference usa.com.

ReferenceUSA contains directory listings for more than 12 million businesses and 120 million households in all zip code areas of the United States and is available by subscription.

Education Directories

Frequently, information is requested about schools and universities. General education reference books with health care facilities and the professional health associations formed by these schools and their administrators provide timely and accurate information about their programs, admission requirements, and curricula. Some examples follow.

12.40 *Directory of American Medical Education.* Washington, DC: Association of American Medical Colleges, 1996–. Annual. Preceding title: *AAMC Directory of American Medical Education.*1900s–1995. Available: www.aamc.org.

12.41 *Graduate Medical Education Directory.* Chicago, IL: American Medical Association, 1993–. Annual. Continues: *Directory of graduate medical education programs.* Available: www.ama-assn.org/go/freida.

12.42 *Medical School Admission Requirements, United States and Canada.* Washington, DC: Association of American Medical Colleges, 1951–. Annual. Formerly: Admission Requirements of American Medical Colleges, Including Canada, 1951–1964/65.

12.43 *Peterson's 2000 U.S. and Canadian Medical Schools: A Comprehensive Guide to All 159 Accredited Medical Schools.* Princeton, NJ: Petersons Guides, 2000; CD-ROM edition (December 1999).

12.44 *Peterson's Guide to Nursing Programs: Baccalaureate and Graduate Nursing Education in the U.S. and Canada.* Princeton, NJ: Petersons Guides/American Association of Colleges of Nursing, 1994–. Annual.

12.45 *The ADEA Official Guide to Dental Schools*, 40th ed. Washington, DC: American Dental Education Association, 2002. Preceding title: *Admission Requirements of U.S. and Canadian Dental Schools.*1975–2001.

The *Directory of American Medical Education* provides a geographical listing of medical schools that are institutional members (U.S.) or affiliate institutional members (Canadian) of the Association of American Medical Colleges (AAMC). The *Directory* includes comprehensive information on the medical school and includes name, address, type of institution (public or private), total enrollment, a detailed list of the clinical facilities, university officials from the president of the university to all of the university associate vice presidents, medical school administrative staff from the medical school dean to all of the associate deans, directors, and department and division or section chairs. Other sections of the *Directory* provide information on the AAMC organizational structure and activities, Council of Deans, Council of Academic Societies, Council of Teaching Hospitals and Health Systems, Steering Committees of AAMC Groups, Organization of Student Representatives, and other members. An index to individuals mentioned in all sections of the *Directory* is also included.

The *Graduate Medical Education Directory* provides medical students with a list of accredited graduate medical education programs in the United States. Section one includes graduate medical education information. Section two provides comprehensive descriptions of accredited residencies in graduate medical education with the requirements of each of the specialties and subspecialties as set forth by the Accreditation Council for Graduate Medical Education. Section two also details the requirements for the length of the residency program, the requirements of the institutions (medical school) affiliated with the residency program, personnel, and even curricular content for each specialty and subspecialty (almost 400 pages). Section three is an alphabetical list of the specialties and subspecialties. Within each specialty, programs are listed in alphabetical order by state and city. It provides only brief information on each specific program but orients each program within its specialty (almost 600 pages). Section four includes the new and withdrawn programs since the last edition of the *Directory.* Section five lists graduate medical education teaching institutions. Two appendices provide information on specialty programs, specialty board certification requirements, and lists of medical schools in the United States. *GMED Companion: An Insider's Guide to Selecting a Residency Program* includes information for foreign-born medical graduates, appointment to the U.S. Armed Service programs, electronic application, and the National Residency Matching Program. *AMA-FREIDA* (American Medical Association Fellowship and Residency Electronic Interactive Database Access) is available from the AMA Web site. Users can search all ACGME accredited programs by specialty, subspecialty, state, program size, and educational requirements. All program listings include program director's name and address, program length and number of positions available, resident to faculty ratios, work schedule, policies, and educational environment.

The *Directory of American Medical Education* and the *Graduate Medical Education Directory* provide very different approaches, but contain essential information on residency programs. The *Directory of American Medical Education* includes detailed information about medical schools that are members of Association of American Medical Colleges. On the other hand, the *Graduate Medical Education Directory* provides extensive information on the residency program requirements of each of many specialties and subspecialties and lists brief information about the residency programs, but covers all of the specialties and subspecialties.

Medical School Admission Requirements includes comprehensive admissions information on every AAMC-accredited United States and Canadian medical school. The AAMC represents 125 accredited U.S. medical schools and 16 accredited Canadian medical schools in the directory.

Peterson's 2000 U.S. and Canadian Medical Schools includes information on faculty, enrollment costs, financial aid, resource and hospital affiliations, medical degree clerkships, and student body profiles.

Peterson's Guide to Nursing Programs: Baccalaureate and Graduate Nursing Education in the U.S. and Canada is published by Peterson's, the leading publisher of college guides, in collaboration with the American Association of Colleges of Nursing (AACN) and is a comprehensive guide to accredited baccalaureate, master's, doctoral, postdoctoral, and joint-degree nursing education programs. The 2002 guide profiles more than 2,000 nursing programs offered by nearly 700 colleges and universities and includes entrance qualifications, degree requirements, costs, RN and LPN fast-track opportunities, accelerated programs for nonnursing graduates, part-time opportunities, continuing education, and distance learning options. Other sections provide advice on how to select a program, tips for nurses returning to school, guidance on financial aid and scholarships, and information for international nursing students.

ADEA Official Guide to Dental Schools, published by American Dental Education Association, is an authoritative guide to information on the 55 U.S. and 10 Canadian dental schools. The guide provides information to familiarize the student with the dental profession and discusses an overview of the dental profession, including benefits of being a dentist and descriptions of the varied areas of specialization and practice options, admission criteria, academic background generally needed, guidelines to help students determine which schools are the best match, and financial tips. Entries include information on the characteristics of each program, including specialties and strengths, admission requirements and student selection factors, application timetables, estimated expenses, financial aid available, comparison of applicants and matriculated students, and contact information for admission.

12.46 *World Directory of Medical Schools*, 7th ed. Geneva: World Health Organization, 2000. Available: www.who.int/health-services-delivery/med_schools.

12.47 *World of Learning*, 53rd ed. London: Europa, 2003.Available: www.europapublications.co.uk.

The World Directory of Medical Schools, published by the World Health Organization, provides information based on a WHO questionnaire sent to governments and individual schools with medical schools in 157 countries and areas. Information on criteria for practicing medicine in 14 countries without medical schools is provided. The World Directory is arranged by country, providing the names and addresses of each school. Other pertinent information includes the date instruction began, admission requirements, length of medical studies, degrees awarded, language of instruction, and number of students admitted and graduated. The World Health Organization electronically publishes the World Directory of Medical Schools (base year 2000 with updates) and includes additions or other changes to the base-year file.

The *World of Learning* contains full directory information for over 30,000 universities, colleges, libraries, archives, learned societies, research institutes, and so forth in more than 180 countries throughout the world. Every important library is covered with details of the number of volumes held and outstanding features of the collection. Each entry includes address, telephone number, Web site address, date of foundation, membership (learned societies), and learned journals published by the institution. For each institution there is a list of key academic staff and officials and also the name and subjects taught by professors at major institutions. A section lists 400 major international organizations concerned with worldwide education with an index of the institutions and organizations. The World of Learning ONLINE is available by subscription through Europa Publications as a fully searchable multiuser product that is updated throughout the year.

Internet Sources

The following Internet sources also provide directory information.

12.48 Accreditation Council for Graduate Medical Education. Chicago, IL: ACGME. Available: www.acgme.org.

12.49 International Medical Education Directory (IMED). Philadelphia, PA: Foundation for Advancement of International Medical Education and Research (FAIMER), 2002. Available: http://imed.ecfmg.org/pfmain.asp.

12.50 MedicalStudent.com. Curated by Michael P. D'Alessandro. Available: www.medicalstudent.com.

12.51 National Library of Medicine, Medical Research Libraries by State. Besthesda, MD: National Library of Medicine. Available: www.nlm.nih.gov/libraries/state.html.

The Accreditation Council for Graduate Medical Education is a private professional organization responsible for the accreditation of nearly 7,800 residency education programs.

The International Medical Education Directory (IMED) is available online from the Educational Commission for Foreign Medical

Graduates Web site. It provides up-to-date information on medical schools worldwide that are recognized by the appropriate government agency in each country, generally the Ministry of Health. A medical school is listed by the Foundation for Advancement of International Medical Education and Research (FAIMER) only when confirmation that it is a recognized medical school has been received. Searches can be performed by region, country, and/or school name. In addition to the usual directory information for name, address, phone/fax numbers, Web and e-mail addresses, each listing includes former official name(s) of the school, degree awarded, graduation years, year instruction began, language of instruction, duration of curriculum, entrance examination requirement, eligibility of foreign (nonnational) students, and total enrollment. Updates are received from each country's Ministry of Health.

MedicalStudent.com, curated by Michael P. D'Alessandro, M.D., provides a digital library of authoritative medical information for all students of medicine. Selection for inclusion in the digital library is based on four standards: authorship, including the author's name, affiliation, and credentials; attribution of facts through the listing of references; disclosure of site ownership and sponsorship; and currency of the site by listing dates of content posting and updating. The site must be free to use, in part or in whole.

The National Library of Medicine, Medical Research Libraries by State site provides a directory of medical libraries in the United States that are resource libraries under NLM's National Network of Libraries of Medicine (NN/LM).

The biographical sources and directories listed above are only a few of the vast number available. In the United States, regions, states, counties, and cities often issue directories of physicians, other health personnel, services, and organizations. A library should maintain directories of these local resources first, for a great number of its directory questions will undoubtedly be for local people and places. Again, the telephone directory can be an invaluable resource, and a library should maintain current telephone books for its immediate and surrounding communities.

320

Hospital and Clinic Directories

12.52 *AHA Guide to the Health Care Field.* Chicago, IL: American Hospital Association, 1973–. Annual. Formerly: *Guide* issue of *Hospitals. AHAData.com.* Available: www.ahadata.com.

12.53 *Guide to Canadian Health Care Facilities. Guide des e'tablisse-ments de soins de sante' du Canada.* Ottawa, ON: Canadian Healthcare Association, 1993–. Vol. 1–. Formed from: Canadian hospital directory 1953–1992.

The *AHA Guide* is essential, particularly for up-to-date information on hospitals, multihospital systems, and health-related organizations. The 2002–2003 edition has three major sections identified by tabs and a separate table of contents. The Hospitals section lists American Hospital Association (AHA)-registered hospitals in the United States and associated areas by city within state, U.S. government hospitals outside the United States, and includes an index of hospitals arranged alphabetically by hospital, an index of health care professionals, and a list of AHA associate members.The lists provide a variety of information about each hospital, including the address, telephone number, and chief administrator. Additional coded information indicates the hospital's facilities, service, governing structure, size of staff, and accreditation by the Joint Commission on Accreditation of Healthcare Organizations (JCAHO). Brief statistical information on utilization data (beds, admissions, census, outpatient visits, births), expenses (total, payroll) and personnel are also provided. The Health Care Systems, Networks and Alliances section is an alphabetical listing of health care systems and their hospitals, a list of the names and addresses of networks and their hospitals, and multistate alliances and their members. The Health Organizations, Agencies and Other Health Care Providers section has four categories including national, international and regional organizations; U.S. government agencies; state and local organizations and government agencies; and other health care providers. Information from AHAData.com is available for purchase and provides the ability to download slices of data from the AHA Annual Survey Database. For example, introductory information and sample pages are available in PDF and HTML format. Information is available in an online session where users may select, customize, purchase, and download information about any or all of the more than 6,000 U.S. hospitals.

The *Guide to Canadian Health Care Facilities* provides information for each health care facility and is arranged geographically within sections by town or city and includes name, address, telephone numbers, ownership and operating body, the year of establishment, number of beds and bassinets, personnel, and the annual budget for a few entries. The amount of information varies per entry.

Internet Sources

12.54 *AHD.com.* Louisville, KY: American Hospital Directory, Inc. Available: www.ahd.com.

12.55 *Best Hospitals Finder. U.S. News & World Report.* Washington, DC: U.S. News & World Report. Available: www.usnews.com /usnews/nycu/health/hosptl/tophosp.htm.

12.56 *HospitalWeb.* Boston, MA: Massachusetts General Hospital, Department of Neurology. Available: http://neuro-www.mgh.harvard.edu/hospitalweb.shtml.

12.57 *MEDLINEplus: Specialized Hospitals and Clinics.* Bethesda, MD: National Library of Medicine. Available: www.nlm.nih.gov/medlineplus/directories.html.

12.58 *Quality Check.* Oakbrook Terrace, IL: Joint Commission on Accreditation of Healthcare Organizations. Available: www.jcaho.org/qualitycheck/directry/directry.asp.

AHD.com provides online data for over 6,000 hospitals. Information is built from Medicare claims data, cost reports, and other public-use files obtained from the federal Centers for Medicare and Medicaid Services (CMS, formerly HCFA). The directory also includes AHA Annual Survey Data licensed from *Health Forum*, an American Hospital Association company. Summary hospital data are provided free as a public service. Detailed information about hospitals is available only to subscribers.

Best Hospitals Finder from *U.S. News & World Report* ranks medical centers in different specialties. Centers are searchable by subject. Annoying advertisements pop up intermittently.

HospitalWeb from the Massachusetts General Hospital, Department of Neurology, provides hospital Web pages on the U.S. Hospitals on the World Wide Web page by state and Global Hospitals on the World Wide Web page (not including U.S.A.) by country.

MEDLINEplus: Specialized Hospitals and Clinics from the National Institutes of Health and other trusted sources includes 32 sources and is updated daily. The site lists links to Internet sites to locate general and specialized hospital and clinics.

Quality Check from the Joint Commission on Accreditation of Healthcare Organizations provides information on nearly 18,000 health care organizations.

Miscellaneous and Meta Directories

Many Internet sites compile extensive lists of directories of health-related Web sites. Fortunately, many of these are from trusted sources such as medial schools, hospital libraries, and governmental agencies. A few examples are provided, but a search of the following National Library of Medicine Web site (Available: www.nlm.nih.gov /libraries/state.html) directs the searcher to other medical school libraries, many of which are good sources for meta directories. Many medical school libraries provide a "reference shelf" or list of references that includes links to a number of useful online directories. Examples of health sciences library–sponsored sites are the University of Iowa's Hardin Meta Directory of Health Sources, which is a "list of lists" on health-related subjects. The subject pages indicate the length of lists in each subject. HealthWeb is a collaborative project of the health sciences libraries of the Greater Midwest Region (GMR) of the National Network of Libraries of Medicine (NN/LM) (Available: http://nnlm.gov/gmr/) and member libraries. The HealthWeb User Guides provide information on the Web for locating, evaluating, and using health-related Internet resources. MedWeb is maintained by the staff of the Robert W. Woodruff Health Sciences Center Library at Emory University. The University of Florida's Internet Resource Library has extensive links to health topics. From a hospital library, the National Jewish Medical and Research Center's Gerald Tucker Memorial Medical Library (Available: http://library.nationaljewish .org/index.html) provides a wide variety of information including consumer health resources and information pathfinders.

The following meta directories are examples from the United Kingdom. Each provides extensive categorized lists of sites.

12.59 *National Electronic Library for Health.* London and Leeds, U.K.: National Health Service. Available:www.nelh.nhs.uk.

12.60 *OMNI (Organising Medical Networked Information).* Nottingham, U.K.: University of Nottingham, Greenfield Medical Library. Available: http://omni.ac.uk.

National electronic Library for Health from the National Health Service is a meta directory from the United Kingdom. Similarly, OMNI is a U.K. gateway to high-quality Internet resources in health and medicine and was developed by experts based at the University of Nottingham Greenfield Medical Library in partnership with key organizations throughout the United Kingdom and beyond.

Two of following Web sites present directories of medical images, and the other gives a directory of instructions to authors.

12.61 *Public Health Image Library.* Atlanta, GA: Centers for Disease Control and Prevention. Available: http://phil.cdc.gov /Phil/default.asp.

12.62 *HONmedia.* Geneva: Health on the Net Foundation. Available: www.hon.ch/HONmedia.

12.63 *Instructions for Authors in the Health Sciences.* Toldeo, OH: Mulford Library, Medical College of Ohio. Available: www.mco.edu/lib/instr/libinsta.html.

Public Health Image Library from the Centers for Disease Control and Prevention provides an extensive directory of still images, image sets, and multimedia files.

HONmedia is a repository of 3,300 medical images and videos offered by Health On the Net Foundation, a nonprofit, nongovernmental organization.

Instructions for Authors in the Health Sciences, sponsored by Raymond H. Milford Library, Medical College of Ohio, provides links to Web sites that provide instructions to authors for over 3,500 journals in the health and life sciences. All links are to publishers and organizations with editorial responsibilities for the titles.

References

1. Katz WA. Ready reference sources. In: *Introduction to reference work. Volume one: basic information services*, 8th ed. New York: McGraw-Hill, 2002:280.
2. Dee CR. The information needs of rural physicians: a descriptive study. *Bull Med Libr Assoc* 1993; 8(3):263.
3. Boorkman JA. Directories and Biographical Sources. In: Roper F, Boorkman JA, eds. *Introduction to reference sources in the health sciences.* Metuchen, NJ: Scarecrow Press, 1994:238.
4. Katz WA, op. cit.
5. Balay R. *Guide to reference books*, 11th ed. Chicago, IL: American Library Association, 1996.
6. Walford AJ. *Walford's Guide to reference material.* London: The Library Association, 2000.

CHAPTER 13

HISTORY SOURCES

Lucretia W. McClure

"The library is the historian's laboratory," and in health sciences libraries, the historian may be a resident, a student, a physician, or an individual interested in a particular topic or person in the fields of medicine or science. Gnudi goes on to say the historian must have the scholarly reference works that form the "working apparatus" of this laboratory [1].

The purpose of this chapter is to provide a sampling of the resources that hold the information necessary to the users seeking historical facts and knowledge. The earlier editions of this book included chapters on history sources by Judith A. Overmier [2]. They continue to be relevant and useful. This chapter will focus on new resources as well as those that may be found in a general collection. Many libraries in the health sciences do not have formal history of medicine departments or collections; yet users come with history-related questions. There are a surprising number of books, journals, materials in electronic format, and so forth, that may be useful in answering questions of a historical nature. Librarians must develop a creative mode of thinking when searching for answers in general works.

The Nature of Questions

Many of the questions fall into these categories: biographical, bibliographical, dates and facts, and illustrations. These are the "Who was it?" "What did he do?" "When did it happen?" "Do you have a picture of it?" questions. The development of the Internet brings a new dimension to the librarian's ability to find historical information. Once it was necessary to have the volumes at hand in order to search. Today, the library can supplement its print resources with an array of digital locations. Because the Internet changes rapidly, only a sample of Web sites will be provided because new URLs appear and disappear daily.

The librarian in a small medical, hospital, or special library now has more opportunity than ever to search for the answers to historical questions. When the search of print resources proves unfruitful, the Web opens doors to the home pages of libraries with spectacular history of medicine collections. These libraries often have librarians with extensive knowledge of the history of medicine who may provide assistance. The history of medicine organizations have Web sites as well as electronic discussion lists and all may be tapped for guidance and help.

Biographical Sources

One of the most frequently asked questions is about the individual physician or scientist. Often the person asking has sketchy information at best. Knowing the dates of birth or death, an institution from which the individual was graduated or taught, or a medical specialty can give the librarian a lead to an obituary or an announcement of an honor. The following are examples of resources of biographical information.

13.1 Hafner AW, ed. *Directory of Deceased American Physicians, 1804–1929; a genealogical guide to over 149,000 medical practitioners providing brief biographical sketches drawn from the American Medical Association's Deceased Physician Masterfile.* Chicago, IL: American Medical Association, 1993. 2 vol.

13.2 *The New York Times Obituaries Index.* New York: New York Times, 1970–1980. v.1, 1858–1968; v.2, 1969–1978.

13.3 Magill FN, ed. *The Nobel Prize Winners: Physiology or Medicine.* Pasadena, CA: Salem Press, 1991–. v.1, 1901–1944; v.2, 1944–1969; v.3, 1969–1990.

13.4 *JAMA: The Journal of the American Medical Association.* Chicago, IL: American Medical Association, 1919–. v.1–.

13.5 Sammons VO. *Blacks in Science and Medicine.* New York: Hemisphere, 1990.

13.6 Bullough VL, Church OM, Stein AP. *American Nursing; A Biographical Dictionary.* New York: Garland, 1988–1992. 2 vol.

13.7 Scrivener L, et al. *A Biographical Dictionary of Women Healers: Midwives, Nurses, and Physicians.* Westport, CT: Oryx Press, 2002.

13.8 Thacher J. *American Medical Biography.* Boston, MA: Richardson & Lord, 1828. 2 vols. in 1. Reprint: New York: DaCapo, 1967.

13.9 Atkinson WB. *The Physicians and Surgeons of the United States.* Philadelphia, PA: Robson, 1878.

13.10 Kelly HA. *Cyclopedia of American Medical Biography: Comprising the Lives of Eminent Deceased Physicians and Surgeons from 1610–1910.* Philadelphia, PA: Saunders, 1912. 2 vol.

13.11 Kelly HA, Burrage WL. *American Medical Biographies.* Baltimore, MD: Norman, Remington, 1920.

13.12 Kelly HA, Burrage WL. *Dictionary of American Medical Biography.* New York: Appleton, 1928.

13.13 Holloway LM. *Medical Obituaries: American Physicians' Biographical Notices in Selected Medical Journals before 1907.* New York: Garland, 1981.

Each of these tools provides information for those seeking biographical material. The AMA *Directory of Deceased American Physicians* includes indexes of African American practitioners, female practitioners, and self-designated eclectic, homeopathic, and osteopathic practitioners. *The New York Times Obituaries Index* provides the date of death and location of an obituary. Finding the death date of an individual is often the key to locating further information (i.e., an obituary, and so forth). *The Nobel Prize Winners: Physiology or Medicine* provides comprehensive information on a laureate's life and career, along with description of the speeches and commentary that accompany the awarding of the Nobel Prize.

One of the most useful sources for information is *The Journal of the American Medical Association* (*JAMA*). The journal indexes list names of physicians under the terms Deaths or Obituaries, leading to brief obituaries that provide basic information. Specialty journals often have extensive obituaries of their noted members, and the transactions of many societies write elaborate memoirs of cherished members.

More than 1,500 African-American physicians, scientists, and other professionals are listed in *Blacks in Science and Medicine*. Bullough's *American Nursing* directory includes biographies of 175 women and two men in nursing who were deceased or born before 1890. The *Dictionary of Women Healers* is another source for information on women in a variety of health professions.

The biographical tools for American physicians of an earlier age begin with Thacher. His work was followed by Atkinson, Kelly, and others. All are of value when searching for biographies and/or portraits of important practitioners. Holloway's work includes brief biographical information as well as sources of obituaries for some 17,350 physicians deceased before 1907.

13.14 Rosen G, Caspari-Rosen B, coll. and arrang. *400 Years of a Doctor's Life.* New York: Schuman, 1947.

13.15 Comroe JH, Jr. *Retrospectroscope: Insights Into Medical Discovery.* Menlo Park, CA: Von Gehr Press, 1977.

Popular biographies or sources such as Rosen's *400 Years* portray physicians through short sketches or personal experiences. Other titles such as Comroe's *Retrospectroscope* offer background information concerning various discoveries, thus shining light on the scientist or physician seeking answers.

Other good biographical information may be found in alumni directories, local newspapers, and historical society publications. Major textbooks often have biographical information concerning those who developed a treatment or device or who made significant breakthroughs in medicine or science. The standard medical, nursing, and dental directories are also useful in finding basic information about individuals. Databases such as MEDLINE as well as the print *Index Medicus* for earlier years are good sources for obituaries of well-known individuals in science and medicine. The *Journal of Medical Biography*, started in 1993 by the Royal Society of Medicine in London, has biographies of both patients and physicians.

Biographical Web Sites

With the advent of the Internet, a whole realm of resources has been developed. Never before has so much information been available at the touch of a keyboard. The caveat is, of course, to be certain of the creator of the information and to view all sites with a healthy skepticism. Among the useful sites are the following:

13.16 *Biography and Genealogy Master Index.* Farmington Hills, MI: Gale Group. Available: http://galenet.gale.com /a/acp/db/bgmi.

13.17 *Whonamedit.com.* Oslo: Whonamedit.com Available: www.whonamedit.com.

13.18 *Profiles in Science.* Bethesda, MD: National Library of Medicine. Available: www.profiles.nlm.nih.gov.

13.19 *The Social Security Death Index*. Provo, UT: MyFamily.com, Inc. Available: http://ssdi.genealogy.rootsweb.com.

13.20 *American National Biography Online*. New York: Oxford University Press, 2000. Available: www.anb.org.

The Web tools listed above offer a great variety of coverage. The Gale resource lists persons from all time periods, geographical locations, and fields of endeavor. The Whonamedit source lists eponyms from A to Z, includes biographies by country, lists female entries, traces the eponym to the article by the named author, and identifies the source of an obituary.

The National Library of Medicine is producing the Profiles in Science database, listing prominent twentieth-century biomedical scientists. The listing may be reviewed chronologically or alphabetically and many have pictures and papers. The Death Index lists more than 70 million names, including dates of birth and death, social security number, last known residence, and date of last benefit. The American National Biography includes some 18,000 men and women who have influenced and shaped American history and culture.

There are many such sources on the Internet today, and it is likely that many more will appear. A search may start with putting an individual's name on a search engine to bring forth an array of sites. Comparing the information with one of the standard biographical tools is one way to ensure that the information is accurate.

Portraits and Illustrations

While many of the biographical sources include portraits of the individuals, there is need for resources that point to the printed source or institutional location of portraits of widely known scientists, physicians, nurses, or others in the health field. Several works that include anatomical illustrations are also listed.

13.21 *Portrait Catalog of the Library of the New York Academy of Medicine*. Boston: G. K. Hall, 1960. 5 vol. Suppl. 1, 1959–1965; Suppl. 2, 1966–1970; Suppl. 3, 1971–1975.

13.22 Berkowitz JS. *The College of Physicians of Philadelphia Portrait Catalogue.* Philadelphia, PA: The College, 1984.

13.23 Burgess R. *Portraits of Doctors and Scientists in the Wellcome Institute of the History of Medicine. A Catalogue.* London: Wellcome Institute for the History of Medicine, 1973.

13.24 Roberts KB, Tomlinson JDW. *The Fabric of the Body: European Traditions of Anatomical Illustration.* Oxford: Clarendon Press, 1992.

13.25 Porter R. *The Cambridge Illustrated History of Medicine.* Cambridge: Cambridge University Press, 1996.

13.26 Netter FH. *The Ciba Collection of Medical Illustrations, A Compilation of Pathological and Anatomical Paintings.* Summit, NJ: Ciba Pharmaceutical Products, 1959–1993.

The New York Academy of Medicine Library's catalog is the most comprehensive source for portraits. Included are the library's holdings of more than 14,000 original portraits, paintings, woodcuts, engravings, and photographs. In addition, it provides nearly 300,000 citations to portraits in journals and books, both primary and secondary sources. The College of Physicians and the Wellcome catalogs are examples of sources for portraits or paintings from these institutions.

Illustrations of a medical nature are often requested by historians, scholars, writers, and students. *The Fabric of the Body* is an anthology of anatomical illustrations from the medieval period to the present day. It includes text about the anatomists, their collaborators, and their books. It is also about the context in which anatomical illustrations were prepared and distributed. The work features some of the most beautiful and renowned anatomical illustrations. Porter's work uses illustrations to further describe the sections on disease, hospitals and surgery, medical science, and so forth. The Ciba collection includes eight volumes, some with many parts, illustrating various parts of the body such as nervous system, respiratory system, reproductive system, and so forth.

Images On the Web

The Internet offers a wide range of sites with images and portraits. One has only to enter the words "medical illustrations" in a search engine to find dozens of possibilities. The National Library of Medicine has two important offerings.

13.27 *Images from the History of Medicine* (*IHM*). Bethesda, MD: National Library of Medicine. Available: http://wwwihm.nlm.nih.gov.

13.28 *The Visible Human Project.* Bethesda, MD: National Library of Medicine. Available: www.nlm.nih.gov/research /visible/visible_human.html.

13.29 *Online Portrait Gallery of the Moody Medical Library, University of Texas Medical Branch at Galveston.* Galveston, TX: University of Texas. Available: www.utmb.edu.

13.30 Wellcome Trust. *History of Medicine.* London: Wellcome Trust. Available: www.wellcome.ac.uk.

13.31 *The Whole Brain Atlas.* Cambridge, MA: Harvard School of Medicine. Available: www.med.harvard.edu:80/AANLIB /home.htm.

The National Library of Medicine's database has nearly 60,000 images from the Library's historical and photographs collection. It includes portraits, photographs, fine prints, caricatures, genre scenes, posters, and other graphic art illustrating the social and historical aspects of medicine from the Middle Ages to the present. The Visible Human Project is the creation of complete, anatomically detailed, three-dimensional representations of the normal male and female bodies.

Many libraries have mounted portraits and images from their collections on the Web. Two examples are the thirty-nine portraits from the 6,000 images relating to the history of the biomedical sciences in the Moody Medical Library and the Wellcome Trust's site that includes a medical photographic library with exquisite images from the library's collections.

The Whole Brain Atlas produced by Keith A. Johnson and J. Alex Becker is a source providing central nervous system imaging which integrates clinical information with magnetic resonance, computed tomography, and nuclear medicine images.

Medical Instruments

Libraries receive many requests to identify medical instruments as well as to provide illustrations of scalpels, obstetric tools such as forceps, artificial hearts, and so forth. Two examples, one print and one from the Internet, are representative of available sources.

13.32 Edmonson JM. *American Surgical Instruments: The History of Their Manufacture and a Directory of Instrument Makers to 1900.* San Francisco, CA: Norman Publishing, 1997.

13.33 Shultz SM. *Sources for Identification of Antique Medical Instruments in Print and on the Internet.* York, PA: WellSpan Health. Available: www.priory.com/homol/ant.htm.

Edmondson's work is a comprehensive directory of surgical instrument makers in the United States prior to 1900 with some 280 illustrations. The Web site includes a bibliography of books and articles on antique instruments, Internet sites, catalogs, and dealers.

Readers should be cautioned to note the copyright restrictions for use of images from both print and Web sources.

Discoveries/Chronologies

Questions concerning medical discoveries and happenings are among the most frequent. These questions take the form of who made a scientific discovery, when did an event take place, and were there controversies. The following tools provide answers.

13.34 Morton LT, Moore RJ. *A Chronology of Medicine and Related Sciences.* Aldershot, Hants, England: Scolar Press, 1997.

13.35 Friedman M, Friedland GW. *Medicine's 10 Greatest Discoveries.* New Haven, CT: Yale University Press, 1998.

13.36 Schmidt JE. *Medical Discoveries: Who and When; A Dictionary Listing Thousands of Medical and Related Scientific Discoveries in Alphabetical Order* . . . . Springfield, IL: Thomas, 1959.

Morton's work begins with 3000 BC and runs through 1996. Only 236 pages brings one to 1850; from 1851 to 1996 requires 430 pages. The Friedman work is a more detailed review of major discoveries whereas Schmidt's work is an easy to use dictionary with brief statements.

Chronology Web Sites

There are dozens of Internet sites devoted to medical discoveries, both general and by specialty. The following example is from the National Institutes of Health:

13.37 *NIH Chronology of Events.* Bethesda, MD: National Institutes of Health. Available: www.nih.gov/about/almanac /historical/chronology_of_events.htm.

Bibliographies/Library Catalogs

The advent of the Internet and the ease and speed of citation retrieval has changed the way individuals search for information. While the MEDLINE database is a boon to searchers for literature from 1957 onward, historians and scholars as well as students need resources that cover the literature of earlier centuries. Medicine has an array of print resources that serve users well.

13.38 *Index-Catalogue of the Library of the Surgeon-General's Office.* Washington, DC: Government Printing Office, 1880.

61 volumes in 5 series: 1880–1895; 1896–1916; 1913–1932; 1936–1955; 1959–1961.

13.39 *Current Work in the History of Medicine.* London: Wellcome Institute for the History of Medicine, 1954–1999. Available: http://library.wellcome.ac.uk.

13.40 Norman J, ed. *Morton's Medical Bibliography: An Annotated Check-List of Texts Illustrating the History of Medicine (Garrison and Morton)*, 5th ed. Aldershot, Hants, England: Gower, 1991.

13.41 Hoolihan C, comp. and annot. *An Annotated Catalogue of the Edward C. Atwater Collection of American Popular Medicine and Health Reform.* Rochester, NY: University of Rochester Press, 2001–.

13.42 Washington University (Saint Louis, MO), School of Medicine Library. *Catalog of the Bernard Becker, M.D. Collection in Ophthalmology*, 2nd ed. St. Louis, MO: Washington University School of Medicine Library, 1983.

13.43 Wygant LJ, comp. *The Truman G. Blocker, Jr., History of Medicine Collections: Books and Manuscripts.* Galveston, TX: University of Texas Medical Branch, 1986.

13.44 *A Catalogue of Printed Books in the Wellcome Historical Medical Library.* New York: Martino Publishers, 1995–.

The publications of the National Library of Medicine, the largest medical library in the world, are the most comprehensive for users working in the history of medicine. The *Index-Catalogue* is the monumental work established by John Shaw Billings in 1880 which includes the holdings of the Surgeon-General's Library, now the National Library of Medicine. The dates of the volumes do not reflect the dates of the items; the first three series cover the books, articles, pamphlets, and dissertations from 1500 through the 1926. A project to digitize the

Index-Catalogue is underway, and its completion will provide an enormous database for older materials.

The *Index Medicus,* the index to the most important and most used journals in medicine, is also useful in the search for articles of an earlier time. Published under various titles, this print source includes obituaries. A complete description of *Index Medicus* will be found in Chapter 4. It should be noted here that MEDLINE does include the citations formerly in the Histline database. The print version of Histline, the *Bibliography of the History of Medicine,* was published by NLM from 1964 to 1993.

Current Work in the History of Medicine is an index to periodical articles on the history of medicine and includes a list of books received in the Wellcome Library. The Wellcome Library now publishes *Current Work in the History of Medicine* as the Wellcome Bibliography for the History of Medicine on its Web site.

In addition to the bibliographies cited above, there is a definitive bibliography now in its fifth edition. *Morton's Medical Bibliography* is a heavily used resource listing nearly 9,000 publications, classed by subject, that were of significance in the development of Western medicine. Translations and reprint editions are noted. The first four editions were produced by Leslie T. Morton, beginning in 1943. He based the work on a list of milestones in the development of medicine compiled by Fielding H. Garrison and which was printed in the *Index-Catalogue,* volume 17:89–178, 1912. Morton undertook the task of expanding and updating the list after Garrison's death, hence the designation Garrison and Morton.

Many libraries have published catalogs of collections on special topics that can be of great help to historians and others searching for works on one subject. The Atwater collection on popular medicine and the Becker collection on ophthalmology are good examples of topical bibliographies. The Wellcome and the Blocker catalogues reflect the holdings of the libraries.

Histories

Histories of medicine provide a wide range of information. Some are general, covering the entire realm, others focus on an aspect or specific time period. Following are examples of a variety of histories.

13.45 Kiple KF, ed. *The Cambridge World History of Human Disease.* Cambridge; New York: Cambridge University Press, 1993.

13.46 Bynum WF, Porter R, eds. *Companion Encyclopedia of the History of Medicine.* New York: Routledge, 1993. 2 vol.

13.47 Kohn GC. *Encyclopedia of Plague and Pestilence.* New York: Facts on File, 1995.

13.48 Major RH. *History of Medicine.* Springfield, IL: Thomas, 1954. 2 vol.

13.49 Sigerist HE. *A History of Medicine.* New York: Oxford University Press, 1951–61. 2 vol.

13.50 Castiflioni A; Krumbhaar EB, trans. *A History of Medicine,* 2nd ed., rev. and enl. New York: Alfred A. Knopf, 1958.

13.51 Garrison FH, ed. *An Introduction to the History of Medicine, With Medical Chronology, Suggestions for Study, and Bibliographic Data,* 4th ed., reprinted. Philadelphia, PA: Saunders, 1966.

Histories abound in the fields of medicine and science. The Cambridge volume includes essays on distribution of diseases, medical traditions, various organs, and organ systems as well as a section on "Major Human Diseases Past and Present" arranged alphabetically by disease. The *Companion Encyclopedia* is a two-volume work arranged by topics whereas the *Encyclopedia of Plague and Pestilence* outlines and provides a timeline for specific epidemics.

Many older volumes of history continue to be of use. While they vary in style and organization, all serve as a starting point for those interested to learn from and about the past. The titles by Major, Sigerist, and Castiglioni have served generations of readers. The Garrison history includes a medical chronology and suggestions for study; a great book for anyone who wishes to use such a resource as a study guide with answers.

History of Medicine Journals

Many journals contain historical articles along with their general topics. There are also journals devoted to the history of medicine. A number of the titles are now online.

13.52 *Bulletin of the History of Medicine.* Baltimore, MD: Johns Hopkins University Press; American Association for the History of Medicine, 1939–. 7–. Available: http://muse .jhu.edu/journals/bulletin_of_the_history_of_medicine.

13.53 *Gesnerus.* Basel: Schwabe; Swiss Society of the History of Medicine, 1943–. 1–.

13.54 *Isis.* Chicago, IL: University of Chicago Press for the History of Science Society, 1913–. 1–. Available: www.journals .uchicago.edu/Isis/home.html.

13.55 *Journal of the History of Medicine and Allied Sciences.* London: Oxford University Press, 1946–. 1–. Available: http: //www3.oup.co.uk/jalsci.

13.56 *Medical History.* London: Wellcome Trust Centre for the History of Medicine, 1957–. 1–.

History of medicine journals provide the works of today's medical and scientific historians. All of the journals cited contain articles and book reviews. The *Journal of the History of Medicine and Allied Sciences* also carries a list of recent dissertations in the history of medicine. The titles cover the social, cultural, and scientific aspects of medical history as well as the other disciplines that impinge on it.

Tools for the Librarian

Librarians must deal with questions concerning the book as a physical object as well as the content it contains. Many questions arise about the cost of books and other publications as well as how to care for books, determination of quality over time, and how to become a collector. Librarians must know and understand the structure of bibliography and be prepared to answer questions concerning collations, watermarks, signatures, and so forth. Medical publishing and medical literature are topics of great interest to historians and scholars, and the library will find the following array of sources to be a good basis for collecting in this area.

13.57 *American Book Prices Current.* New York: Bancroft-Parkman, 1894/95–. Vol. 1–.

13.58 *Bookman's Price Index.* Detroit, MI: Gale, 1964–. Vol. 1–.

13.59 Carter J. *ABC for Book Collectors,* 7th ed. New Castle, DE; New York: Oak Knoll Press, 1998.

13.60 McKerrow RB. *An Introduction to Bibliography for Literary Students.* Winchester: St. Paul's Bibliographies; New Castle, DE: Oak Knoll Press, 1994.

13.61 Thornton JL. *Thornton's Medical Books, Libraries, and Collectors; A Study of Bibliography and the Book Trade in Relation to the Medical Sciences,* 3rd rev. ed. Aldershot, Hants, U.K.: Gower, 1990.

13.62 Blake JB, Roos C. *Medical Reference Works, 1679–1966, A Selected Bibliography.* Chicago, IL: Medical Library Association, 1967. Three supplements: 1970–1975.

Library users as well as librarians are interested in the prices of book they wish either to purchase or donate. The *American Book Prices Current* and *Bookman's Price Index* are useful for this purpose as are recent catalogs from rare-book dealers. The world of the "book," its production, description, format, and terminology are identified in Carter's *ABC for Book Collectors* and in McKerrow's classic work on bibliography. The development of medical literature and the book trade are examined in Besson's revision of Thornton's *Medical Books*. Blake and Roos provide the standard list of medical reference works dating from 1679 through 1975.

13.63 Brooks C, Darling PW. *Disaster Preparedness.* Washington, DC: Association of Research Libraries, 1993.

13.64 Waters P. *Procedures for Salvage of Water-Damaged Library Materials,* 2nd ed. Washington, DC: Library of Congress, 1979.

13.65 Harvey DR. *Preservation in Libraries: Principles, Strategies, and Practices for Librarians.* London; New York: Bowker-Saur, 1993.

13.66 Horton C. *Cleaning and Preserving Bindings and Related Materials,* 2nd ed., rev. Chicago, IL: Library Technology Program, American Library Association, 1969.

Acquiring is only the first step in collection management. The volumes held in both special and general collections must properly be housed, handled, and, when necessary, repaired or restored. Preservation is an essential part of the library's responsibility for its collections. The books on disaster preparedness, water damage, and preservation are full of information to help librarians deal with the protection of their collections.

Rare book librarianship has many facets because of the great variety of formats collected in history of medicine libraries. Users of the collections are also varied as individuals interested in history and historical research range from students to scholars, laymen to health professionals, historians of medicine to those in different disciplines.

Good overviews of the kinds of work expected from rare book/history librarians as well as the wide range of resources needed can be found in the series of handbooks published by the Medical Library Association. The titles given in the "Readings" section below will acquaint librarians with background and guidelines.

References

1. Gnudi MT. Building a medical history collection. *Bull Med Libr Assoc* 1975 Jan.; 63(1):42–46.
2. Overmier JA. History sources. In: Roper FW, Boorkman JA, eds. *Introduction to reference sources in the health sciences*, 3rd ed. Metuchen, NJ: Scarecrow Press, 1994:257–270.

Readings

1. Annan GL. Rare books and the history of medicine. In: Doe J, ed. *A handbook of medical library practice*. Chicago, IL: American Library Association, 1943:256–370.
2. Cavanagh GST. Rare books, archives, and the history of medicine. In: Annan GL, Felter JW, eds. *Handbook of medical library practice*, 3rd ed. Chicago, IL: Medical Library Association, 1970:254–283.
3. Zinn NW. Special collections: history of health science collections, oral history, archives, and manuscripts. In: Darling L, ed. *Handbook of medical library practice*, 4th ed. Chicago, IL: Medical Library Association, 1988:469–572.

Chapter 14

Grant Sources

Jo Anne Boorkman

In today's economy, there is an increasing opportunity for health sciences librarians to play an important role in assisting health professionals and institutions to meet their funding needs, whether the library user is researching the availability of support for a research project, a travel grant, "bricks and mortar" funding for a major construction project, or seed money to start a new program. In order to offer effective service, the librarian must be familiar with the complex structure of the grant-making world along with the equally complex array of information sources in this area.

There is a wide range of information sources available that deals with the different grant-making organizations. Sources vary in terms of funding sectors included, comprehensiveness, level of specificity, format, disciplines covered, and frequency of updating. The grant seeker's primary purpose is to locate appropriate funding agencies likely to be interested in a specific project. This task will involve surveying federal programs in the relevant field and, if advisable, examining the foundation and corporate arenas through a geographic or subject approach to identify likely contributors. The grant seeker will need to discern how closely the proposed project matches a foundation's or agency's interests and funding patterns.

There are three types of publications that will be useful in this process, regardless of which sector the applicant ends up approaching. These include grantsmanship guides, directories, and indexes. This chapter will concentrate on directories that encompass both government and private funding sources.

Multisector Directories

14.1 *Annual Register of Grant Support.* New Medford, NJ: Information Today, 1969–. Annual. Continues *Grant Data Quarterly.* Los Angeles, CA: Academic Media, 1967–1968. Available: www.infotoday.com.

Now in its 36th edition (2003), this multidisciplinary directory covers more than 3,500 support programs and fellowships of government agencies, public and private foundations, corporations, community trusts, unions, educational and professional associations, and special interest organizations. While not comprehensive, this directory contains entries for various special interest organizations, such as the American Diabetes Association, that are not found in some of the other major sources. It provides a good place to start. The directory has a classified arrangement organized by 11 major subject areas with 61 subcategories and four indexes: subject, organization and program, geographic, and personnel. The introduction discusses types of grant-supporting organizations, and there is a chapter on program planning and proposal writing. The "Life Sciences" chapter includes medicine and other health sciences specialties.

14.2 *Directory of Research Grants.* Phoenix, AZ: Oryx Press, 1975–. Annual. Available: www.grantselect.com.

14.3 *Directory of Biomedical and Health Care Grants.* Phoenix, AZ: Oryx Press, 1985–. Annual. Available: www.grantselect.com.

These two sources are part of an array of grant-oriented Oryx Press products. The *Directory of Research Grants,* now in its 28th edition in 2003, is more comprehensive and includes more than 3,700 listings of research programs from 1,880 U.S. and foreign governments, foundation, and corporate sponsors. Entries are alphabetically arranged with subject, sponsoring organization, and sponsoring type (e.g., nonprofit organization, foundation) indexes. The *Directory of Biomedical and Health Care Grants* lists slightly over 3,000 funding programs, with the same format and indexes as *Directory of Research Grants.* The 18th edition is due in October 2003. Entries include information: from 1) the sponsor's update of previously published program statements included in prior editions of GRANTS publications; 2) questionnaires sent to sponsors whose programs were not included in previous editions; 3) other materials published by the sponsor and furnished by Oryx. Updated information for U.S. government programs includes new and revised program information published in the latest edition of the *Catalog of Federal Domestic Assistance* [Introduction].

The GRANTS database from which these publications are printed is available through DIALOG as well as the publisher. Larger libraries that serve clientele with broad subject interests will be more interested in having the *Directory of Research Grants* available; smaller libraries with clientele strictly in the health sciences will find the *Directory of Biomedical and Health Care Grants* more appropriate because it singles out those sponsoring organizations that support the health care fields specifically. Both publications include a section "A guide to Proposal Planning and Writing," by Jeremy Miner and Lynn Miner.

Federal Funding Sources

One caveat for grant seekers is that sources of federal funding should be explored before turning to foundations. This sequence is necessary because foundations tend to avoid duplicating federal programs and because the federal government still plays a major role in the total funding picture, in spite of well-publicized federal spending cutbacks.

The grant seeker will find some significant differences between the application process for private and federal funds. Federal agencies usually have standardized application forms whereas foundations tend to provide the grant writer with only general application guidelines allowing more flexibility in the proposal. Furthermore, as a matter of public policy, all federal grant opportunities are announced in advance while printed material about foundation and corporate giving may be scarce—especially for small grant-making organizations.

Because two major, comprehensive government publications on federal support exist, reference service in this area of funding could be viewed as a deceptively simple enterprise. For contract opportunities, one would consult the *Commerce Business Daily* (*CBD*), which is now available on the Web as CBDNet (http://cbdnet.access.gpo.gov) and for grants, the hefty *Catalog of Federal Domestic Assistance* (*CFDA*), which is also available on the Web (www.cfda.gov). However, this approach discounts the fact that government programs are in a constant state of flux with changing funding levels, program status, and application procedures prevailing. Furthermore, a variety of materials published by individual federal grant-making agencies supplement program information in the *CFDA*. Then, too, the commercially produced sources on government funding should be consulted. Some of these publications are informative and help the grant seeker cope with the changing federal scene; others are simply duplicated government publications being sold at inflated prices.

Effective information service in the federal funding arena begins with a basic knowledge of the agency supporting biomedical projects. The Public Health Service supports the bulk of biomedical investigations. There is a number of major grant-making agencies within the Office of Public Health and Science of the U.S. Department of Health and Human Services (Available: www.hhs.gov/grants/index.shtml). These include:

- Agency for Healthcare Research and Quality (AHRQ)
- Agency for Toxic Substances and Disease Registry (ATSDR)
- Centers for Disease Control and Prevention (CDC)
- Food and Drug Administration (FDA)
- Health Resources and Services Administration (HRSA)
- National Institutes of Health (NIH)
- Substance Abuse and Mental Health Services Administration (SAMHSA)

With its mission to improve human health through research, the National Institutes of Health programs provide a broad array of opportunities for funding research oriented toward basic and applied scientific inquiry related to the cause, diagnosis, prevention, treatment, and rehabilitation of human diseases and disabilities; the fundamental biological processes of growth, development, and aging; and the biological effects of the environment. In addition, the National Science Foundation and the Environmental Protection Agency both administer

funding programs of potential interest to the health sciences professional.

14.4   *NIH Guide for Grants and Contracts (Online)*. Bethesda, MD: NIH
       Office of Extramural Research. January 17, 1992–. Formerly:
       National Institutes of Health. *NIH Guide for Grants and Contracts*.
       Washington, DC: U.S. Government Printing Office, 1966–1997.
       No. 26–no.40. Available: http://grants2.nih.gov/grants/guide
       /index.html.

14.5   *Computer Retrieval of Information on Scientific Projects (CRISP)*.
       Bethesda, MD: 1972–. Available: http://crisp.cit.nih.gov.

The *NIH Guide for Grants and Contracts* is the primary source for
NIH awards. It contains relevant NIH policy information as well as new
program announcements. Now available on the Web, the *NIH Guide for
Grants and Contracts* provides a listserv, comprehensive archives, and
program announcements. It is completely searchable from 1992 to the
present. Scanned PDF copies of historical files covering the period
1972–1992 are also available.

The CRISP database provides information on grants and contracts
awarded by the National Institutes of Health, Office of Substance
Abuse and Mental Health Services, Health Resources and Services
Administration, Food and Drug Administration, Centers for Disease
Control and Prevention, Agency for Healthcare Research and Quality,
and the Office of Assistant Secretary of Health (OASH). It provides
another means for determining which agency to approach with a proposal. Basic and Advanced searching is possible and instructions are
provided for searching by keywords or fields. The database is updated
weekly. This information was formerly published in *Biomedical Index
to PHS-supported Research* (National Institutes of Health, Divisions of
Research. Washington, DC: U.S. Government Printing Office, 1988–.
Annual. Formerly: National Institutes of Health. *Research Awards
Index*. Washington, DC: U.S. Government Printing Office,
1976–1987.)

349

Foundation Funding

A private foundation is a nongovernmental, nonprofit organization with funds usually coming from a single source, such as an individual family or corporation. These funds are managed by the foundation's directors or trustees to "maintain or aid educational, social, charitable, religious, or other activities serving the common welfare primarily by making grants to other nonprofit organizations" [1]. In the United States, there are approximately 22,500 private foundations falling into four basic categories: independent, company sponsored, operating, and community. Briefly, independent foundations award grants from an endowment established by a single donor or family and giving may or may not be restricted by geographic or subject area.

Company-sponsored foundations manage funds provided by a profit-making corporation and are inclined to make awards in the neighboring communities of the sponsoring company. An operating foundation usually makes few external grants; instead, it uses endowment funds to conduct its own research or social welfare programs. As the name implies, community foundations are publicly supported and make grants to charitable organizations in the local community.

Unlike the federal government, which generates a constant stream of funding announcements, foundations do not usually issue lists of grants to be awarded in the upcoming months. In fact, depending on the size of the foundation, it may be difficult to locate any specifics at all about an organization's giving priorities.

Tracking down appropriate foundations is not a trivial exercise. No matter what the requirements of a particular proposal, the Foundation Center publications are the most highly recommended resources in the area of grantsmanship. Located in New York City, the Foundation Center's mission is to collect information on private foundations and then distribute this information through its publications and library collections. For reference purposes, the librarian should be aware of this organization's nationwide network of reference libraries where extensive grant information collections are maintained and open to public use. A list of these cooperating collections may be found in any of the Foundation Center reference tools.

14.6 *Foundation Directory.* New York: The Foundation Center, 1960–. Annual. Available: www.fdncenter.org.

14.7 *Foundation Grants Index.* New York: The Foundation Center, distributed by Columbia University Press 1970/71–. Annual. Available: www.fdncenter.org.

The *Foundation Directory* is one of many publications from the Foundation Center. The 2003 25th edition lists the 10,000 largest grant-making foundations of nonprofit, nongovernmental organizations that have private financial backing that ranges from $1 million to $10 million in assets [Introduction]. This edition provides information on over 39,000 grants. This directory is especially useful for individuals seeking funds for research and education. Entries are geographically arranged by state and include the address, date of establishment, donors, trustees, and purpose of the foundation as well as its fields of interest and financial assets. Also included is grant application information. Indexes provide access by:

1. Names of persons associated with the foundations, such as donors, trustees, and administrators.
2. Geographic location.
3. Types of support (e.g., annual campaigns, building funds, conferences, and seminars).
4. Subject.
5. Foundations new to the edition.
6. Foundation names.

The Foundation Directory Online is a searchable, fee-based service with varying subscription levels available. The entire database, representing over 70,000 grant-makers with over 200,000 grants, can be searched in its entirety by subject, foundation name, or grant type. More focused searching of the 20,000 or 10,000 largest foundations is also available. The database is updated biweekly and has links to free Web resources. Annual and multiyear subscriptions are also available.

Corporate Funding

In addition to the independent company-sponsored foundations, corporations also distribute funds through direct giving programs. Since 1935, the Internal Revenue Service has allowed a charitable deduction for corporate contributions up to 5% of net income. Due to the nature of direct corporate giving and the lack of published reference resources in this area, fund-raising from the business sector depends heavily on personal contact.

Given the idiosyncratic nature of corporate philanthropy and the scarcity of published information about corporate giving policies, fund-raising from the business sector is at least as challenging as tracking the small foundation grant. It is common knowledge that most corporations do not employ professionals to operate systematically the company giving program, nor do they have well-defined philanthropic objectives or procedures for grant applications. Companies offer various reasons for this lack of definition in corporate grant programs, ranging from a reluctance to violate corporate confidentiality to the fear of a deluge of applications.

Grant seekers should be aware that even company-sponsored foundations have little autonomy and exist merely to carry out the philanthropic objectives of their sponsoring corporations. No matter how vague or nonexistent their published charitable giving guidelines, corporations tend to fund organizations serving company employees, communities in which the company operates, research in related fields, or projects that will bolster the company's public image [2]. The company's financial outlook and the special interests of the organization's principal officers also play a part in the contributions. The burden of proof is clearly on the grant seeker to demonstrate how a project is related to the company's products and services or how the company's customers, employees, or public image could benefit from funding the proposal. The specialized directories discussed in this section are particularly suited to the corporate funding environment.

14.8   *Corporate Foundation Profiles*. New York: The Foundation Center, 1980–. Irregular.

14.9   *Corporate Giving Directory.* Rockville, MD: Taft Group, 1991–.
Annual. Continues *Taft Corporate Giving Directory.* Washington,
DC: Taft Group, 1984–1990. Continues *Taft Corporate Directory.*
Washington, DC: Taft Corporation, 1981–1984.

Compiled by the Foundation Center, *Corporate Foundation
Profiles* appeared in its 12th edition in 2002. It provides detailed profiles of 181 of the largest company-sponsored foundations that have
made annual contributions over $1.2 million. Each foundation profile
is divided into three sections providing a Foundation Portrait with basic
information about the foundation, including the purpose, giving limitations, and application guidelines; Grant Analysis, providing detailed
information on the foundation's grant program; and Sample Grants,
where recently awarded grants are listed. An appendix provides additional information on 1,131 corporate foundations that provided at least
$66,000 annually in grants.

The *Corporate Giving Directory* profiles the foundations of
America's major corporations and their charitable giving programs.
The directory provides information on corporate giving policies, areas
of funding interest, geographic preference, corporate financial and
product information, types of activities funded, sample grants awarded,
amount and range of grants, and application procedures.

Although this directory is extremely useful for researching the
larger corporate giving programs, the grant researcher may wish to contact smaller corporations in the local area. For this purpose, the library
user should be directed to the customary business reference tools such
as the *Standard and Poor's Register of Corporations* or the *Dun &
Bradstreet Reference Book of Corporate Managements,* both of which
are available online through DIALOG.

Corporate Giving Directory is published by the Taft Group and distributed by Gale. The 25th edition, published in December 2002, profiles 1,000 large corporate foundations that provide over $6 billion in
support annually. Searching is assisted by 14 indexes listing foundations by state, operating location, grant type, recipient type, and non-
monetary support among the categories.

Canadian Sources

14.10 *Canadian Institutes of Health Research (CIHR)/Instituts de recherche en santé du Canada (IRSC).* Ottawa, ON: Canadian Institutes of Health Research. Available: www.cihr-irsc.gc.ca.

14.11 *Canada Foundation for Innovation/Fondation canadienne pour l'innovation.* Ottawa, ON: Canada Foundation for Innovation. Available: www.innovation.ca.

14.12 *Social Sciences and Humanities Research Council (SSHRC)/Conseil de recherches en sciences humains du Canada (CRSH).* Ottawa, ON: Social Sciences and Humanities Research Council. Available: www.sshrc.ca.

14.13 *Natural Sciences and Engineering Research Council (NSERC)/Conseil de recherches en sciences naturelles et en génie du Canada (CRSNG).* Ottawa, ON: Natural Sciences and Engineering Research Council. Available: www.nserc.ca.

14.14 *National Cancer Institute of Canada/Institut national du cancer du Canada.* Toronto, ON: National Cancer Institute of Canada. Available: www.ncic.cancer.ca.

14.15 *Heart and Stroke Foundation of Canada Research Programs.* Ottawa, ON: Heart and Stroke Foundation of Canada. Available: www.hsf.ca/research.

Canadian Institutes of Health Research (CIHR) replaced the former Medical Research Council of Canada (MRCC) in the summer of the year 2000 as the federal government's major funding program for health research in Canada. Between 1960 and 2000, MRCC was the major Canadian source of money to fund health and health care research in Canada; CIHR has now expanded the mandate of MRCC to include support for research infrastructure at postsecondary educational institutions and research hospitals. The new agency has double the money the old one had and will pursue a national health research agenda with input from the federal and provincial governments, the health research community, health charities, and the private sector.

The CIHR Web site brings together the 13 virtual institutes that are part of the CIHR, providing information about the parts as well as the whole. Additionally, the site provides access to information about careers, strategic initiatives of the CIHR, ethics, services, publications, and funding. The "Funding" section lists various funding opportunities available from the CIHR (both the open and strategic competitions of the CIHR). It also brings together a list of external sources of funding: information about many competitions and sources of funding open to Canadian investigators, which are not under the control of the CIHR. All the information and the forms necessary to make application for CIHR funding are accessible through the "Funding" section, and there is an archive of decisions detailing the history of grants awarded by the CIHR. All information on the site is available in both French and English.

The Canada Foundation for Innovation (CFI) is an independent corporation established by the government of Canada in 1997 to strengthen research infrastructure in Canadian universities, colleges, research hospitals, and other not-for-profit institutions, thus promoting research excellence. The CFI works by forming partnerships with institutions in which both partners put up money to fund new programs, the acquisition of equipment, or the creation of new facilities to support research initiatives in the public, private, and voluntary sectors.

The Web site offers access to information about the programs funded already, new initiatives of the CFI, available funds, and information necessary for applications. Partner institutions can obtain institutional reports and gain access to information not available to the public. PDF documents and encryption options are standard features. Information is provided in both official languages of Canada.

The Social Sciences and Humanities Research Council (SSHRC) is another of the federal funding agencies at "arm's length" from the Canadian government. It funds university-based research and training in the social sciences and humanities and promotes "innovative thinking about real life issues, including the economy, education, health care, the environment, immigration, etc." Social Sciences and Humanities Research Council is not likely to fund clinical research, but does support nursing research that makes a contribution to the social sciences and humanities. It also includes psychology and educational psychology, which are sometimes allied with health care.

The Web site for this agency contains a section to assist those pursuing interdisciplinary research identify a funding agency appropriate to their interests and likely to grant them funding. There are the usual sections describing the programs supported by the agency, the funding available, and information on applying for funding and how to manage a grant.

The Natural Sciences and Engineering Research Council (NSERC) supports basic university research in science and technology as well as training of highly qualified researchers. Like SHRC, the interests of NSERC do not include clinical research, but many funded projects involve basic sciences in the health care arena: pathology, anatomy, biochemistry, biology, and psychology, among others.

The Web site provides the standard information about awards administered by the council, with application guidelines and forms. PowerPoint tutorials on the site provide information on how to use the NSERC system and guides to assist with grant writing. A list of successful awards from the past several years is also available.

The National Cancer Institute of Canada (NCIC) acts in concert with its partner, the Canadian Cancer Society, and with The Terry Fox Foundation to provide support for cancer research and related programs undertaken at Canadian universities, hospitals, and other research institutions.

The Web site offers a PDF version of the NCIC manual, *Support for Research and Training*, which fully describes their programs and policies. For those who do not want to download the whole manual, the site provides access to each chapter, also in PDF format. All the forms necessary for application are available on the site as are lists of new grants and awards by competition and year for the past 3 years. Like other sites of this sort, the NCIC offers promotion material such as "News and Views" and "Meet our Researchers."

The mission of the Heart and Stroke Foundation of Canada, as stated on its main site, is "to improve the health of Canadians by preventing and reducing disability and health from heart disease and stroke through research, health promotion and advocacy."

The research site of the Heart and Stroke Foundation is separate from the main site, which is intended for the public, and is directed totally to the researcher. The "Research Programs" site provides access to information about funding opportunities, the HSF Research Fund, peer review, and the results of previous competitions. Guidelines and application forms are available on the site. The site provides a searchable database of over 900 researchers in Canada with an interest in heart disease, stroke, and related diseases who are or have been recipients of grants from the HSF.

14.16 *Canadian Directory to Foundations and Grants.* Toronto, ON: Canadian Centre for Philanthropy, 1996–. Available: www.ccp.ca.

The Canadian Centre for Philanthropy is a membership-based organization that works with charities, governments, and corporations to advance the role and interests of the charitable sector for the benefit of Canadian communities. It publishes the *Canadian Directory to Foundations and Grants,* now in its 16th edition (2002). The directory offers a list of over 1,800 Canadian grant-making foundations whose funds are disbursed to a variety of organizations, along with a much briefer list of U.S. foundations with a history of granting in Canada. The entries for each foundation provide basic contact information, skeletal histories, information about the purpose of the foundation, and funding interests and types of support offered as well as restrictions on support or funding, some financial data, names of officers and directors, and a recent history of grants larger than $1,000, where the information is available. There is a geographic analysis of the size and scope of the foundations listed and their funding, useful in a country as regionalized and as large as Canada is. There are indexes to (or lists of) the top 100 foundations by assets, government foundations, the top 10 family foundations, community foundations, and corporate foundations. The *Canadian Institutes of Health Research*, SSHRC, NSERC, and the like are not included, as they are not foundations. There is also a useful list of foundations with Web sites.

Preliminary material provides help in understanding what a foundation is and how it operates as well as the different types of foundation, so that the applicant has a better chance of developing a successful proposal. There is detailed information for foundations about fund-raising, and similar advice and assistance for individuals wanting to develop proposals to present to foundations with money to grant. A list of grant recipients is also provided.

While *The Canadian Directory to Foundations and Grants* is the only Canadian resource listed here that offers information on more than one funding source, it will be most useful to investigators looking for relatively small amounts of money. Although some of the foundations listed offer as much as $15 million (Canadian) in grants, the majority of the foundations listed have less money than is needed to support major health sciences research.

The Web site offers services for foundations in its "research" section where articles that track topics such as "trends in individual donations" and "insights into Canada's major donors" appear. The free-access portion of the CCP Web site is aimed at foundation executives and board members who want to build and enhance the assets of their foundation. The subscription-based portion is the part that provides information for someone seeking grants or funding.

International Sources

14.17 *The International Foundation Directory.* Detroit, MI: Gale; London: Europa. 1974–. Irregular.

The *International Foundation Directory* emphasizes foundations that operate internationally, but also covers selected national foundations located throughout the world. Arranged by country, the 2003 directory contains 2,200 entries for foundations, trusts, and other similar nonprofit institutions in over 100 countries. Each entry furnishes the organization's name, address, telephone and fax numbers, Internet and e-mail addresses, in addition to a brief history and description of its activities, plus limited financial data. To assure as much accuracy as possible, institutions included in the directory have provided information directly.

Grants to Individuals

14.18 *Foundation Grants to Individuals*. New York: The Foundation Center, 1977–. Biennial. Available: http://gtionline.fdncenter.org.

14.19 *Grants Register*. New York, London: Palgrave Macmillan, 1969/70–. Biennial. Available: www.nature.com/nature/grants.

14.20 *GrantsNet*. Available: www.grantsnet.org.

Foundation Grants to Individuals contains programs arranged by grant type, including such categories as scholarships and loans, fellowships, grants for foreign individuals, general welfare and medical assistance, and grants restricted to company employees. This resource is well indexed and provides the usual descriptive information in each entry along with lists of sample grants awarded. In addition, two informative articles appear in *Foundation Grants to Individuals*—an analysis of federal laws pertaining to this area of grantsmanship and an essay and extensive bibliography covering further sources of information on grants to individuals. Like other databases from the Foundation Center, online access is available by subscription for one month, three months or one year.

Published every 2 years, the *Grants Register* is broader in scope, listing information on more than 4,500 awards and grants from government agencies as well as international, national, and private organizations. Over 80 countries are represented. Compiled for students at or above the graduate level and for others requiring further professional training, this directory includes scholarships and fellowships plus research and travel grants. While this publication emphasizes individuals in need, some of the programs make awards only through sponsoring institutions. Section six of the subject index is devoted to medical and health sciences. The Nature Publishing Group provides the *Grants Register* online under the name International grants finder. The online resource is annually updated.

Sponsored by the Howard Hughes Medical Institute (HHMI) and American Association for the Advancement of Science (AAAS), GrantsNet is available at no charge. It provides funding information for training in biomedical research and science education. The Web site provides tools for customizing, information on how to write a grant proposal, and an index to international grants and fellowships. It is continually updated.

Institutional Databases

14.21 *Community of Science* (*COS*). Baltimore, MD: Community of Science. Available: www.cos.com.

14.22 *Illinois Researcher Information Service* (*IRIS*). Urbana, IL: Univerisity of Illinois, Urbana-Champaign. Available: www.library.uiuc.edu/iris.

14.23 *Sponsored Programs Information Network* (*SPIN*). Albany, NY: InfoEd International. *SPINPlus*. Available: www.infoed.org.

Available by institutional subscription, these databases provide opportunities for researchers to manage their profiles for identifying funding sources, identifying researchers doing similar work, and being alerted to forthcoming funding opportunities.

The Community of Science (COS) provides global information on research and development (R&D) opportunities. A variety of services are provided, including COS Funding Opportunities (updated daily); COS Funding Alert, a weekly e-mail notification service; COS Funded Research, a service for tracking funding histories of research facilities; COS Expertise, profiles for participating individuals and institutions; COS Workbench, access to services and databases; COS Abstract Management System (AMS), online collaborative authoring and submission, peer review, conference or meeting scheduling, and so forth; and access to Bibliographic Databases such as MEDLINE.

A service of the University of Illinois at Urbana-Champaign Library, the IRIS database provides information on funding opportunities in 25 subject areas. IRIS also provides selected searching from such sources as, the *Commerce Business Daily,* fedbizopps.gov, a single government point-of-entry (GPE) for Federal government procurement opportunities over $25,000, and the *Federal Register*. While designed for the University of Illinois community, other institutions can subscribe as well. Profiles can be set up for the IRIS Alert Service.

The Sponsored Programs Information Network (SPIN) is an integrated sponsored programs software that provides current information on funding opportunities from federal, nonfederal, and international organizations. Funding opportunity areas include conference support, curriculum development, fellowships, research grants, Request for Applications (RFAs), Request for Proposals (RFPs), and more. Over 2,500 agencies are profiled, with information provided directly from the sponsoring agency. Database searching is from multiple access points: keyword, location, sponsoring agency, and deadline.

References

1. Introduction. In: *The Foundation Directory*, 14th ed. New York: The Foundation Center, 1992.
2. Kurzig CM. *Foundation fundamentals*, rev. ed. New York: The Foundation Center, 1981:4.

Reference Collection Development Policy

Kornhauser Health Sciences Library, University of Louisville

Reference Collection Development Policy

The Kornhauser Health Sciences Library Reference Collection is a core collection of highly used general and specialized sources of information. The main purpose of a reference collection is convenience. By separating selected, heavily used materials into a distinct location, convenient for all library users at all times, and restricting its use to on-site consultation, users' questions can be answered more efficiently and thoroughly than if the reference materials were available for checkout.

The IES Team will formally review the Reference Collection biennially. The IES Team will formally review the Reference Collection Development Policy biennially.

A. SCOPE AND COVERAGE

1. Titles are included in this collection primarily because they provide access to the journal literature (indexes, abstracts, and electronic databases); provide factual information (directories, handbooks, dictionaries, statistical compilations); or give general

363

background information on a topic (encyclopedias and text-books).

2. Materials are chosen for inclusion in the Reference Collection only if they meet the selection criteria based on authoritativeness, currency, comprehensiveness, and ease of use and value to our user.

B. COLLECTION AREAS

1. Reference materials may be in any format: print, electronic and/or multimedia.
2. Types of material to be added to the collection include, but are not limited to:

a. Abbreviations and Acronym
   - Inclusion: general and periodicals
   - Collection: current editions only
   - Retention: superseded volumes should be discarded or forwarded to new location

b. Abstracts and indexes
   - Retention: retain all volumes for which electronic access is not available

c. Almanacs
   - Collection: current editions only
   - Retention: discard earlier editions

d. Dictionaries
   i. English
      - Inclusion: current
   ii. Health sciences
      - Inclusion: general medical and specialized
      - Collection: most recent editions only
      - Retention: place earlier editions in circulating collection
   iii. English/other languages
      - Inclusion: especially medical or scientific dictionaries in languages our patrons speak or need

iv. Pharmacology and toxicology
- Collection: current editions only
- Retention: earlier editions to circulating collection

e. Directories

i. Audiovisual and computer information resources
- Inclusion: reference directories of multimedia materials and computer software with emphasis on sources related to biomedical sciences, health care, database searching, and information technology
- Collection: current editions only
- Retention: discard earlier editions

ii. Biographical

f. Book catalogs
- Books in Print and WorldCat and/or equivalents available electronically
- Do not collect publishers catalogs

g. Educational information
- Inclusion: sources of current information about medical schools, graduate medical and biomedical education and training programs, medical licensure, residencies, and matching programs
- Collection: current editions only
- Retention: discard earlier editions
- Formats

h. Grant registers
- Inclusion: current sources of grants, loans and scholarships
- Collection: current editions only
- Retention: discard superseded volumes
- Note: direct patrons to Office of Sponsored Programs and their Web page

i. Handbooks
- Inclusion: authoritative handbooks in basic and clinical sciences
- Collection: latest editions only
- Retention: earlier editions in stack

j. Meetings
- Inclusion: scientific and biomedical meetings and conferences
- Collection: retain 2 years only
- Retention: discard earlier information

k. Membership lists
- Collection: latest edition only
- Retention: discard earlier editions

l. Organizations
- Inclusion: hospitals, research facilities, associations
- Collection: latest edition only
- Retention: discard earlier editions

m. Serials directory
- Collection: latest edition only
- Retention: earlier editions discarded or forwarded to new location

n. Supply catalogs
- Exclusion: do not collect

o. Encyclopedias
- Inclusion: general knowledge and basic and health sciences specialty works
- Collection: replace at least every 5 years if necessary
- Retention: discard earlier editions

p. Standards, codes, practice guidelines
- Collection: latest edition only
- Retention: superseded volumes to stacks

q. Statistical compendia
- Inclusion: significant compilations of data on health care, morbidity and mortality (*MMWR* is in journal stacks), socioeconomic factors
- Collection: most recent editions only
- Retention: earlier editions in circulating collection

r. Style manuals
- Inclusion: resume, curriculum vitae, cover letter and personal statement guides

- Collection: latest edition only
- Retention: older edition to stacks

s. Tests and measurements
  - Inclusion: research instruments, psychological, and aptitude tests
  - Retention: retain earlier editions if not cumulative

t. Textbooks
  - Inclusion: most current, significant textbooks in the basic and clinical sciences
  - Collection: latest edition only
  - Retention: earlier editions in circulating collection
  - Note: duplicate circulating collection if necessary

Note: This reference collection development policy is reproduced and modified with permission from the Kornhauser Health Sciences Library, University of Louisville, Louisville, Kentucky. The *Collection Development Policies* of which this is a part is available at: http://library.louisville.edu/kornhauser/info/colldev.doc.

INDEX

369

About the Editors

Jo Anne Boorkman (MS) is Head of the Carlson Health Sciences Library, University of California, Davis, where she also serves as coordinator for health sciences collections. She is a Fellow of the Medical Library Association and a distinguished member of the Academy of Health Information Professionals (AHIP). She is also a Fellow of the Special Libraries Association and is SLA representative to the International Federation of Library Associations (IFLA) Health & Biosciences Section (2003–2007).

Jeffrey T. Huber (PhD) is Associate Professor and coordinator of the Houston Master's program and health sciences curriculum for the School of Library and Information Studies at Texas Women's University, Houston. He recently copublished with M. Snyder "Facilitating Access to Consumer Health Information: A collaborative approach employing applied research" in *Medical Reference Services Quarterly* (21[2]: 29–46, 2002) and is a member of the editorial board for *JMLA, Journal of the Medical Library Association*.

Fred W. Roper (PhD) is recently retired dean of the College of Library and Information Sciences at the University of South Carolina. Active in the Medical Library Association, Special Libraries Association, the American Library Association, and the Association for Library and Information Science Education, he is past president of the Medical Library Association and recipient of its Marcia C. Noyes Award, among other honors.

The Medical Library Association, founded in 1898, is an educational organization of more than 1,100 institutions and 3,600 individual members in the health sciences information field, committed to educating health information professionals, supporting health information

387

research, promoting access to the world's health sciences information, and working to ensure that the best health information is available to all.

LIST OF CONTRIBUTORS

AMELIA (AMY) BUTROS, AHIP
Scripps Institute of Oceanography
Library
University of California, San Diego
La Jolla, CA
(Chapter 9)

JO ANNE BOORKMAN, AHIP, FMLA
Carlson Health Sciences Library
University of California, Davis
Davis, CA
(Chapter 1, Chapter 8, Chapter 14)

MARY L. BURGESS
CDC Information Center
Centers for Disease Control and
Prevention
Atlanta, GA
(Chapter 11)

CHERYL RAE DEE, PhD, AHIP
School of Library and Information
Sciences
University of South Florida
Tampa, FL
(Chapter 12)

MARY L. GILLASPY
Northwestern Memorial Hospital
Chicago, IL
(Chapter 10)

DAVID K. HOWSE
Arizona Health Sciences Library
University of Arizona
Tucson, AZ
(Chapter 4)

JEFFREY T. HUBER
School of Library & Information Studies
Texas Women's University
Houston, TX
(Chapter 2)

LUCRETIA W. McCLURE, AHIP,
FMLA
Rochester, NY
(Chapter 13)

SUSAN (SUE) McGUINNESS
Biomedical Library
University of California, San Diego
La Jolla, CA
(Chapter 9)

GERALD J. PERRY, AHIP
Denison Memorial Library
University of Colorado Health Sciences
Center
Denver, CO
(Chapter 4)

JOCELYN A. RANKIN, PhD, AHIP
CDC Information Center
Centers for Disease Control and
Prevention
Atlanta, GA
(Chapter 11)

FRED W. ROPER, PhD, AHIP, FMLA
College of Library and Information
Science
University of South Carolina
Columbia, SC
(Chapter 3, Chapter 5, Chapter 6,
Chapter 7)

JOAN SCHLIMGEN
Arizona Health Sciences Library
University of Arizona
Tucson, AZ
(Chapter 9)